Neurosurgery and the Clinical Team

Gerald R. Litel, M.D. is in the private practice of neurological surgery in Lake Charles, Louisiana. He received his B.A. from Pomona College in 1959 and his M.D. from Baylor College of Medicine in 1963. He did his neurosurgical residency in the Baylor affiliated hospitals of the Texas Medical Center in Houston, Texas. He is certified by the American Board of Neurological Surgery and holds teaching appointments at both Baylor College of Medicine and Louisiana State University. He was selected for membership to the Alpha Omega Alpha Honor Medical Society at Baylor in 1962.

Patricia E. Mahoney, R.N., M.A. is the Clinical Nursing Specialist–Nursing Care Coordinator of the Neurology-Neurosurgery Service at The New York Hospital–Cornell Medical Center in New York City. She received her B.S.N. from Georgetown University and her M.A. in Nursing from New York University. She is a member of Sigma Theta Tau, the National Honor Society in nursing and has frequently published and lectured on topics in neuro-nursing.

Joyce Keen, M.A. received her master's in Speech-Communications from California State University, Fullerton. She holds a Certificate of Clinical Competency in Speech-Language Pathology and works with Newport Language, Speech, and Audiology Center. She has served as Supervisor of the Speech Pathology Department at St. Jude Hospital and Rehabilitation Center and is on the part-time faculty of the Communication Disorders Department at Chapman College.

Neurosurgery and the Clinical Team

A Guide for Nurses, Technicians, and Students

Gerald R. Litel, M.D.

with contributions by

Patricia E. Mahoney, R.N., M.A.

and

Joyce Keen, M.A.

Springer Publishing Company
New York

To my wife, Colleen,
who continually encouraged me
during the many weeks and months
taken to write this book

Springer Publishing Company, Inc.
200 Park Avenue South
New York, New York 10003

80 81 82 83 84 / 10 9 8 7 6 5 4 3 2 1

Library of Congress Cataloging in Publication Data

Litel, Gerald R
Neurosurgery and the Clinical Team

Bibliography: p.
Includes index.
1. Nervous system—Surgery. I. Mahoney, Patricia E., joint author. II. Keen, Joyce joint author. III. Title. [DNLM: 1. Nervous system—Surgery. WL368 L776c]
RD593.L57 617'.48 80-195
ISBN 0-8261-2970-6
ISBN 0-8261-2971-4 pbk.

Printed in the United States of America

Contents

Foreword

In no surgical field is the help of professional, sophisticated ancillary personnel more needed or appreciated than in neurological surgery. Since the early days of Drs. Cushing, Dandy, etc., neurological surgeons have leaned heavily on their colleagues in nursing and allied fields to aid in the pre- and postoperative care of these cases. The best surgical performance can become a disaster by inadequate follow-up on the ward, and the operative candidate can irreparably deteriorate without alert bedside care and observation prior to surgery. Increasing awareness of these facts has contributed to the development of both nursing subspecialization and modern neurosurgical intensive care units.

A text designed to deliver the necessary information to our colleagues in nursing and other disciplines has been needed but unavailable. Dr. Litel has devoted time and effort to produce a book that, in clear, concise language, fills this void. It should appeal to all those being introduced to neurological surgery because of the strong emphasis on practical issues relating to clinical cases. The material presented provides an excellent base for further study from the special texts and articles related to each subject. Dr. Litel, a clinician of practical excellence who has developed an active service in a community where resident help is not available, is singularly qualified for this task. This book should quickly find a home in the neurosurgical hospital units.

William R. Cheek, M.D.
St. Luke's – Texas Children's Hospital
Houston, Texas

Preface

Throughout my years of neurosurgical practice I have often had the opportunity to lecture to nurses, therapists, and technicians. In doing so I am frequently asked to recommend a book that could be obtained to supplement my lectures. To my surprise I find that very few such books exist, and of those that do, most are overly simple, treating the subject matter superficially and incompletely.

To be sure there are several excellent nursing textbooks, but quite naturally their format is purely nursing. My students, however, want to approach neurosurgery from the perspective of the neurosurgeon. They want to know how I perform a craniotomy or a lumbar laminectomy to remove a ruptured disc. They ask how I would monitor intracranial pressure or how I would manage cerebral vasospasm from a subarachnoid hemorrhage. To answer these questions and many more, I undertook the writing of this book.

The first four chapters, on neuroanatomy and neurophysiology, neuropathology, neurological examination, and neurodiagnostic studies, are presented to provide a foundation for the reader. I have tried to present this information so that it has direct clinical interest and application. These chapters are not intended to replace the many excellent basic textbooks available on these subjects.

The uniqueness of the book is embodied in its remaining chapters. There is a chapter on each of the following subjects: craniotomy, laminectomy, peripheral nerve surgery, miscellaneous neurosurgical procedures, and pain-relieving procedures. In each chapter the surgical procedures and the general technique for each are presented where appropriate variations of approach and technique are discussed and compared. Finally, preoperative and postoperative considerations from the neurosurgeon's standpoint are fully presented. In certain instances the efficacy of medical versus surgical treatment is given.

Chapter 5 was written by Patricia E. Mahoney, R.N., who has wide experience with neurological patients. Mahoney gives the reader insight into the unique nursing problems presented by neurological and neurosurgical patients. This contribution greatly complements my effort to write a clinically oriented book that provides readily available and practical information.

Chapter 11 was written by Joyce Keen, a practicing speech pathologist. Keen's presentation of disorders of communication not only explains concisely and understandably the diversity of communication pathology but gives practical information on how the medical team can assist those afflicted.

Special appreciation must go to Mary Rasberry and Rene Manuel for their assistance in the editing and typing of this book. Also special acknowledgement is extended to Jane Bono, R.N., for her assistance in research for certain materials. Finally I wish to express my thanks to Ursula Springer and all those at Springer Publishing Company for their patience and kindness.

It is my sincere hope that this book will fill a void that previously existed. If it can assist someone in being a better nurse, therapist, technician, or doctor, all our efforts will have been worthwhile.

Gerald R. Litel
Lake Charles, Louisiana

CHAPTER 1

Neuroanatomy and Neurophysiology

The function of the nervous system is to receive stimuli from the environment and to transmit this information to the brain, which in turn formulates and initiates the appropriate body response.

The Nerve Cell

The basic functional unit of the nervous system is the neuron. These highly specialized cells vary in size and shape depending on location and function. They are, however, basically quite similar. They have a cell body that contains a conspicuous nucleus with a nucleolus. The cell body is variously shaped, with several short processes and a single long one. The short ones are called dendrites, and their function is to carry nerve impulses to the cell body. The long process is the axon, and it carries impulses away from the cell body.

The spread of an impulse along an axon or dendrite is an active process. Some understanding of nerve transmission is necessary if one is to have an idea of how the nervous system functions.

A nerve cell in the resting state is said to be polarized. Microelectrodes have shown that the inside of such a cell is negatively charged compared to the outside. In this state there is a high concentration of sodium ions outside the cell, while inside, the concentration of potassium ions is high. If the cell is stimulated sufficiently, electrically or otherwise, there is a rapid influx of sodium ions. This process, which is called depolarization, begins at the point of stimulation and then spreads along the axon or dendrite. It is this spreading wave of depolarization that accomplishes the transmission of an impulse.

The speed of transmission of an impulse varies. Larger fibers transmit with greater speed than smaller ones, and myelinated fibers transmit impulses a good deal faster than unmyelinated ones. Myelin is composed of concentric layers of lipid and protein. It is wrapped around an axon, the way insulation is wrapped around a wire except for segmental gaps called nodes of Ranvier (Figure 1-1), which make the myelinated axon look somewhat like a string of sausages. The process of depolarization skips from one node of Ranvier to the next, making the transmission of an impulse more rapid in the myelinated fiber.

In most instances the transmission of information from one part of the nervous system to another involves more than one neuron. The connection between an axon of one cell and the dendrites of another is called a synapse. When the spreading wave of depolarization comes to the synapse, it causes the release of a chemical substance that flows across the gap of the synapse. This substance has the ability to achieve the threshold of stimulation of the coupled nerve fiber so that further transmission is thus accomplished.

Figure 1-1 Neuron

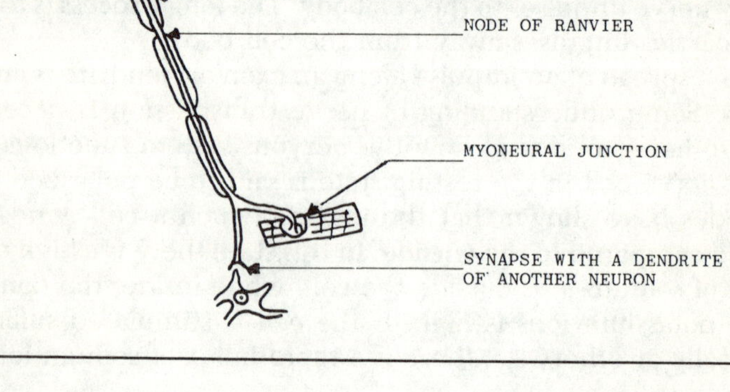

The cell bodies of neurons tend to occur in groups. They occur in sheets, or layers, in the cortex or gray matter. When they are in groups deep in the brain or spinal cord, these groups are referred to as nuclei. A single group is a nucleus. When they are grouped outside of the central nervous system, they are collectively called a ganglion.

The Nervous System

The nervous system is composed of two parts: the central nervous system and the peripheral nervous system. The CNS includes the two large, paired cerebral hemispheres; the brainstem; the cerebellum; and the spinal cord. The peripheral nervous system is composed of the cranial nerves that arise from the brainstem and the spinal nerves that arise from the spinal cord.

The Central Nervous System

The Cerebral Hemispheres

The general shape of the cerebral hemispheres when viewed from the side looks somewhat like a boxing glove. The surface contour, however, is like a walnut. The elevated ridges are called gyri and the valleys are sulci. There are certain long and deep sulci that are called fissures. The fissures tend to be the boundary markers between different sections or areas of each cerebral hemisphere, which are called lobes.

The Rolandic fissure separates the frontal and parietal lobes. The temporal lobe is distinct from the frontal and parietal lobes because of the prominent Sylvian fissure. The boundary between the parietal and occipital lobes is less distinct but is marked by the parieto-occipital sulcus (Figure 1-2).

Although it is possible to attribute certain functions to the different lobes of the cerebrum, it should not be assumed that each lobe acts autonomously. Most if not all of the functions of the brain are achieved by coordinated efforts of several different portions of the brain. The function of the different lobes has been shown best by observing patients who have sustained injury to the specific lobe studied.

Injury to both frontal lobes produces personality changes. Patients with such injuries have short attention spans and often change

Figure 1-2 Side View of the Dominant Cerebral Hemisphere

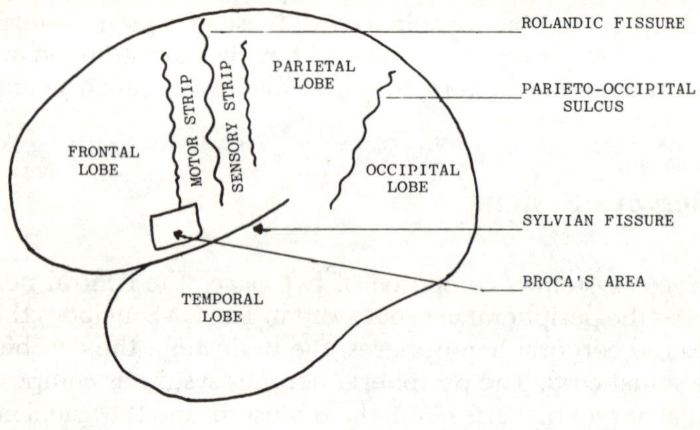

from one activity to another in quick succession. They are often grossly profane with little consideration for others. Though their IQs are little changed, they are unable to plan future events on the basis of past experience. The level of consciousness is frequently quite variable. The patients may be frivolous and silly or apathetic and showing little emotion.

In the posterior portion of each frontal lobe and running parallel to the Rolandic fissure is the motor strip. Neurons located in the motor strip produce movement of the opposite side of the body. These neurons are arranged in definite order according to the portion of the body that they move (Figure 1-3).

Figure 1-3 demonstrates the location of areas of the motor strip concerned with specific muscles or areas of the body. Those sending motor fibers to the mouth and tongue are nearest the Sylvian fissure. Above the tongue region are cells sending fibers to the face, neck, and fingers. Cells responsible for hand movement are next; those sending motor fibers to the trunk, leg, and foot are located at the top of the strip or along that part of the motor strip that swings down between the two hemispheres. It should be noted that there are many more neurons sending axons to the tongue or hand muscles than there are sending axons to all of the muscles of the trunk. It is a rule of thumb that, the more intricate and varied the movements of a body part, the greater the number of motor neurons responsible for those movements.

Broca's area (Figure 1-2), which is the motor speech area, is near the part of the motor strip concerned with the movements of the

Figure 1-3 Cross-section through the Motor Strip of the Cerebral Hemispheres, Showing the Relative Location of Specific Functions

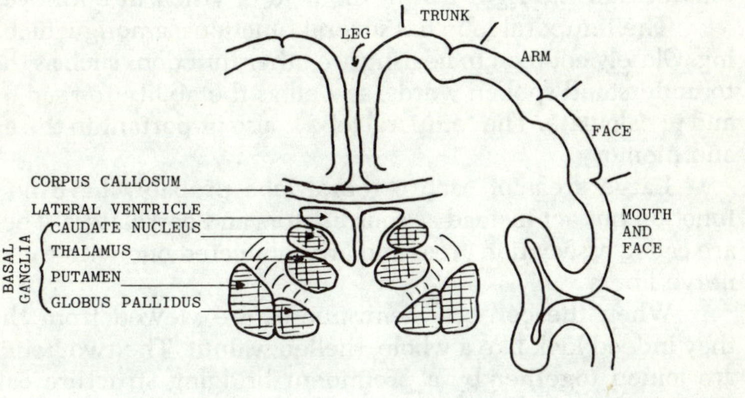

tongue, pharynx, and larynx. It acts to plan and coordinate the muscles used in speech. Injury produces a motor or expressive aphasia, so that patients know what they wish to say but cannot say it. Broca's area is found in the dominant cerebral hemisphere. The dominance of a cerebral hemisphere is determined, for the most part, by inheritance. Most people are right handed with the left cerebral hemisphere dominant. It is estimated, however, that many people who are left handed still have the speech center in the left cerebral hemisphere.

The sensory cortex is in the parietal lobe. Like the motor strip the sensory cortex runs parallel to the Rolandic fissure (Figure 1-2). It is nearly a mirror image of the motor strip because of the similar arrangement of cells. Thus those cells concerned with sensation of the lips and mouth of the opposite side of the body are nearest the Sylvian fissure. Then in an orderly fashion, the other parts of the opposite side of the body are represented. The sensory cortex receives incoming information concerning the elementary sensations of pain, touch, pressure, heat, and cold.

The remainder of the parietal lobe that lies behind the sensory cortex plays a more abstract role in sensation. It discriminates between hot and cold or between rough and smooth. It distinguishes weight, shape, form, and texture, thus making it possible to think in a three-dimensional manner. Patients with injuries to the parietal lobe may fail to put their arms in their jackets, not because of paralysis, but because their arms are not a part of their body images.

The occipital lobe is for practical purposes concerned entirely with vision. One occipital lobe gives sight in the opposite half of the visual field of both eyes. Thus injury to the left occipital lobe causes blindness in the right half of the field of vision in both eyes.

The temporal lobe has several functions, among which is hearing. Closely coupled to hearing are other functions such as the ability to understand spoken words, as well as the ability to read, to write, and to calculate. The temporal lobe is also important in the emotions and memory.

Large areas of each cerebral lobe probably have no specific function but act instead as coordinators and correlators. These areas are called association areas and are connected one with the other by nerve fibers.

When the cerebral hemispheres are viewed from the front, they indeed look like a whole, shelled walnut. The two hemispheres are joined together by a prominent bridging structure called the corpus callosum (Figure 1-3).

If one takes a knife and cuts across the two cerebral hemispheres one sees the brain's internal features. First is the thin outer layer of each cerebral hemisphere, which has a gray or dark color. This layer, called the cortex, contains many millions of neuron cell bodies. Beneath the cortex the brain is distinctly white. This white portion is composed of millions of myelinated axons (nerve fibers) whose cell bodies lie in the cortex. Axons with similar functions (e.g., transmitting impulses for movement) tend to run in close proximity and are known collectively as nerve or fiber tracts. Many of these tracts have specific names and are mentioned later.

Deep within each cerebral hemisphere one sees definite islands of gray matter. Each has a specific name and function, but generally speaking they serve as way stations for nerve tracts running to and from the spinal cord, cerebellum, and brainstem. Collectively called the basal ganglia, they include the thalamus, the caudate nucleus, the putamen, and the globus pallidus (Figure 1-3).

Finally, within each cerebral hemisphere one sees an empty cavity called the lateral ventricle (Figure 1-4). On the floor of each lateral ventricle is a delicate frondlike structure called the choroid plexus, which produces much of the cerebrospinal fluid. The paired lateral ventricles communicate with a midline space called the third ventricle. A small tubular structure, called the aqueduct of Sylvius, then connects the back part of the third ventricle with the fourth ventricle, which is located in the cerebellum. Normally cerebrospinal fluid flows in this direction, in other words, from the lateral to the third and then to the fourth ventricles. The CSF then leaves the fourth ventricle to enter the subarachnoid space.

Figure 1-4 Ventricular System Shown within the Substance of the Brain

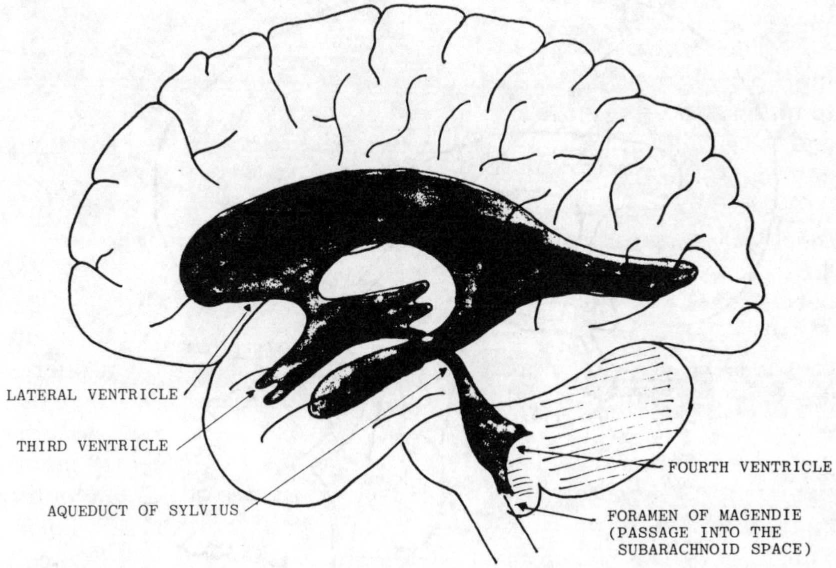

The Brainstem

The brainstem is continuous with the underside of the cerebral hemispheres (Figure 1–5). Its most anterior portion is the hypothalamus. This structure forms the walls and floor of the third ventricle. An extension called the infundibulum goes from the floor of the third ventricle to the pituitary gland. In the hypothalamus, specific nuclei (groups of neurons) have been identified that control the body's glandular structures by producing hormones that affect pituitary, thyroid, adrenal, and sex gland (testicle and ovary) function. Other nuclei of the hypothalamus play roles in the body's temperature control, appetite, urine output, and emotion.

The midbrain is continuous with the posterior portion of the hypothalamus. This portion of the brainstem contains great fiber tracts that begin in the cerebral hemispheres and go to other parts of the brainstem as well as to the spinal cord. It also contains tracts that ascend to the cerebral hemispheres from the spinal cord.

A cross-section of the midbrain reveals several important structures (Figure 1–6). In the upper portion is seen the aqueduct of Sylvius, which is the slender passageway through which CSF flows from the third to the fourth ventricle (Figure 1–4). Surrounding the

Figure 1-5 Longitudinal Section of the Brainstem

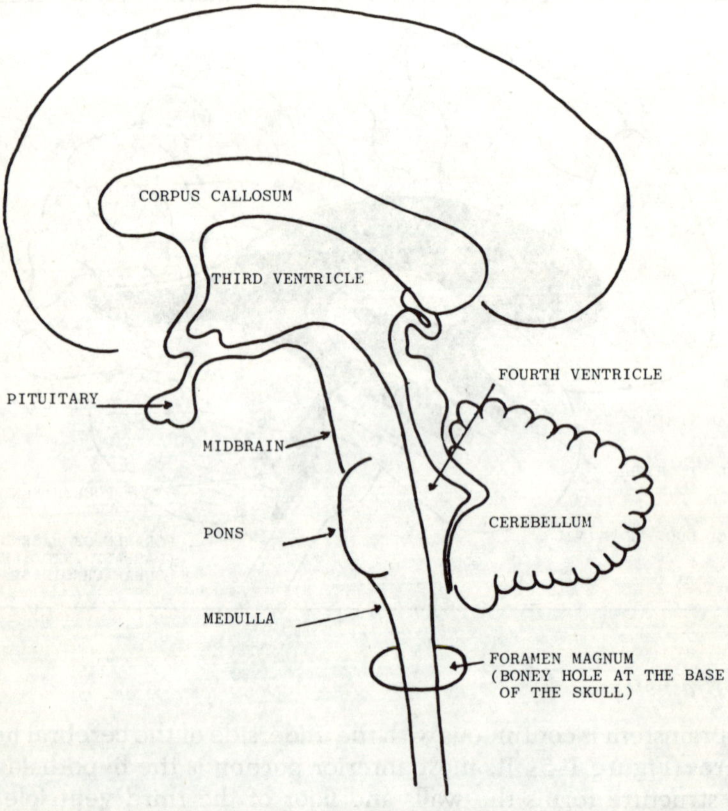

aqueduct is the central gray, which contains several ill-defined nuclei containing neurons of varied shapes and sizes. Similar groups of nuclei are found in the pons and the medulla oblongata (Figure 1–5). Collectively these nuclei make up the reticular activating system, which plays a role in maintaining the state of consciousness.

Below the aqueduct and adjacent to the central gray in the midbrain cross-section are the two paired nuclei of the third cranial nerve. In the third cranial nerve nuclei are the cell bodies of the neurons whose axons travel in the third nerve to the eyes. These axons go to the upper eyelid, the pupil of the eye, and some of the eye muscles that move the eyeball. On each side of the central gray are two important ascending nerve tracts, the medial lemniscus and the spinothalamic tract. The two paired red nuclei lie below the central gray; the third-nerve fibers travel through them on their way

Figure 1-6 Cross-section of the Midbrain

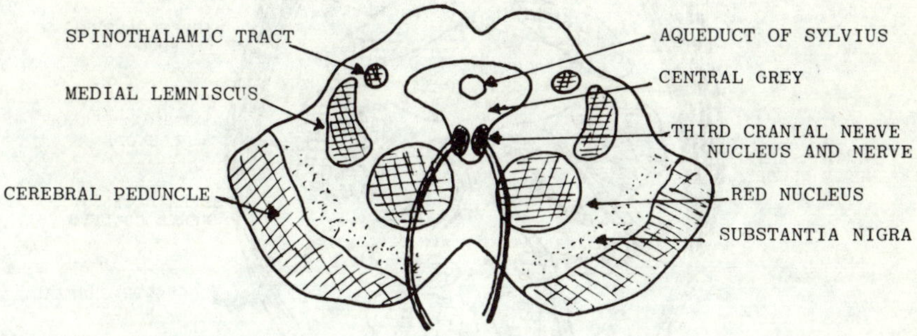

to the eye. The red nuclei have important connections with the cerebellum. Finally one sees the two large cerebral peduncles, which contain tracts from the motor cortex going to the brainstem and the spinal cord.

If a cross-section of the midbrain is made a bit lower, one sees the fourth cranial nerve nuclei. These two nuclei have the same relationship with the central gray that the third-nerve nuclei have. The fourth nerve also goes to the eye but to a single muscle that helps move the eyeball.

The pons is the next portion of the brainstem one encounters moving from front to back along the brainstem (Figures 1–5 and 1–7). The pons carried the same ascending and descending tracts that one sees in the midbrain. It is distinctive, however, because it forms the floor of the fourth ventricle and it has the cerebellum sitting on top of it. The cerebellum attaches to the brainstem by the cerebellar peduncles. There are three peduncles on each side, the middle peduncle being the largest. The peduncles are fiber tracts that run to and from the cerebellum.

Several cranial nerve nuclei are found in the pons. On each side of the fourth ventricle are the vestibular nuclei, which play a role in our balance. They receive nerve fibers from the inner ear by way of the eighth cranial nerve. The sixth cranial nerve nucleus (abducens) lies in the pons just under the floor of the fourth ventricle. Fibers from this nucleus go to the eye muscle called the lateral rectus. Deep

Figure 1-7 Cross-section of the Pons

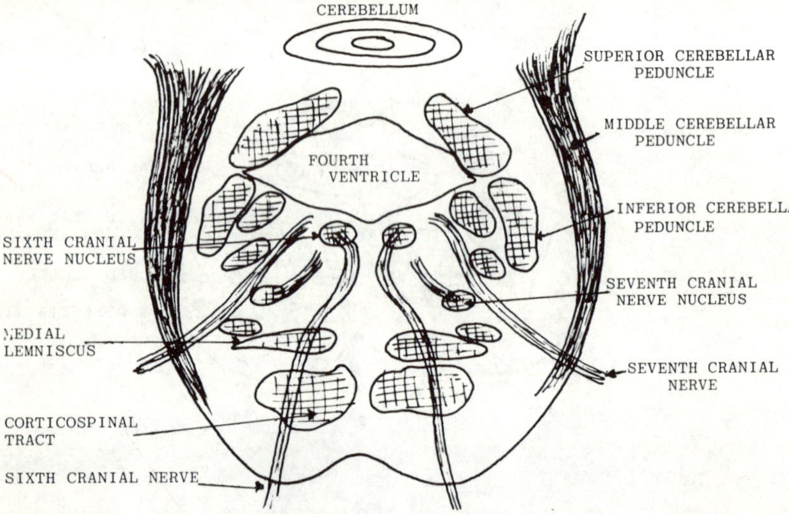

in the pons are two other cranial nerve nuclei, the seventh cranial nerve nuclei and the sensory portion of the fifth cranial nerve. The seventh cranial nerve nuclei contain neuron cell bodies whose axons make up the seventh cranial nerve (facial) and which go to the face muscles. These muscles are the ones that give us our facial expression. The sensory nucleus of the fifth cranial nerve, located in the pons, is the one that receives fibers carrying sensation from the face.

The medulla is the backmost portion of the brainstem (Figures 1–5 and 1–8). It goes through the foramen magnum (the large hole in the base of the skull) and is continuous with the upper portion of the spinal cord. Like the pons and the midbrain, there are many tracts running up and down its length. The more important tracts include the spinothalamic tracts, and the lemnisci. The remaining cranial nerves originate from nuclei located in the medulla. For example there are the hypoglossal nuclei, from which the two twelfth cranial nerves originate. There are other nuclei that contribute fibers that run in the ninth, tenth, and eleventh cranial nerves.

The Cerebellum

The cerebellum is the prominent structure seen on the back of the brainstem (Figure 1–5). It attaches to the brainstem at the level of the

Figure 1-8 Cross-section of the Medulla

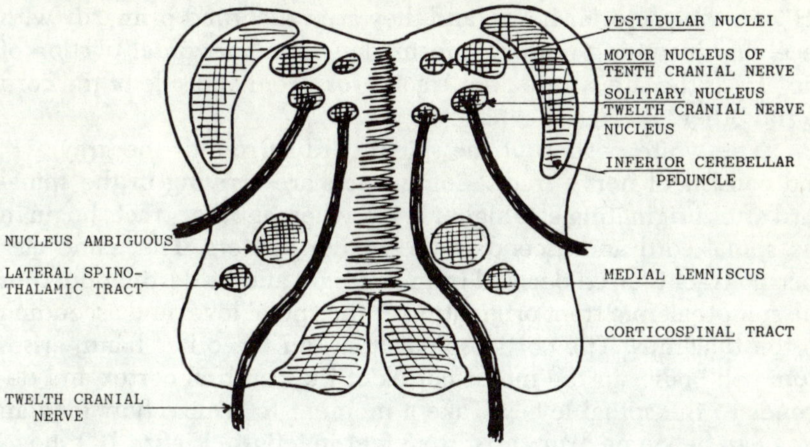

pons and the upper medulla by the three cerebellar peduncles on each side. In doing so, it forms the sides and roof of the fourth ventricle.

The surface of the cerebellum is marked by several parallel grooves called folia. The cerebellum has lobes, but they are less distinct than those of the cerebral hemispheres. From the standpoint of function, the midline portion, called the vermis, coordinates the trunk of the body, whereas the two large hemispheres on each side of the vermis coordinate the extremities, particularly the hands.

The cerebellum has a cortex that, like the cerebral cortex, is gray in appearance and contains the cell bodies of neurons. In the cerebellar cortex there is a unique neuron called the purkinje cell. Beneath the cortex there is white matter that consists of myelinated nerve fibers. Deep within the cerebellum there are nuclei that receive various incoming nerve tracts and that send tracts elsewhere, such as to the red nucleus and the thalamus.

The Spinal Cord

The spinal cord is continuous with the medulla and lies within the spinal canal. A cross-section of the spinal cord reveals its distinctive features (Figure 1–9). One notes immediately that the relationship of the gray and white matter in the spinal cord is the reverse of that seen in the cerebrum and the cerebellum. The gray matter of the cord is the "H" shaped portion in the cord's center. The larger ventral portions are called the ventral horns and contain pyramid-shaped neurons called anterior horn cells. The dorsal portions of the "H" are the posterior horns, and they are concerned primarily with receiving incoming sensory information. The horizontal portion of the "H" is the site where fiber tracts cross from one side of the cord to the other.

The white portion of the spinal cord surrounds the gray "H" and consists of nerve tracts. Some tracts are arriving in the spinal cord after originating at a higher level, whereas other tracts begin in the spinal cord and ascend to the higher centers. The name of a specific tract is often derived from its origin and its destination: thus the spinothalamic tract originating at the spinal level and ascending to the thalamus. The corticospinal tract, on the other hand, arises from cell bodies in the motor cortex of the cerebral cortex and descends to the spinal levels. Take a moment to realize how long an axon can be. Some axons are 2 to 3 feet in length. Figure 1–9 shows the names and locations of other important tracts in the spinal cord.

The Peripheral Nervous System

The peripheral nervous system is that portion of the nervous system beyond the confines of the CNS; it goes, therefore, to all parts of the body. It is divided into two parts, the cranial nerves and the spinal nerves. It is the sensory portion of the peripheral nervous system that is given the responsibility of receiving stimuli and transmitting the information to the brain. The CNS, having been provided this information, formulates and initiates the appropriate body response. Then it becomes the responsibility of the motor portion of the peripheral nervous system to carry out this response by transmitting commands to the muscles, glands, and so forth.

The Sensory Tracts of the Spinal Cord

In the skin there are specialized structures that respond to specific sensory stimuli. Some respond to pressure, others to cold, others to heat, and others to pain. Whereas the functions of these receptors are easily appreciated, there are other receptors located in the joints, tendons, and muscles of the body whose function is less obvious. These receptors send to the CNS information about the position of a joint or limb, the speed of movement of a joint, or the tension exerted on a tendon or muscle. Although this sensory information does not for the most part reach our consciousness, it is vital informa-

Figure 1-9 Schematic Cross-section of the Spinal Cord, Showing the Relationship with the Sympathetic Chain

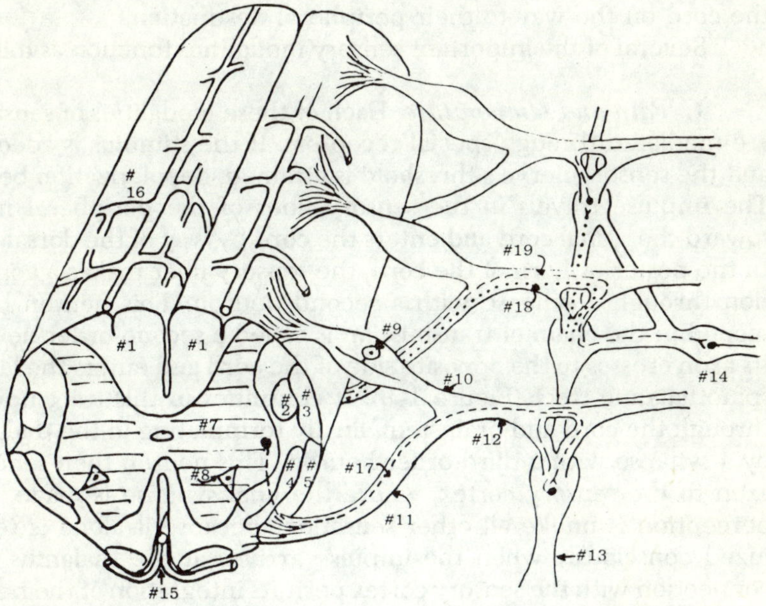

1. DORSAL COLUMNS
2. LATERAL CORTICOSPINAL TRACT
3. DORSAL SPINOCEREBELLAR TRACT
4. LATERAL SPINOTHALAMIC TRACT
5. VENTRAL SPINOCEREBELLAR TRACT
6. VENTRAL SPINOTHALAMIC TRACT
7. "H" SHAPED PORTION CONTAINING MANY NEURONS
8. ANTERIOR HORN CELL (MOTOR CELL)
9. SENSORY CELL IN DORSAL ROOT GANGLION
10. DORSAL ROOT (CARRIES SENSORY FIBERS)
11. VENTRAL OR ANTERIOR ROOT (CARRIES MOTOR FIBERS)
12. SPINAL NERVE
13. SYMPATHETIC CHAIN AND GANGLIA ATTACHED TO THE SPINAL NERVES
14. DISTAL SYMPATHETIC GANGLION
15. ANTERIOR SPINAL ARTERY AND BRANCHES
16. POSTERIOR SPINAL ARTERY AND BRANCHES
17. PATHWAY OF SYMPATHETIC FIBER GOING INTO SPINAL NERVE AT THE SAME LEVEL
18. PATHWAY OF SYMPATHETIC FIBER WITH MULTI LEVEL SYNAPSE AND DESTINATION
19. PREGANGLIONIC FIBER FORMING SYMPATHETIC NERVE WITH SYNAPSE AT A DISTAL SYMPATHETIC GANGLION

tion without which we could not walk at night, for we would not know which leg was in front of the other. Still more receptors are located in the body organs, such as the lungs, the walls of the intestines, and the bladder.

All receptors have a particular strength of stimulation that must be achieved before they respond. If this threshold is attained, a wave of depolarization begins in the nerve connected to the receptor, and the information is sent to the CNS. The impulse that arises from the receptor travels toward the spinal cord in sensory fibers located within a peripheral nerve. Prior to entering the spinal cord each peripheral nerve divides into a dorsal and a ventral root. The sensory nerve fibers enter the cord through the dorsal root. The cell bodies of the sensory nerves are located within the dorsal root ganglia (Figure 1–9). The ventral root carries motor nerve fibers that are leaving the cord on the way to their peripheral destination.

Several of the important sensory modalities function as follows:

1. *Pain and temperature.* Each of these modalities of sensation are mediated through special receptors. If the stimulus is adequate and the sensory nerve's threshold is attained, depolarization begins. The impulse travels in the sensory fiber of the peripheral nerve toward the spinal cord and enters the cord by way of the dorsal root. In the posterior horn of the cord, the sensory fiber makes a connection through a synapse with a second neuron. This neuron being second in the chain of transmission is called a second-order neuron. Its axon crosses to the opposite side of the cord and enters the lateral spinothalamic tract (Figure 1–9). It continues in this tract upward through the cord and brainstem, finally terminating in the thalamus by a synapse with a third-order neuron. This neuron then sends an axon to the sensory cortex, where the final synapse is made. Pain perception is unlike all other sensations because it alone is recognized consciously when the impulse arrives at the thalamus. The connection with the sensory cortex permits integration of the painful stimulus with other sensory stimuli.

2. *Touch.* This modality of sensation is conveyed to the sensory cortex by two different spinal cord pathways. The impulse begins when the touch receptor is stimulated; it travels in the peripheral nerve and enters the cord via the posterior root. In the posterior horn of the cord, a synapse may be made with a second-order neuron, or the fiber of the first-order neuron may enter the posterior (dorsal) columns of the cord (Figure 1–9). If a synapse is made, the axon of the second-order neuron crosses to the opposite side of the cord and enters the ventral spinothalamic tract. This tract ascends the cord and the brainstem and ends in the thalamus. A synapse with the third-order neuron is made with the impulse going then to the sensory cortex. If the other route is taken, the central branch of the first-order neuron (cell body located in the dorsal root ganglion) ascends the spinal cord in the dorsal column on the same side of the cord it enters. In the medulla a synapse is made with the second-order neuron located in the nucleus gracilis. The axon of this neuron crosses to the opposite side of the medulla and ascends the brainstem in the medial lemniscus making a synapse with a third-order neuron in the thalamus. This neuron in turn sends its axon to the sensory cortex.

3. *Conscious proprioception.* Receptors in joints, tendons, and muscles give rise to information, such as vibration sense and joint position sense, that is sent to the parietal lobe. This information reaches the parietal lobe in a manner similar to the modality of touch; that is, it ascends the posterior columns and the medial lemnisci.

4. *Unconscious proprioception.* Much of the proprioceptive information originating from receptors in joints, tendons, and muscles does not reach the conscious level. It instead goes to the cerebellum, where it is used to facilitate and coordinate movements of the body. There are two pairs of tracts in the spinal cord that carry proprioceptive information to the cerebellum. Sensory nerve fibers carrying this information from their peripheral receptors enter the cord via the dorsal roots and then ascend the cord in either the dorsal spinocerebellar tract or the ventral spinocerebellar tract on the same side of the spinal cord (Figure 1-9). The dorsal tract enters the cerebellum by way of the inferior cerebellar peduncle and terminates either in various cerebellar nuclei or the cerebellar cortex. The ventral tract enters the superior cerebellar peduncle, but unlike the dorsal tract, it would cross the midline to terminate in nuclei or the cortex of the opposite side of the cerebellum.

The final goal for this information has been shown to be either the sensory cerebral cortex or the cerebellum, but sensory information is also required by other parts of the CNS. Thus, as the various tracts ascend the spinal cord and brainstem, fibers leave the tracts going elsewhere.

The Reticular Activating System

The reticular activating system (mentioned in the discussion of the midbrain) consists of groups of ill-defined nuclei containing neurons of varied type and shape that are found throughout the brainstem. This system receives input from the cranial nerves and from the ascending sensory tracts of the cord. Experiments have shown that the reticular activating system is responsible for activating the cerebral cortex. In other words it keeps the cortex "awake." The connection between the reticular activating system and the cortex is achieved by many synapses that create in effect a reticulothalamic tract and from the thalamus, a multisynaptic thalamocortical tract. It has been shown that many anesthetics act at the level of the reticular formation. Without the constant arousal influence from the reticular activating system, the cerebral cortex goes to sleep.

The Motor Tracts of the Spinal Cord and Brainstem

Let us turn now to the voluntary motor pathways of the peripheral system. The discussion of the frontal lobe included a description of the motor strip and its topographical arrangement according to body parts. From the large motor cells (Betz's cells or pyramidal cells) in the motor strip, axons arise that converge in the white matter to form the principal descending motor tracts of the brain. The major tract is the corticospinal or pyramidal tract. It descends through the brainstem on the same side from which it arises. Then, in the lower medulla, most of the fibers cross to the other side and continue in the spinal cord. When an axon running in this tract reaches its destination in the cord, the axon leaves the corticospinal tract and enters the anterior horn of the gray matter. Here it makes a synapse with an anterior horn cell. The motor neuron in the cortex that sent the original axon is considered the upper motor neuron, while the anterior horn cell becomes the lower motor neuron. The axon of the lower motor neuron or anterior horn cell leaves the cord through the ventral root, which joins the dorsal root, making up the spinal or peripheral nerve. The axon from the anterior horn cell travels in its peripheral nerve to a muscle. The anterior horn cells that send their axons to the muscles of the upper extremity are located in the cervical portion of the spinal cord; those sending axons to the legs are in the lumbar and upper sacral portions of the cord.

The corticobulbar tract and the corticomesencephalic tract are two other descending motor tracts that should be mentioned. The corticobulbar tract begins with the corticospinal tract but ends in the brainstem. It goes to the motor nuclei of cranial nerves V, VII, IX, X, XI, and XII. Most of the fibers of the corticobulbar tract cross over to enter nuclei (cranial nerve nuclei) of the opposite side of the brainstem, though some remain uncrossed. This tract goes to nuclei III, IV, and VI, which are the nuclei that control the movement of the eye.

Motor impulses along these tracts cause muscular activity. For example, a wave of depolarization, begun in the motor cortex, travels in the corticospinal tract to the appropriate anterior horn cell. Transmission across a synapse stimulates the anterior horn cell to depolarize; this sends the nerve impulse along a peripheral nerve to the muscle. The connection between the nerve fiber and muscle is achieved by a unique structure called the myoneural junction, which is like the synapse between two nerves because, as the impulse arrives at the myoneural junction, a chemical substance called acetylcholine is released. This substance spreads to the receptor site of the muscle fiber and causes it to depolarize. When this has been accomplished acetylcholine is deactivated by an enzyme called acetylcholinesterase, which splits it into acetic acid and choline. The wave of depolarization in the muscle spreads along a membrane in the muscle called the sarcolemma. When this occurs energy is released that causes the muscle fiber to contract.

The number of muscle fibers served by a single axon varies in each muscle. Those muscles that perform gross movements have several fibers per axon, whereas muscles such as those that move the eye have few muscle fibers per axon. Once the threshold for contraction of a muscle fiber is reached, the fiber contracts as hard as it can—an example of the all-or-none concept. Just how hard an entire muscle contracts depends on how much effort is required to perform a specific action. This obviously requires judgment, which is done by the higher centers in the CNS. The variation of strength that a muscle produces depends on the number of muscle fibers called into action at the time. Hence the maximum strength of a muscle would be evident if all of its component fibers contracted at once.

The mechanism of contraction of muscle is not fully understood, but it appears that a muscle fiber shortens when certain muscle proteins slide past one another. Figure 1-10 illustrates how the actin and myosin proteins slide in the process of contraction. When the fiber is shortened chemical bridges occur between the two proteins. This holds the proteins in the shortened configuration and permits the buildup of tension so the fiber can perform the action required of it. When the fiber relaxes the chemical bridges disappear, and the proteins slide back to the longer position. Calcium is vital in the process of muscle contraction.

Figure 1-10 Diagrammatic Illustration of Muscular Contraction

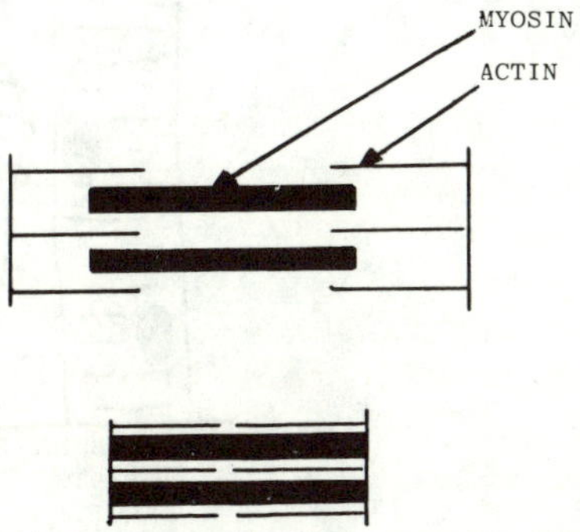

Within muscles and situated among muscle fibers are special receptors that monitor the length of muscle fibers and play a role in maintaining muscle tone. A muscle at rest is never flabby; it has a definite firmness. The firmness is called muscle tone. This quality is a state of readiness on the part of the muscle. The receptors in the muscle are called muscle spindles (Figure 1-11). They lie parallel to the muscle fiber and are attached to it, so that if the fiber is stretched the muscle spindle is also stretched. There is a sensory nerve

Figure 1-11 Muscle Spindle

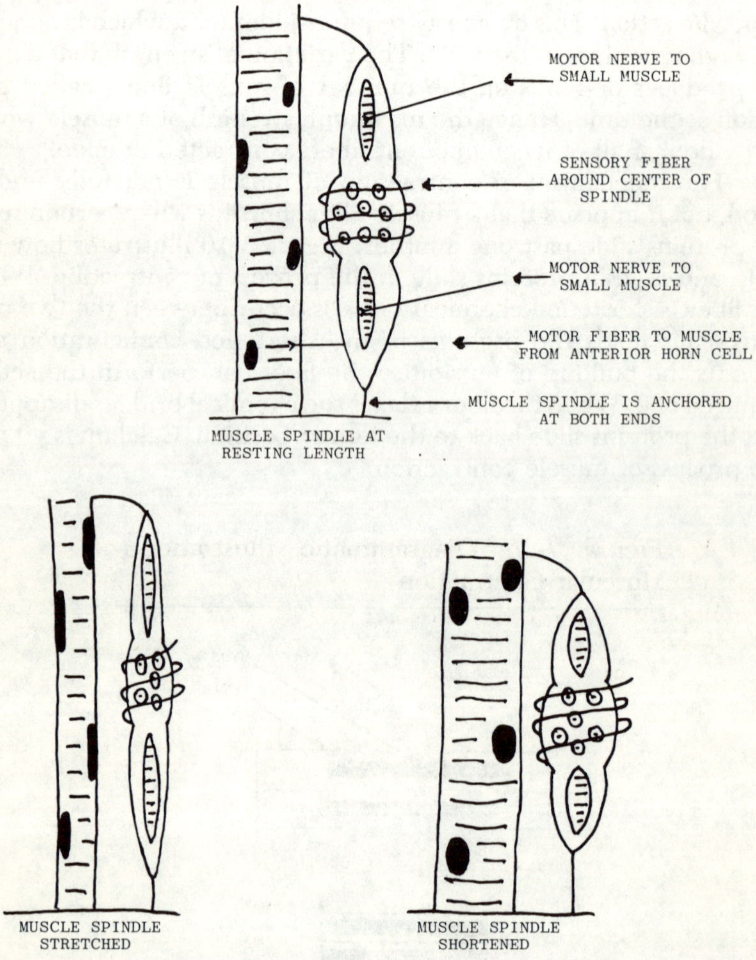

wrapped around the center of the spindle that carries information regarding spindle length to the spinal cord. The cell body of this sensory nerve is in the dorsal root ganglia just like the other sensory nerves already discussed. The central process of this type of sensory neuron goes to an anterior horn cell (motor cell) and if necessary stimulates it to send a motor impulse to the muscle fibers telling them to contract or shorten. We have all experienced this process when we slip unexpectedly: Certain muscles in our legs are momentarily stretched, but before we can consciously realize what has occurred, we have regained our balance. Another example is the deep-tendon reflex that occurs when the tendon at the knee is tapped with a reflex hammer. The rapid tap stretches the muscle in the front part of the thigh (the quadriceps). This is picked up by the muscle spindle, and its sensory fiber sends an impulse to the anterior horn cells, which in turn send an impulse through motor fibers to the quadriceps. This muscle is stimulated to contract, and we see the leg kick. This circuit is called the reflex arc and is the basis of all deep-tendon reflexes.

Another important anatomic feature of the muscle spindle is the presence of two very small muscle fibers that begin at each end and run toward the center of the spindle. The center of the spindle contains nuclei, and this is the site where the sensory nerve attaches. Small motor nerves come from the spinal cord and go to the two muscle fibers. These motor nerves do not arise from the large motor neurons in the spinal cord but from smaller ones close by. We can now see that, if the two small muscles in the spindle contract, the center will be stretched just as it would if the entire muscle were stretched. The sensory nerve responds, the anterior horn cells send motor impulses to the muscle fibers, and the muscle contracts. The amount of contraction is not great in this instance and the limb does not move, but the muscle fibers do tighten. This resultant muscle shortening or firmness is called muscle tone. It is possible that the tremors seen in some neurological disease result from an imbalance in this system.

This discussion of muscular contraction and the schematic illustration pertain to skeletal or striated muscle. Skeletal muscles are those of the arms and legs as well as of the trunk. There are two other kinds found in the human body: the heart or cardiac muscle and the smooth muscle that is in the wall of the digestive tract, in blood vessels, and in the reproductive organs. Smooth muscle and cardiac muscle also have nervous control and have the ability to contract. They are, however, largely without voluntary control.

The Cranial Nerves

The cranial nerves, along with the spinal nerves, comprise the peripheral nervous system. There are twelve pairs of cranial nerves that arise from the brainstem. They are numbered, beginning with the olfactory nerves and ending with the hypoglossal nerves.

Olfactory nerve. The first pair of cranial nerves are the olfactory nerves. The sensory neuron that responds to an odor is located in a specialized mucosa (lining membrane) in the roof of each nostril. These neurons have two processes. One goes to the surface of the mucosa; the other, the central process, enters the intracranial space by passing through a very thin bony plate (cribriform plate) that lies between the brain and the roof of the nostril. The central processes then enter the olfactory bulb and synapse with another neuron. Axons from the second-order neuron run in the olfactory tract to the brain. The final destination of these axons is either the anterior hypothalamus or the temporal lobe.

The loss of the sense of smell is called anosmia and is common with head injuries. The delicate central processes of the sensory neurons are easily torn even with mild trauma. Fractures often occur across the cribriform plate because the bone is so thin. If the dura is torn adjacent to the cribriform plate fracture, spinal fluids may leak through the nose. This is called CSF rhinorrhea.

Optic nerve. The second pair of cranial nerves are the optic nerves, and they are concerned exclusively with vision. The human eye may be compared to a camera, for it has a lens, an aperture for light control, and film. The aperture is the variably sized pupil, and the film is the retina. In the retina are special receptors called rods and cones that have the ability to absorb light. The rods, responsible for night vision, produce gray images; the color images of day vision depend on the cones' function. In these receptors are chemical substances that are changed in a reversible manner when light hits them. The resultant chemical change causes depolarization of optic nerve fibers and, therefore, initiates a nervous impulse. The impulse first travels in the optic nerve to the optic chiasm and then along the optic tract to the lateral geniculate body, which lies near the posterior part of the thalamus. In the lateral geniculate body, a synapse is made with another neuron, which sends its axon to the visual cortex (occipital lobe) by way of the optic radiations (Figure 1-12).

As can be seen in Figure 1-12 the image (arrow) falls on the left half of each retina. The nerve fibers that arise from the left half of each retina go first in their respective optic nerves, but at the chiasm, the fibers from the right eye cross and then run in the left optic tract.

Figure 1-12 Visual Pathways

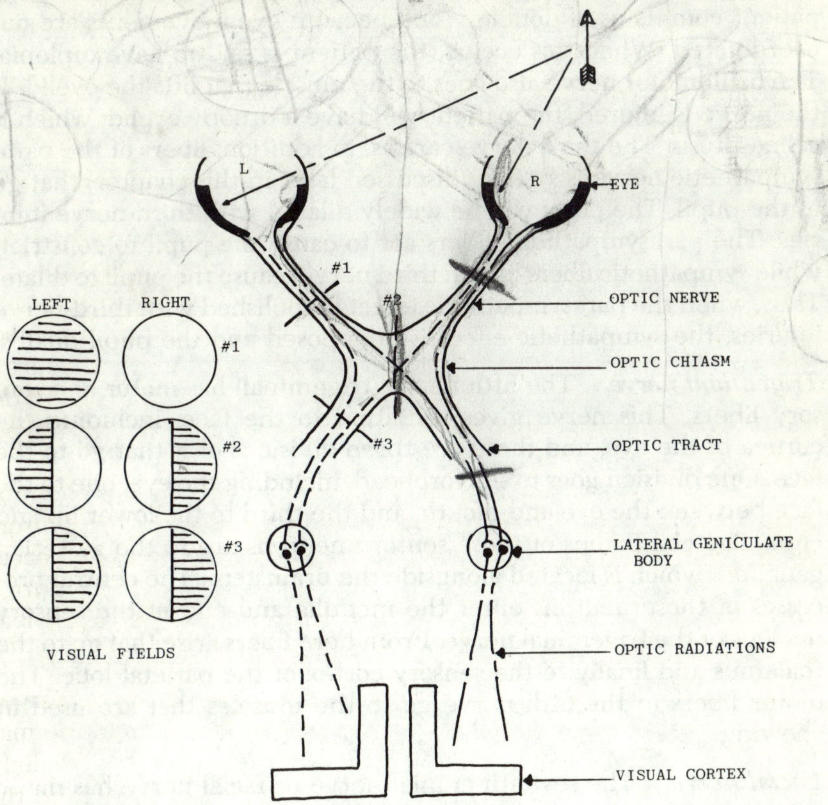

It is the rule that the axons arising from the medial or nasal (nose) half of each retina cross in the chiasm running in the opposite optic tract. We can see then that the left visual cortex serves the right half of each visual field. In other words, if the left visual cortex is destroyed by a brain tumor, our patient will be unable to see to the right in either eye. This is illustrated in the Visual Field 3 in Figure 1-12. If injury is sustained by one optic nerve at the point marked by dotted line 1, the patient is blind in the left eye; Visual Field 1 illustrates this. If the chiasm is injured at the point marked by dotted line 2, a field defect illustrated by Visual Field 2 will be seen.

Oculomotor, trochlear, and abducens nerves. Cranial nerves III (oculomotor), IV (trochlear), and VI (abducens) all go to the muscles that move the eye. The sixth nerve goes to a single muscle that moves the eye outward. The third and fourth nerves control the rest of the eye movements. If one of these nerves is injured or diseased, the patient complains of double vision because eye movements are not coordinated. When this occurs, the patient is said to have diplopia. The oculomotor nerve also goes to the muscle that lifts the eyelid. If the nerve is injured, the patient will have a droopy eyelid, which is called ptosis. The third nerve carries, in addition, fibers of the parasympathetic nervous system (discussed later in this chapter) that go to the pupil. The pupil will be widely dilated with third-nerve injuries. The parasympathetic fibers act to cause the pupil to constrict, while sympathetic fibers (not in third nerve) cause the pupil to dilate. Thus, when the parasympathetic effect is abolished with third-nerve injuries, the sympathetic effect is unopposed and the pupil dilates.

Trigeminal nerve. The fifth nerve (trigeminal) has motor and sensory fibers. This nerve gives sensation to the face, including the cornea of the eye, and there are three divisions of it that go to the face. One division goes to the forehead, including the eye, one to the face between the eye and mouth, and the third to the lower lip and chin. The cell bodies of these sensory neurons are in the gasserian ganglion, which is located alongside the brainstem. The central processes of these neurons enter the medulla and end in the sensory nucleus of the trigeminal nerve. From here fibers arise that go to the thalamus and finally to the sensory cortex of the parietal lobe. The motor fibers in the fifth nerve go to the muscles that are used in chewing.

Facial nerve. The seventh cranial nerve or facial nerve has many functions. It sends motor fibers to muscles of the face that are used in expression. It also sends fibers to some of the glands that produce saliva, to the tear or lacrimal gland in the eye, and to glands in the mucous membranes of the nose. The facial nerve also has a sensory component that carries the sense of taste from the front two-thirds of the tongue.

When the facial nerve is involved with disease or injury, the prominent feature is facial paralysis. The patient is unable to smile or close the eye on the affected side. If the paralysis is on the right side of the face, when the patient smiles, the mouth will pull to the left. This is because the muscles of the left side of the face contract with the smile, drawing the mouth to the left. There are two types of facial palsies (paralysis). One is the central facial palsy, and the other is a peripheral facial palsy. If one is observant it is easy to distinguish between the two. The facial nerve leaves the intracranial space by way of a small foramen (hole) near the jaw joint (temporomandibular joint). It then divides into several branches that spread out going to the various muscles of expression in the face.

A patient with a peripheral facial nerve palsy will not be able to move any of the muscles on the involved side of the face. A patient with a central facial nerve palsy is able to wrinkle the brow somewhat, but the muscles below the eye and around the mouth are paralyzed. The peripheral seventh-nerve paralysis involves the nerve directly and may occur with fractures of the skull and with tumors, but most often it occurs with no obvious cause, in which case it is called Bell's palsy. Most patients who develop Bell's palsy recover, though some may not. More serious than the cosmetic problems of Bell's palsy is the injury that can result from inability to close the eye when sleeping, such as corneal scratches from the bed sheets. The tear gland may be involved, too, so the eye becomes dry and irritated. Infection of the eye occurs.

Disease or injury to the cells in the motor strip is responsible for the occurrence of a central facial paralysis. Remember that not all of the corticobulbar tract crosses to the opposite motor nuclei of the cranial nerves. The muscles of the brow in fact get motor input from both motor strips. The muscles of the lower face, however, are under the control of the opposite motor strip alone. Thus if the left motor strip is injured, the right lower face will be paralyzed, but the upper facial muscles move because of the still-functioning right motor strip.

Acoustic nerve. The eighth cranial nerve has two components, the cochlear nerve for hearing and the vestibular nerve, which assists with balance and coordination.

The cochlea is a spiral seashell-like receptor located deep within each ear, and its function is to receive sound vibrations. Within its coiled length are rows of small hairlike projections that respond to specific frequencies. In the center of the cochlea is the ganglion containing neuron cell bodies that send nerve processes to each hairlike structure and a longer process to the cochlear nuclei in the medulla by way of the cochlear nerve. From these nuclei, fibers go to various points in the brainstem and to the primary auditory cortex found in the superior temporal gyrus of each temporal lobe. Each ear is represented by both temporal lobes; therefore deafness does not result if a single auditory cortex is destroyed. In addition to deafness that occurs with cochlear disease, a patient may complain of noises in the ear. These noises vary, being described as sounding like such things crickets, rushing water, whistles. Patients are said to have tinnitus when these noises occur.

The receptors for the vestibular portion of the acoustic nerve are also located deep within each ear. They are special organs that monitor the position of the head as well as movement of the head. Nerve fibers connect them with the vestibular nuclei that are found in the medulla. Two prominent tracts arise from the vestibular nuclei. They are the vestibulospinal and the vestibulomesencephalic tracts. The names indicate that each tract arises from the vestibular nuclei, the first going to the spinal cord and the second to the brainstem. They function by producing changes in the posture of the body, depending on the position of the head and neck. There is a similar effect on the movement of the eyes. Disease of the vestibular apparatus may produce a rapid to-and-fro movement of the eyes that is called nystagmus.

Glossopharyngeal nerve. The ninth cranial nerve is called the glossopharyngeal nerve. It has nerve fibers that carry the sensation of touch, temperature, and pain from the back of the tongue, the tonsils, and the throat (pharynx). It also carries the fibers of taste from the back one-third of the tongue. The motor component of significance in the glossopharyngeal nerve goes to the parotid gland on each side, producing saliva. The glossopharyngeal nerve's function is closely aligned with that of the tenth cranial nerve.

Vagus nerve. The vagus nerve is the tenth cranial nerve. This nerve functions primarily as a part of the parasympathetic nervous system (discussed later in this chapter). It carries fibers of sensation from the larynx, the pharynx, the trachea, the esophagus, and the thoracic and abdominal viscera (organs). Other fibers in the vagus nerve transmit impulses that arise in taste buds on the epiglottis. The motor components of importance go to the various organs of the chest and abdomen as well as to the muscles of the larynx (voice box) and the pharynx.

Spinal accessory nerve. The spinal accessory nerve is the eleventh cranial nerve. It has two parts: the cranial and the spinal portions. The cranial part joins the vagus nerve and goes to the muscles of the larynx. Injury to the nerve going to the larynx produces hoarseness. The spinal portion of the eleventh cranial nerve goes to some of the muscles in the neck and shoulder.

Hypoglossal nerve. The last pair of cranial nerves are the hypoglossal or twelfth cranial nerves. These nerve fibers arise in the medulla and go to the muscles in the tongue. Injury to one of the hypoglossal nerves causes loss of muscle bulk or atrophy on the side of the nerve injury.

The Autonomic Nervous System

A very special portion of the nervous system called the autonomic nervous system is divided into the parasympathetic and sympathetic divisions. The discussion to this point has been concerned with the motor supply to skeletal muscles or with sensory fibers arising from receptors in the skin or joints or from specialized receptors such as the ear or eye. The autonomic nervous system has an influence on many different structures including the eye and the cardiovascular, respiratory, digestive, glandular, urinary, and reproductive systems.

Parasympathetic Division

The parasympathetic division leaves the CNS through a cranial and a sacral outflow route (Figure 1-13). The cranial outflow is a part of the cranial nerve system. The third cranial nerve sends parasympathetic fibers to the muscles in the eye that make the pupil become smaller. The seventh and ninth cranial nerves send motor fibers to the saliva glands. The major cranial nerve that carries parasympathetic fibers is the tenth (vagus) cranial nerve. This nerve has a long course through the neck, the chest, and throughout the abdomen. It goes to the air passages of the lung, to the heart, and then into the abdomen, going to the stomach, bile ducts, pancreas, kidney, and intestines. When the parasympathetic fibers reach their destination, they liberate acetylcholine. As a result, these fibers are said to be cholinergic. Many medicines produce effects similar to the parasympathetic nervous system and are called cholinergic drugs.

The sacral outflow of the parasympathetic system is by way of sacral nerve roots S_2, S_3, and S_4. The axon arises from neurons in the gray matter at these cord levels. They exit the cord in the ventral roots and then join nerves going to the bladder, colon, rectum, and sex organs.

Sympathetic Division

The fibers of the sympathetic nervous system arise from neurons located in the gray matter of the cord from the first thoracic level through the third lumbar level (Figure 1–9). They leave the cord through the ventral roots at each cord level and then enter the spinal nerves.

Within just a short distance, the sympathetic fibers leave the spinal nerves and enter special ganglions of the sympathetic nervous system. There is a sympathetic ganglion for each level of the cord that gives rise to the sympathetic fibers, and there are others that are

Figure 1-13 Parasympathetic Nervous System

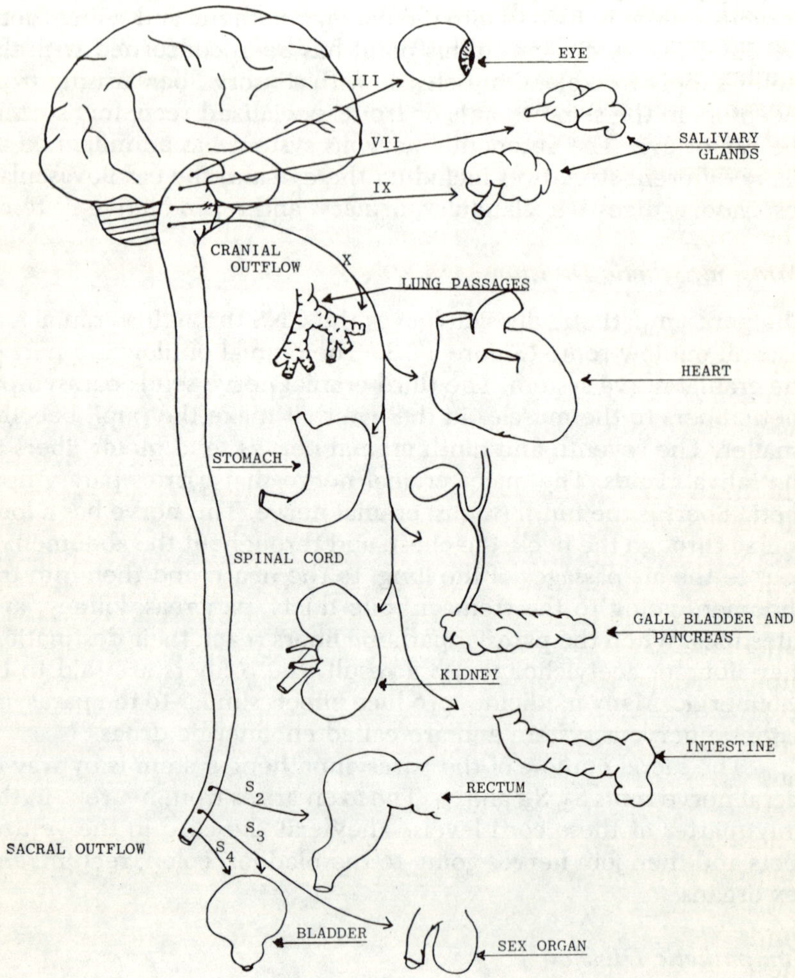

located in the cervical and the sacral regions. The sympathetic ganglia lie next to the vertebrae on each side of the spine and are connected to each other forming a long chain. The two sympathetic chains extend from the base of the skull to the sacrum. After the sympathetic fiber enters the ganglia, it may form a synapse with another neuron. When this occurs the entering neuron is called the preganglionic fiber; the second neuron gives rise to the postganglionic fiber. The postganglionic fiber then joins the same spinal nerve that contained the preganglionic fiber and, therefore, travels to its destination. The preganglionic fiber may, on the other hand, run up or down the sympathetic chain, finally making a synapse in another ganglion from which the postganglionic fibers arise. The preganglionic fibers may also choose to leave the sympathetic chain and join similar fibers from adjacent levels, making up purely sympathetic nerves. These preganglionic fibers eventually enter a sympathetic ganglion (separate from the chain) that is near its destination. The synapse is then made with the postganglionic neuron, which gives rise to the postganglionic fiber that then goes to the specific organ.

The postganglionic fibers of the sympathetic nervous system liberate at their terminal ends a chemical substance similar to adrenalin. Therefore sympathetic fibers are adrenergic fibers. Any medication that produces similar effects is called an adrenergic drug.

Fibers of the sympathetic nervous system are distributed widely throughout the body (Figure 1–9). Fibers arise from the cervical portion of the sympathetic chain forming a loose network that goes with the carotid arteries in the head. They go to sweat glands of the face, to the muscle in the eye and to the muscle that raises the eyelid. If the sympathetic fibers that enter the head are injured, the patient has a lack of sweating on that side of the face (anhidrosis), the pupil is smaller than the opposite pupil, and there is a droop of the eyelid (ptosis). This combination is called Horner's syndrome. Sympathetic fibers go to the blood vessels throughout the body and act to cause them to constrict. This may cause an increase in the blood pressure. Many of the drugs to lower blood pressure have their site of action at this level. Whether sympathetic fibers have any significant effect on cerebral blood vessels is doubtful. If there is any effect it is certainly not as significant as elsewhere in the body. Other sympathetic fibers go to sweat glands, respiratory passages, heart, intestines, bladder, and sex organs.

Nerve supply to the adrenal gland is a special function of the sympathetic nervous system. This gland releases adrenalin and, as a result, supplements the action of the sympathetic nervous system elsewhere in the body. This response is maximal in rage, fear, or extreme pain. In these instances all function in the intestinal tract ceases; blood is shunted to muscles, the heart rate increases, the lung passages dilate to permit the flow of more air, and the spleen contracts, forcing more blood into circulation. The body is in this way made ready to fight or to take flight.

It can be seen that many organs have both parasympathetic and sympathetic nervous supply. In general when there is such a dual supply, the parasympathetic and sympathetic effects are opposite one another.

Overall Nervous System Function

Having discussed the various parts of the nervous system, we can appreciate its beauty by considering it as a whole. Let us begin by restating the first paragraph of this chapter: The function of the nervous system is to receive stimuli from the environment and to transmit this information to the brain, which in turn formulates and initiates the appropriate response. Thus, by receptors such as those for hearing, vision, taste, smell, pain, touch, temperature, and joint position sense, our body constantly monitors the environment. The information gathered is transmitted to the CNS by the cranial nerves and the spinal nerves. Once this information reaches the CNS it is sent throughout the nervous system to those parts that require this specific information to function. Incoming sensory information is dispersed in many ways: (1) the simplest is the reflex arc in which the sensory fiber connects directly by a synapse to a motor neuron. This is illustrated by the jerks of the leg when the patellar tendon at the knee is tapped by the reflex hammer; (2) the sensory information coming in by way of the sensory nerves may make synapses with several neurons locally, or it may travel up or down the cord or brainstem making synapses with neurons at other levels on the same or opposite side. Connections of this kind permit various spinal reflexes that are considerably more complex than the simple reflex arc. One sees such a reflex when one touches something hot with one's hand. The hand is withdrawn before one is consciously aware of the heat. This reflex requires not one muscle but several working together. Another example is illustrated when one steps on a sharp object with bare feet. The foot is rapidly withdrawn, while the opposite leg straightens to support the entire weight of the body.

One can easily appreciate that spinal reflexes involve intricate movements, but more astounding is the split-second integration and response required. The sensory input sets the wheels in motion, but it is the magnificence of the computer of the CNS that makes the proper response a reality. The final output of the computer consists of positive (facilitory) and negative (inhibitory) commands. In the case of touching a hot object with one's hand, the facilitory command goes to those motor neurons that control muscles that can withdraw the hand. The inhibitory portion of the command goes to those neurons that if activated would interfere with the withdrawal of the hand. The inhibitory command tells those neurons to relax and not interfere with the movement.

The last example illustrates an important concept that must be appreciated. This is the concept of facilitory and inhibitory forces that interplay in all nervous system function. Thus, a single motor neuron may receive many inhibitory signals and many facilitory signals. The resultant action of the neuron depends on the quantity and quality of each. To develop the concept of facilitation and inhibition a bit further, consider a neuron receiving a facilitory signal from one part of the nervous system. This signal, however, is not strong enough to reach the threshold required to activate the neuron. If, however, a signal of similar magnitude arrives simultaneously from elsewhere, the two signals together reach the required threshold for action by the neuron. Therefore, subliminal facilitation and inhibition play a very important role in nervous system function.

Consider now the vast amount of sensory information received by the brain through the cranial nerves and the sensory tracts of the spinal cord. Recall that much of this information reaches our consciousness but a significant amount of it does not. The following outline lists the sensory information received by the brain and how it is used to our benefit:

1. Visual sensation
   a. Survey of the environment and orientation
   b. Assistance in most activities of motion such as eating, dressing, and walking
   c. Communication by reading, interpretation of gestures, etc.
   d. Pleasure through art forms and the beauty of nature
   e. Protection by avoiding dangerous situations
2. Auditory sensations
   a. Communication by speech and other spoken media
   b. Pleasure through music, poetry, etc.
   c. Protection, such as warning shout from a friend or the sound of an approaching car
   d. Orientation of the head and the body relative to the earth and local environment
3. Smell and taste sensations
   a. Pleasure by the enjoyment of favorite foods
   b. Protection by identifying dangerous foods that are spoiled or contaminated
   c. Protection by identifying smoke or toxic airborne substances

d. Rudimentary assistance in finding food
e. Assistance in mating (in animals)

4. Vestibular sensations (inner ear)
   a. Orientation of the head and the body relative to the earth and local environment
   b. Identification and quantitative judgment of the effects of acceleration, deceleration, and rotation on the head and body
5. Touch and pressure
   a. Characterization of objects in the environment by texture, firmness, flexibility, contour, and shape
   b. Assistance in use of objects such as a pencil or in turning the pages of a book
6. Temperature
   a. Protection by identifying potentially harmful temperature states, both hot and cold
   b. Pleasure through enjoyment of the warmth of the sun and the coolness of a breeze
   c. Characterization of objects
7. Pain
   a. Protection by identification of harmful and potentially destructive situations or objects
8. Joint position sensation
   a. Conscious information about the position of our limbs relative to the rest of the body
   b. Conscious orientation of the entire body to the environment
   c. Unconscious information to the cerebellum about body and limb position used to corrodinate movement
9. Sensation from receptors in joints monitoring motion, velocity, and tension, and receptors in tendons and muscles monitoring tension and velocity
   a. Conscious and unconscious information needed for coordination of intricate movements
   b. Orientation of body parts
10. Visceral sensations and sensations from special organs
    a. Hunger pangs, motivating search for food
    b. Alerting of body to needs for urination and bowel movement
    c. Sexual organ stimulation, producing orgasm and fertilization
    d. Abdominal cramps and nausea, alerting the brain to illness
    e. Breathlessness, air hunger, and chest pain, alerting brain to possible cardiopulmonary disease

It is readily apparent that the amount of sensory information provided to the brain is vast in quanity and widely varied in type.

The healthy brain is able to effectively manage this data in the following manner:

1. Disregard irrelevant information
2. Monitor the incoming information for additional pertinent information
3. Direct sensory systems to obtain further needed information, for example, prompting motor movements such as turning the head
4. Correlate incoming information with relevant thoughts derived from past experiences, training, and education

As the brain scans the incoming sensory information for pertinent data, priorities may suddenly change. The attentive bird watcher in the rain forest of the Amazon quickly changes priorities upon hearing the roar of a tiger. The healthy brain is at attention, and although directed by the motivation of the moment, it is alert to other eventualities.

Motivation is determined by the needs and drives of the organism at a particular moment in time. Needs and drives depend on both internal and external factors. Internal factors include not only basic drives like hunger and thirst but the consequences of emotional states like grief and joy. The external factors have already been covered in the list of the various sensory modalities, but they include the threat of harm and orientation to the environment.

It appears that the motor system is of secondary importance to the sensory system. It serves to move the various sensory receptors to enable them to obtain needed sensory information. It may also be directed to act (walk, sit, or lie) if necessary to achieve the final needs as determined by the sensory system and the state of motivation.

The greatest ability of the human brain is its capacity for abstract thinking. This ability is illustrated by our achievements in mathematics, physics, and philosophy. A peek at the brilliance of Einstein, Newton, Beethoven, and Hume gives us but a hint of the brain's capabilities.

Cerebrosinal Fluid, Its Production and Circulation

Cerebrospinal fluid is colorless. It is produced by the choroid plexus located in each of the brain's ventricles. The amount of fluid present in the ventricular system and the subarachnoid is about 130 cubic centimeters, but the volume produced in a 24-hour period is approximately 600–700 cubic centimeters. It is therefore readily apparent that CSF circulation is a very dynamic system with fluid being constantly produced and absorbed.

There are two theories about the production of CSF by the choroid plexus. One theory considers CSF to be merely a filtrate that flows passively from the blood in the choroid plexus into the ventricles. The other views the production of CSF to be an active secretory process by the choroid plexus.

The normal flow of CSF after production may be seen by referring to Figure 1–4. It flows from both lateral ventricles into the third ventricle. Next, it passes into the fourth ventricle by way of the aqueduct of Sylvius. From the fourth ventricle the spinal fluid enters the subarachnoid space. In this manner the entire brain and spinal cord are bathed in cerebrospinal fluid. The absorption of the CSF is accomplished by the arachnoid villi (arachnoid granulations). These delicate structures are out-pocketings of the arachnoid that protrude into the dural venous sinuses. It is at this point that the fluid in the subarachnoid space passes through the thin-walled arachnoid villi to enter the venous blood.

The Skull and Vertebral Column

The brain and spinal cord are contained within the bony skull and the vertebral column. The skull in the adult is a firm structure called the calvarium. The skull of an infant, however, is pliable because the bones that make up the calvarium are not fused and they are thin. This permits the calvarium to expand as the brain grows. The junction between the individual bones of the calvarium is called a suture line. The suture line becomes a firm bony bridge between adjacent bones by 18 months of age. At the point where suture lines intersect one another there is a soft spot called a fontanel (Figure 1–14).

The contour of the base of the inside of the calvarium is tiered (Figure 1–15). Each tier is called a fossa. The anterior fossa contains the frontal lobes; the middle fossa is filled by the temporal lobe. The posterior fossa contains the cerebellum, pons, and medulla.

In the base of the calvarium are holes called foramina through which the cranial nerves pass. The largest foramen is the foramen magnum which contains the junction between the medulla and the upper cervical spinal cord (Figure 1–15).

The adult calvarium is quite thick in most places and provides very adequate protection to the brain. The vertebral column, on the other hand, has to be somewhat less protective so that mobility can

Figure 1-14 Bony Skull

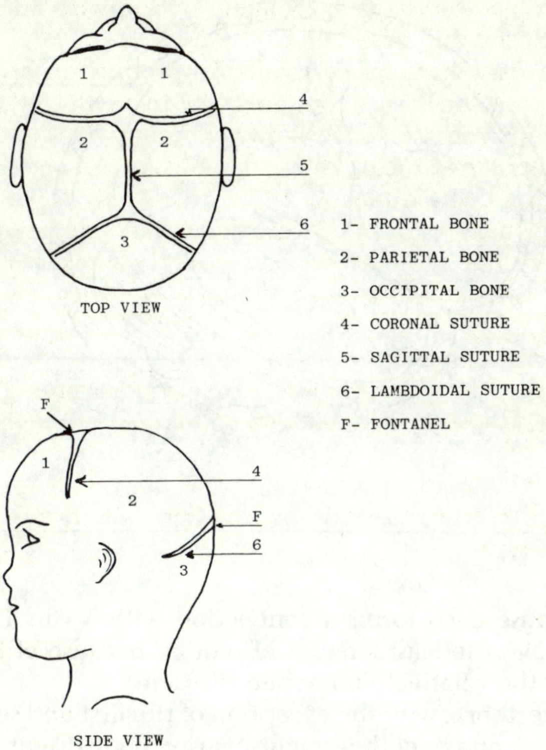

be achieved. The vertebral column consists of individual vertebrae stacked one upon the other. A disc, which has a shock-absorbing function and which permits motion, lies between adjacent vertebrae. There are seven cervical vertebrae, twelve thoracic, five lumbar, and five sacral. The sacral vertebrae are usually fused into a solid structure called the sacrum. The sacrum and the variably shaped coccyx form the tail bone.

Most of the vertebrae have essentially the same structures. The cervical vertebrae are smaller and more delicate. They afford the greatest range of motion, but they are less strong and more easily fractured than the thoracic or lumbar vertebrae. The lumbar vertebrae are the largest because they must support the weight of the trunk, head, and upper extremities; yet they do afford a fair range of motion as one can see by our ability to bend and twist the lower back. The thoracic vertebrae are intermediate in size, but they are

Figure 1-15

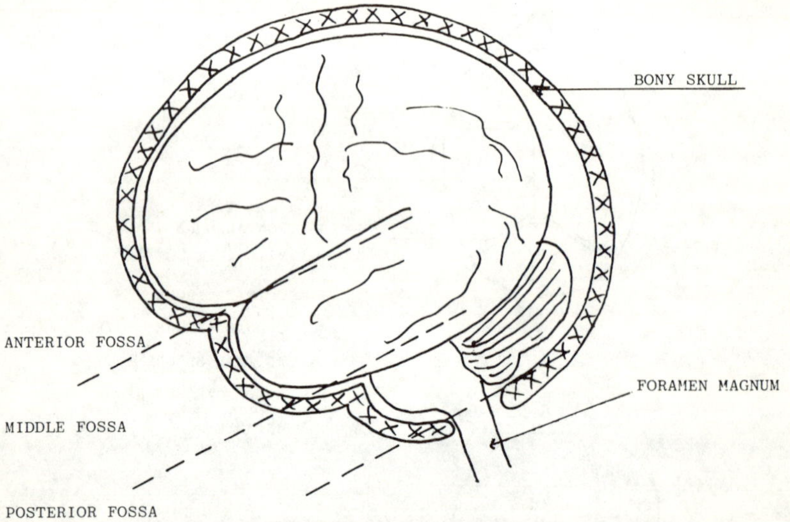

unique because each forms a connection with a rib. The thoracic vertebrae have the least amount of motion because of the stability imposed by the relatively immobile rib cage.

Each vertebra, with the exception of the first and second cervical vertebrae, consists of the weight-bearing body (Figure 1–16). The discs that lie between the bodies are firmly held in that position by strong ligments. Extending backward from the body are two pedicles, which give support to the lamina and spine. These latter two structures of the vertebrae surround a circular space called the spinal canal. The spinal canal is, therefore, a cylindrical space that extends from the base of the skull to the sacrum. The spinal cord lies within the spinal canal. An opening called a foramen is present at each level and on each side of the spinal canal. The nerves that originate from the spinal cord pass through these foramina (Figure 1–16).

The spinal cord runs in the spinal canal from the base of the skull to about the second lumbar vertebra. The cord ends at this level; however, nerve roots that arise from the end of the cord continue running in the spinal canal. The nerves coming from the terminal cord look in the aggregate like the tail of a horse. This appearance has resulted in the name cauda equina. The first two cervical vertebrae are unique in structure and in function. The first cervical vertebra (C_1), which is called the atlas, is a bony ring. The skull sits on the

Figure 1-16 Vertebral Column with Relationship of the Spinal Cord and Nerves Illustrated

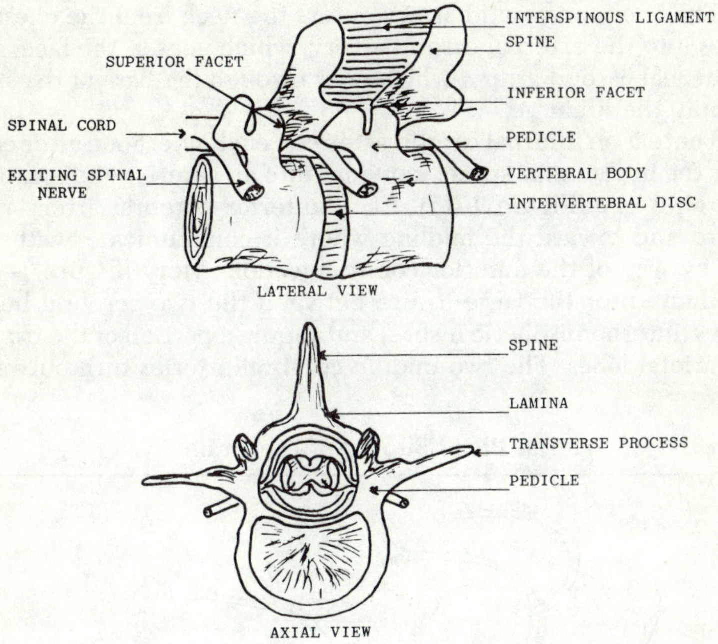

atlas at two points called the atlanto-occipital joints. The motion possible at these two joints is manifest when we move our head to signify "yes."

The second cervical vertebra (C_2) is called the axis. It has an upward vertical bony projection called the odontoid process, which forms a joint with the inside front of the atlas. The motion it makes possible is a rotational movement around the odontoid. The motion permitted at this joint is the motion made when we shake our head signifying "no." The underside of C_2 sits on C_3, with an intervening disc.

Blood Supply of Brain and Spinal Cord

The blood supply of the brain is provided by four arteries that arise from the great vessels leading from the heart. Most of the cerebral hemispheres are supplied by the carotid system, which is the anterior circulation of the brain. The posterior circulation is provided by the vertebrobasilar system, which serves the brainstem, the cerebellum, and the occipital lobes of the cerebrum.

The common carotid artery enters the neck from the chest. It divides into the external carotid artery, which goes to the face, and the internal carotid artery, which goes through the base of the skull to supply the brain.

There is an internal carotid artery on each side. Soon after each enters the intracranial space, it divides into an anterior and a middle cerebral artery (Figure 1–17). Each anterior cerebral artery runs forward and toward the midline where it communicates with the other by way of the anterior communication artery (Figure 1–17). Both then enter the large fissure between the two cerebral hemispheres (interhemispheric fissure) and supply a portion of the frontal and parietal lobes. The two middle cerebral arteries turn outward,

Figure 1-17 Arterial Blood Supply of the Brain

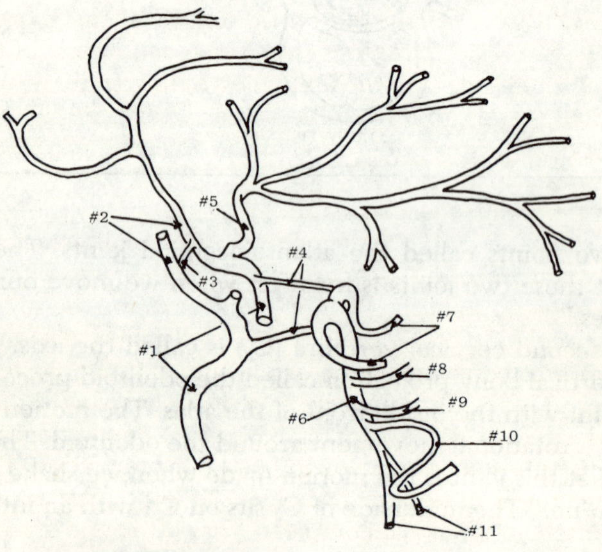

1. INTERNAL CAROTID ARTERIES
2. ANTERIOR CEREBRAL ARTERIES
3. ANTERIOR COMMUNICATION ARTERY
4. POSTERIOR COMMUNICATING ARTERIES
5. RIGHT MIDDLE CEREBRAL ARTERY
6. BASILAR ARTERY
7. POSTERIOR CEREBRAL ARTERIES
8. LEFT SUPERIOR CEREBELLAR ARTERY
9. LEFT POSTERIOR SUPERIOR CEREBELLAR ARTERY
10. LEFT POSTERIOR INFERIOR CEREBELLAR ARTERY
11. VERTEBRAL ARTERIES
12. CIRCLE OF WILLIS FORMED BY #2,3,4 AND 7

entering the Sylvian fissure on each side. Here they divide into several branches that supply most of the outer surface of each cerebral hemisphere. They supply most of the frontal, parietal, and temporal cortex. The branches of both the anterior and middle cerebral arteries that run on the surface of the cortex are called cortical arteries.

Numerous small blood vessels arise near the origin of both the anterior and the middle cerebral arteries. They are collectively called the lenticulostriate arteries and provide blood supply to the basal ganglia, which are located deep within each hemisphere (Figure 1–17).

The posterior circulation of the brain begins with two vertebral arteries which, like the common carotids, arise from the great vessels in the chest. Each vertebral artery ascends the neck lying close to the cervical spine. They then enter the intracranial space of the posterior fossa by passing through the foramen magnum (Figure 1–17). Shortly thereafter they join and form the basilar artery, which runs in front of the brainstem. The basilar artery ends by branching into the two posterior cerebral arteries. These two arteries run back and around the midbrain, supplying each occipital lobe and the under surface of each temporal lobe. Along the entire length of the basilar artery, several paired arteries arise to furnish the blood supply of the brainstem and cerebellum. Like the lenticulostriate arteries of the carotid system, small vessels arise from the basilar artery and form proximal portions of each posterior cerebral artery to course deep within the adjacent brain.

Near the origin of each posterior cerebral artery there arises the posterior communicating artery. These two small arteries run forward and connect to the internal carotid of that side (Figure 1–17). They, therefore, establish a connection between the anterior and posterior circulation of the brain. Figure 1–17 illustrates that a functioning anterior communicating artery and the two posterior communicating arteries form a circle called the circle of Willis.

If the circle of Willis is intact, blood may flow if necessary from posterior to anterior or anterior to posterior circulation. Blood may also flow from left to right or from right to left. Unfortunately, very often the circle of Willis is incomplete. Very often one of the communication arteries is absent.

The blood supply of the spinal cord is accomplished by a single anterior spinal artery and by paired posterior spinal arteries (Figure 1–9). The anterior spinal artery is formed by the joining of two vessels, each of which arises from the vertebral arteries. The anterior spinal artery runs the length of the spinal cord and sends branches into the cord and branches along the outer sides, forming a rich network of vessels. Figure 1–9 shows how most of the blood supply of the spinal cord is via the anterior spinal artery. The posterior spinal arteries course along the back side of the spinal cord and supply the posterior columns of the cord. The posterior spinal arteries are not as well defined as the anterior spinal artery and are more like a network of vessels that run the length of the cord. Small arteries of variable size enter the spinal canal on the nerve roots and join the posterior spinal arteries.

The Blood-Brain Barrier

It has long been realized that many substances in the blood fail to pass into the substance of the brain as readily as they do into other organs of the body. Therefore the concept of the existence of an actual barrier interposed between the blood and the brain substance was born. Anatomically the barrier would consist of: (1) the cells that compose the walls of the capillaries, (2) a basement membrane that invests the capillaries, and (3) the processes of adjacent astrocytes. It is unlikely that these make a very formidable barrier on a physical basis alone.

More likely, the barrier is physiological rather than anatomic. Carbon dioxide, oxygen, and water cross the barrier with little difficulty. Glucose also passes across with ease; most proteins can not. Electrolytes, like sodium and potassium ions, can cross the barrier to enter the brain substance but they enter it more slowly than they enter other body tissues. It has been noted that lipid-soluble substances cross the barrier easier than those that are not fat soluble. In addition, small molecules cross with greater ease than large ones. The latter observation would suggest some kind of a physical barrier.

The blood-brain barrier of a young child is more permeable than the barrier of an adult. Therefore some drugs tolerated by an adult will produce toxicity in a child.

Injury or disease may alter the blood-brain barrier. For example, penicillin normally does not cross the blood-brain barrier; but with inflammation that occurs with bacterial meningitis, it crosses with relative ease.

The Meninges

The meninges or covering membranes of the brain include the outermost layer called the dura mater, the delicate middle layer called the arachnoid, and the pia mater, which is densely adherent to the brain and spinal cord. The arachnoid and pia mater are commonly called the leptomeninges.

The dura mater, usually called the dura, lines the inside of the skull and then, in a cylindrical form, enters the spinal canal and ends at the sacrum (Figure 1–18). In the skull, the dura is closely applied to the bone of the skull. In young people the dura comes away from the bone easily, but in elderly people it often adheres very tightly to the bone. The epidural or extradural space (between dura and bony skull) in the head is only a potential space. It may, however, become a real space when bleeding outside of the dura occurs, producing the very lethal epidural hematoma. In the spinal canal the epidural space is an actual space containing fat and veins.

The dura contains the venous drainage of the brain, which is comprised of the dural sinuses (Figures 1–18, 1–19). Veins on the surface of the brain leave the surface, bridge the subarachnoid space, and enter the sinuses. The midline superior sagittal sinus runs under

Figure 1-18 Contour of the Dura, Containing the Brain and Spinal Cord, after Removal of the Bony Skull and Vertebral Column

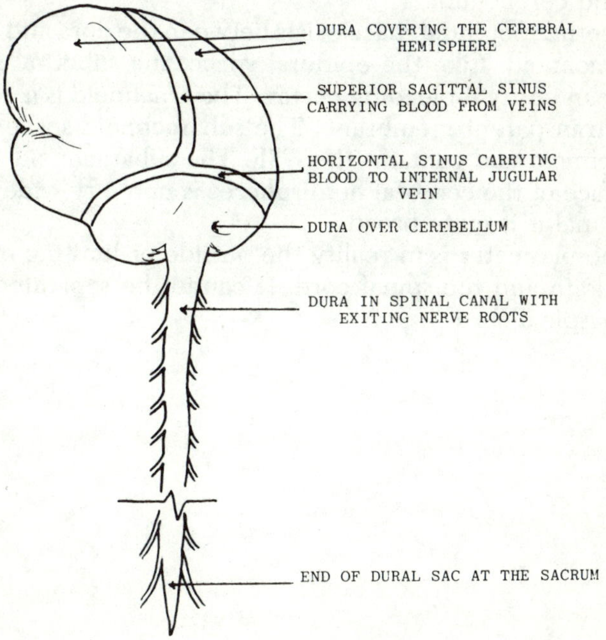

Figure 1-19 Cross-section through the Sagittal Sinus

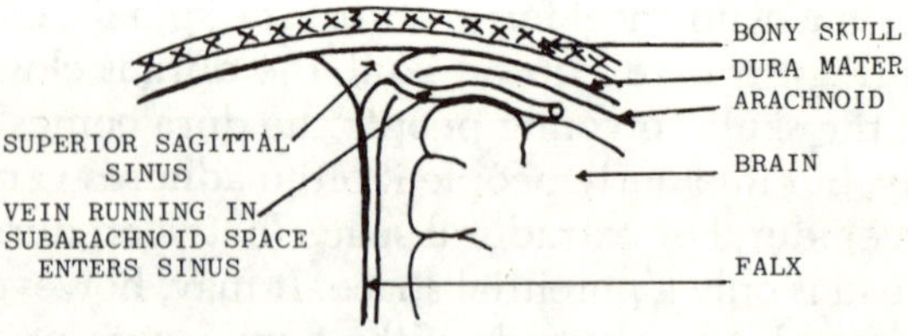

the sagittal suture line of the skull. Posteriorly it divides into two horizontal or transverse sinuses that eventually carry the blood to the internal jugular vein on each side of the neck. There are other dural sinuses on the floor of the intracranial space that also carry venous blood from the brain.

The dura, as illustrated in Figure 1–19, extends like partitions between certain portions of the brain. The dural partition that lies in the fissure between the cerebral hemispheres is called the falx. Another dural partition called the tentorium lies between the cerebrum and cerebellum.

Another potential space exists between the dura and the underlying arachnoid. Like the epidural space, the subdural space may become an entity if bleeding occurs. The arachnoid is a delicate but strong, transparent membrane. The subarachnoid space lies under the arachnoid and contains the CSF. The subarachnoid space over the surface of the cerebral hemispheres is not very wide but in the spinal canal it is quite broad.

The pia mater is in reality the outside or limiting membranes of the brain and the spinal cord. It cannot be separated from the brain or spinal cord.

CHAPTER 2

Neuropathology

The study of neuropathology is the study of diseases that involve the nervous system. Disease of the nervous system, or of any other body system, is the result of the action from certain injurious agents or factors. It is the effect of the agent on the component cells of the system that results in disease. The injurious factor is, to be sure, not a singular entity but includes those that produce vascular disease, trauma, infection, degeneration, toxins, developmental malformations, and neoplasms. Though the nature of the agents is manifold, the diseased cells have limited ways in which to react. Thus the pathologist who looks at a microscope slide of a diseased organ may have some difficulty determining the specific nature of the injurious factor producing the disease.

The effects of injurious factors are applied for a variable time and at a variable intensity. It is the sum of these two variables that determines whether disease occurs or not; certainly it determines a cell's ability to recover or not to recover. One must appreciate the fine line that exists between a cell's survival and its death.

The earliest visible change in an injured cell occurs in the cytoplasm because of alteration of certain biochemical processes. The cell responds by swelling because of an increase in cellular water. If the extent of injury is more severe, there will be an abnormal accumulation of substances in the cytoplasm. The staining qualities of the altered cytoplasm probably indicate coagulation and denaturation of certain proteins. With very serious cellular injury, there are changes involving the nucleus. The nucleus may shrink and appear wrinkled (pyknosis) or it may rupture and become fragmented (karyorrhexis).

Changes in the nucleus indicate severe injury and recovery is not likely.

If the cell dies, the process called necrosis follows. The type of necrosis varies somewhat, depending on the injurious agents and the organ involved. If the cellular death is due to failure of its blood supply, coagulation necrosis occurs. Only the ghosts of the dead cells remain with inner details absent. Eventually, however, all parts of the dead cells are removed and repair follows. Liquefaction necrosis, more commonly seen when cell death occurs in the brain, is complete destruction of the entire cell and its membrane.

The final stage in a disease process, if death of the organism does not occur, is the recovery or reparative stage. The amount of repair and the quality of recovery depend on the severity of the injury. If the injury is slight, cellular recovery occurs; but if it is severe, cellular death and necrosis follow.

In terms of ability to regenerate, there are three types of cells in the body: labile cells, stable cells, and permanent cells. Labile cells are those that normally regenerate, replacing cells with short lifespans. Such cells are found in the skin or in the lining passages of the lungs or intestinal tract. Stable cells ordinarily do not regenerate, but they retain their ability to do so. Cells of this type are included in most glandular organs. Permanent cells seldom if ever regenerate, and as a result, if they are destroyed, they are lost forever. Permanent cells are brain cells and muscle cells.

To this point discussion has centered on the effects of disease on the functional cells of an organ, such as the cells of the liver, kidney, or brain. Each organ also has a unique architecture or framework called the stroma that provides the supportive structure within which the functional cells are found. In disease, the stroma is not immune to the effects of the injurious agent, though it is usually more resistant than the functional cells. Therefore to some degree the ability of an organ to recover from disease depends on the degree of stromal injury. Thus if the injury is to a tissue with labile cells and the stroma is not injured, then near-perfect recovery can be expected. The opposite extreme would be injury and death of permanent cells and destruction of the stroma. The permanent cells could not regenerate, and the stromal recovery would be without architecture or form. To this result we might apply the term *scar.*

Diseases of the Central Nervous System

The response of the nervous system to disease is not unlike the response of the other body systems. The major functional cell of the CNS is the neuron (Figure 2–1). In some acute disease states, the first visible change in the neuron occurs 6 to 12 hours following injury. The cell becomes swollen and there is loss of Nissl substance. The nucleus also swells and is displaced toward the cell membrane. Reversibility is probably possible to this point. Progression, however, produces a change in the staining qualities of the cytoplasm, which is followed by disintegration of the nuclear membrane. Another type of acute change in the neuron is seen when the blood supply of the brain is interrupted. The cell becomes shrunken and the nucleus appears shriveled. The cytoplasm stains a homogeneous (basophilic) purple. In chronic disease states, the neuron decreases in size (atrophies). The membrane of the cell and of the nucleus become irregular. Both the nucleus and the cytoplasm stain darker. In specific diseases certain substances such as lipids accumulate abnormally in the cytoplasm, or the cell may absorb iron or calcium on its surface.

Figure 2-1 Major Cells of the Central Nervous System

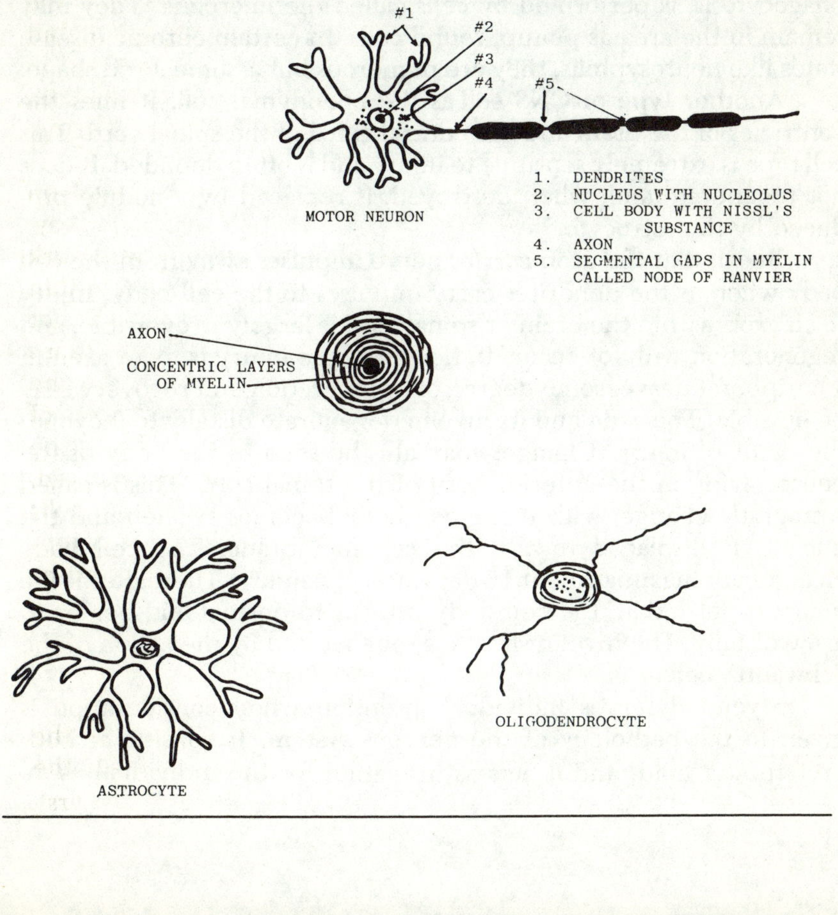

The stroma of the CNS is called the glia. It includes two cell types, the astrocyte and the oligodendrocyte. These cells perform supportive, reparative, and probably some metabolic function. Like stroma elsewhere, the glia is susceptible to injurious factors.

In response to injury the cell body of the astrocyte swells; if the injury is lethal the cell body disintegrates. Liquefaction necrosis follows the death of the cell. If the astrocyte can withstand the insult, it begins to produce and lay down fibers as a part of the reparative process. If the astrocyte is destroyed, fibroblasts enter the area, restoring some supportive framework.

The other type of glial cell, the oligodendrocyte, is found normally in two locations: around the cell body of the neuron, where it assists in metabolic functions, and in the white matter of the CNS lying along myelinated nerve fibers, where it produces and maintains myelin. The oligodendrocyte is very sensitive to toxic and to metabolic injury, and it becomes swollen in response to it.

When a cell dies and disintegrates, it is often engulfed as a part of the reparative process. In the CNS this process, commonly called phagocytosis, is performed by cells called the microglia. They may remain in the area as plump, round cells. In certain chronic disease states like neurosyphilis, they are numerous but assume a rod shape.

Another type of CNS cell is the ependymal cell. It lines the ventricles of the brain and the central canal of the spinal cord. This cell type is extremely sensitive to injury and is often denuded. It does not regenerate and, when destroyed, is replaced by a nodule produced by the astrocyte.

Recall that the axon carries nerve impulses away from the cell body whereas the dendrites carry impulses to the cell body. Injury to an axon within the brain or spinal cord is largely irreversible, and regeneration will not occur. If, however, the injury is to an axon in a peripheral nerve, some degree of regeneration and recovery may be possible. The axon and its myelin degenerate distally to (beyond) the point of injury. Changes may also be seen in the body of the neuron lying in the anterior horn of the spinal cord. This is called retrograde change; with it the cell body becomes swollen and the nucleus is displaced toward the cell membrane. The cell body changes are maximal about 12 days after the injury. Thereafter if the injury is not lethal, the cell body returns to normal and begins to grow distally. The myelin sheath is regenerated by the action of the Schwann's cell.

Myelin deserves individual attention when consideration is given to the pathology of the nervous system. It consists of both protein and lipid, and it acts as insulation for the individual axon.

Diseases like multiple sclerosis attack myelin as their primary effect. The myelin breaks down, causing disturbed function of the fiber it insulated. In other disease states in which axon injury is primary, the myelin breaks down as a secondary result.

Turning now to a more detailed consideration of the various causes of disease in the nervous system, bear in mind that the discussion is broad, covering the characteristics and principles of specific disease categories. Keeping these categories in mind will facilitate the management of a large amount of information.

Vascular Disease

Vascular disease of the brain is disease of the blood vessels supplying blood to the brain. There are numerous causes of cerebral vascular disease, arteriosclerosis (hardening of the arteries) being the most important. Other causes result from abnormal development of artery walls or from the actual occurrence within the brain of malformed groups of blood vessels.

In the process of arteriosclerosis, which begins at an early age and continues throughout life, a fatty material is deposited under the inner lining of the cerebral arteries. These deposits, called plaques, tend to occur where arteries branch. As the plaques enlarge, the hole (lumen) in the vessel becomes smaller. Eventually, the vessel lumen is too small to permit adequate blood flow, and often the decreased flow results in the blood actually clotting. The process of clotting is called thrombosis. In either of the above situations, the brain cells suffer from lack of oxygen. If the cells are not killed by this insult, we say they have suffered ischemia, or that an ischemic episode has occurred (Figure 2–2). If there is cellular death as a result of thrombosis or frequent ischemic episodes, we use the term *infarction.* Thus, cerebral artery thrombosis usually causes cerebral infarction.

In addition to plaque formation, arteriosclerosis also results in weakening of the walls of cerebral arteries. In the presence of hypertension (high blood pressure), the arteriosclerotic vessels may rupture so that massive bleeding occurs (Figure 2–2). A cerebral hemorrhage of this type is a particularly serious event which results in death in most instances. The brain injury that occurs with a spontaneous intracerebral (within-the-brain) hemorrhage results from destruction of brain tissue by the enlarging clot, from the interruption of blood flow, and from a marked increase in pressure inside of the head (intracranial pressure).

Embolization is another disease phenomenon associated with arteriosclerotic cerebrovascular disease. The inner lining (intima) of

Figure 2-2 Disease Phenomena Associated with Arteriosclerosis

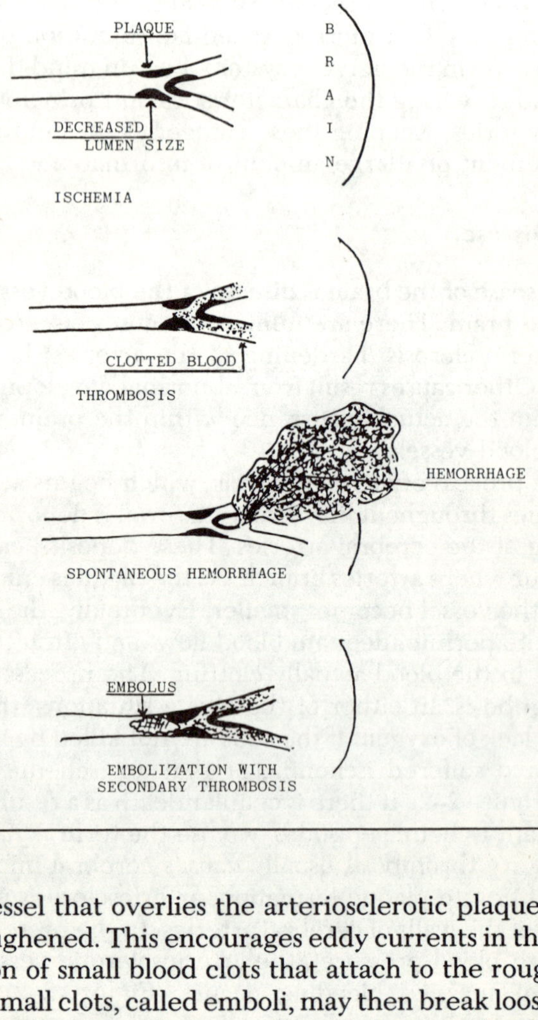

the blood vessel that overlies the arteriosclerotic plaque frequently becomes roughened. This encourages eddy currents in the blood and the formation of small blood clots that attach to the roughened surface. These small clots, called emboli, may then break loose and enter the bloodstream, where they travel until they reach a blood vessel that is too small to permit further passage. Blood flow ceases beyond that point, and as a result thrombosis occurs and infarction quickly follows (Figure 2–2). Emboli can also arise in the heart and frequently do so after a heart attack, so that cerebral embolization with infarction is a common problem following heart attacks.

The formation of a cerebral aneurysm (ballooning of the artery wall) is another type of cerebrovascular disease (Figure 2–3). Aneurysms occur for three reasons. Most commonly they occur because of failure in the development of the muscular layer in the wall of a cerebral artery. The vessel wall balloons outward forming the aneurysmal sac. These aneurysms are called congenital or Berry aneurysms. Arteriosclerotic aneurysms may also occur as a result of the ballooning of the weakened arterial wall. Aneurysms of this type tend to be small and are often deep within the brain. Their rupture causes the spontaneous intracerebral hemorrhage already discussed. Finally, infected emboli that arise from diseased heart valves may lodge in small cerebral arteries. The resulting infection weakens the

Figure 2-3

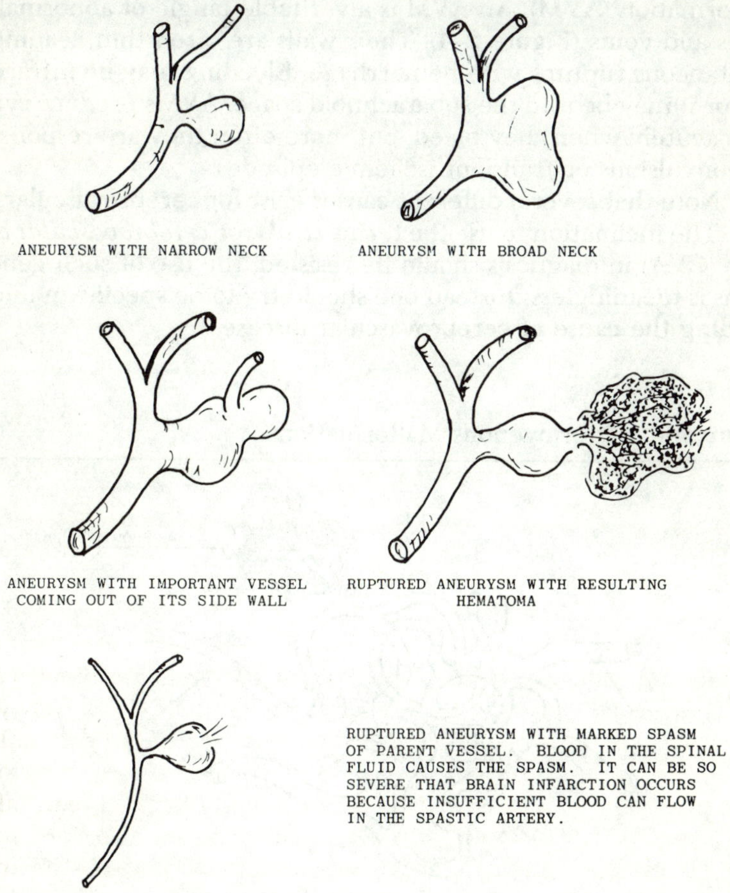

vessel wall, so that aneurysmal dilatation occurs. These aneurysms are called mycotic aneurysms.

Aneurysms cause symptoms in most cases when they rupture. The resulting blood mixes with the cerebrospinal fluid, and therefore this type of hemorrhage is called a subarachnoid hemorrhage (the CSF is located in the subarachnoid space). If the bleeding ceases, the patient may survive, but death is common owing to continued hemorrhage and massive clot formation. Another problem occurring with subarachnoid hemorrhage is the phenomenon of vascular spasm (Figure 2–3). It appears that in some manner the blood in the CSF causes the cerebral vessels to go into spasm. When this occurs, the blood flow through the vessels is so drastically reduced that severe ischemia or even cerebral infarction can occur.

Another kind of vascular lesion is the cerebral arteriovenous malformation (AVM). An AVM is a veritable tangle of abnormal arteries and veins (Figure 2–4). Their walls are often thin, leading to spontaneous rupture with hemorrhage. Bleeding may be intracerebral or it may be into the subarachnoid space. AVMs produce symptoms acutely when they bleed, but more often they are responsible for convulsions or transient ischemic episodes.

Note that several different causes exist for cerebrovascular disease. The inclination to use the terms *stroke* or *cerebrovascular accident* (CVA) in diagnosis should be resisted; the use of such general terms is meaningless. Instead one should try to be specific in understanding the cause of cerebrovascular disease.

Figure 2-4 Arteriovenous Malformation

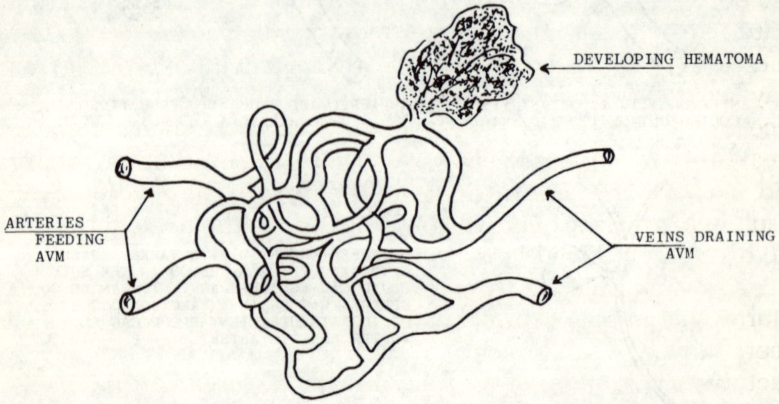

Trauma

The advent of the automobile and other forms of mechanized transportation has placed trauma near the top of the list as a cause of serious disability and death. The potential sources of trauma in our modern society are many and varied. There is the trauma to the brain or spinal cord that may occur when the head hits the windshield. There is the trauma inflicted on the brain by depressed fragments of a skull fracture or by any object that may penetrate the skull. There is the trauma to the brain that occurs at birth as the head molds to the contour and size of the birth canal. There are the traumata of ultrasound, radiant energy, or excessive atmospheric pressure. Finally, there is the trauma inflicted on the brain by the expanding mass of a hematoma or brain tumor.

Exhaustive clinical and laboratory studies have been made in the effort to understand the mechanism of head injury. Picture a person driving a car at a set rate of speed. A collision occurs; the car stops but the person's head continues forward briefly, hitting the windshield. The skull stops with the impact, but the brain, which is surrounded by CSF, continues the forward motion for a very brief second. The tips of the frontal and middle lobes of the brain strike the bony confines of the skull (calvarium) and are injured. Consider next a person being hit on the back of the head by a hammer. The calvarium starts to move forward while the brain, for a split second, remains stationary. The moving skull strikes the occipital lobe tips, causing injury. Now both the brain and skull move forward. The victim falls to the ground, hitting the front of the head. The brain is again injured as it strikes the already-stationary skull. There is therefore injury to the brain at the site of impact (the hammer blow) and also on the opposite side or frontal portion of the brain. The injury that occurs opposite the hammer blow is called a contrecoup lesion. These examples illustrate how a closed-head (nonpenetrating) injury may occur. They are overly simplified, for they illustrate only linear acceleration and linear deceleration. To be sure, linear force is of great importance; usually, however, there are, in addition, rotational and shear forces that contribute to the injury. The rotational forces result in the tearing of nerve fibers and also in the stretching or even the breaking of blood vessels.

One can imagine the vast types of injury or combinations of injuries that might occur in head trauma. First, there may be a scalp laceration and a skull fracture. The fracture may be a simple linear fracture, or fragments of the fracture may be forced inward, lacerating the dura and brain. This kind of fracture is called a compound depressed skull fracture when it is associated with a laceration of the adjacent scalp. Such a fracture may be complicated by infection or hemorrhage if dural blood vessels or brain blood vessels are interrupted. If there is no fracture, the brain at the site of the blow may still be seriously injured with cerebral contusions (bruises) or cerebral lacerations. Either may result in cell death, local necrosis, and scar formation. The formation of intracranial hematomas as a consequence of head injuries is very common. Three types of intracranial hematomas occur (Figure 2–5).

Figure 2-5

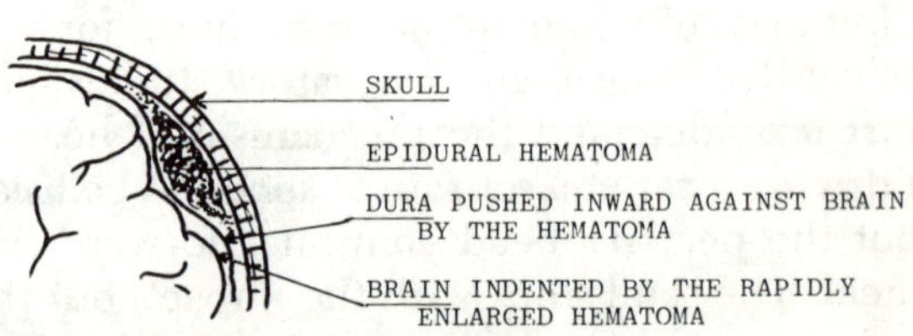

EPIDURAL (EXTRADURAL) HEMATOMA

BLEEDING IS FROM A TORN ARTERY IN THE DURA. BLEEDING IS BRISK WITH A RAPIDLY ENLARGING VOLUME OF BLOOD

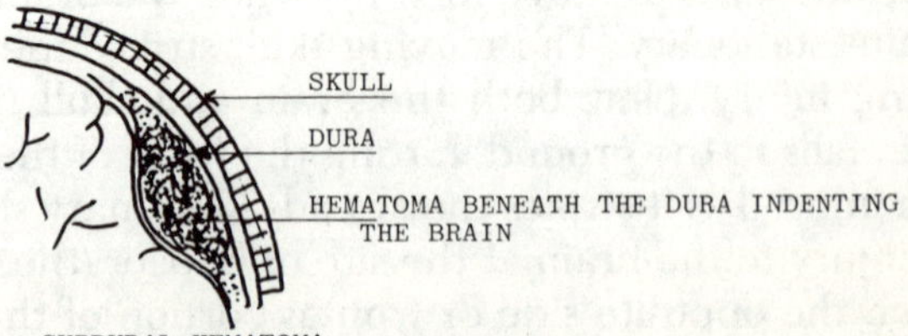

SUBDURAL HEMATOMA

BLEEDING USUALLY FROM A TORN VEIN

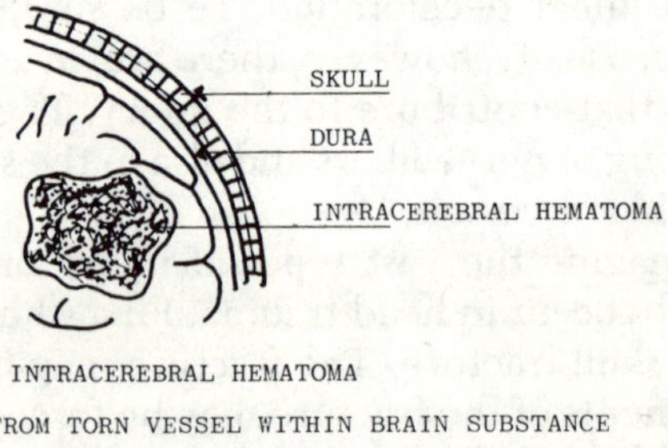

INTRACEREBRAL HEMATOMA

BLEEDING FROM TORN VESSEL WITHIN BRAIN SUBSTANCE

The epidural (outside-the-dura) hematomas result when the meningeal arteries are lacerated. The formation of this hematoma is very rapid because the source of blood is an artery. Patients with developing epidural hematomas may lapse into coma so rapidly they may die before they get to the hospital. An epidural hematoma represents one of the true neurosurgical emergencies.

The subdural hematoma forms between the dura and the brain, and there are both acute and chronic forms. The acute subdural hematoma occurs in very severe head injuries and carries with it a very high mortality rate. The source of bleeding may be from a torn dural sinus or large cortical vein. The chronic subdural hematoma may form after an insignificant trauma, and it occurs especially in the elderly, in people with a poor nutritional state, like the alcoholic, or in patients with bleeding tendencies. The source of bleeding is often from a cortical vein or veins that bridge the gap between the cortex and the dura. Bleeding is slower and the brain has more time to compensate for the expanding mass. Such hematomas may not produce symptoms for several weeks.

The intracerebral hematoma occurs in head trauma associated with brain laceration, or when intracerebral vessels are ruptured by the mechanical forces already described. This hematoma may cause death from increased intracranial pressure if the mass is large.

Brain swelling or cerebral edema often is a consequence of closed-head injuries. The edema may be localized or diffuse. We have seen how the astrocyte swells in response to an injurious agent; it is this intracellular accumulation of fluid in the astrocyte that causes brain swelling. Brain swelling may be so severe that the resultant intracranial pressure will cause death. One of the principle efforts of a neurosurgeon treating a head injury is to counteract the swelling tendency by using dehydrating agents.

It is helpful to realize that trauma to the CNS may produce serious disability or death in two ways: First, the degree of trauma may be so great that there is immediate destruction of vital neural structures (neurons, etc.). Second, the trauma may produce a lesion that causes increasing intracranial pressure, as in the case of a developing hematoma or brain swelling. Keep in mind that the growth of a brain tumor will also increase intracranial pressure.

The effects of increasing intracranial pressure are the same regardless of cause. The rapidity with which the pressure develops is of great importance. In the slowly developing or chronic state, very large masses can be tolerated. The best example is the brain tumor called the meningioma. Its growth is slow, and the brain has time to compensate for its increasing size. An opposite example is the very rapid accumulation of the epidural hematoma. The first effects are local, with pressure on brain cells immediately adjacent to the hematoma. Soon, the size of the clot is such that there is shifting of large parts of the brain. This results in forces that may break nerve pathways; stretch, occlude, or rupture blood vessels; and press the shifting brain against bony edges of the inside of the skull. When the pressure is quite severe, the brainstem is affected. This results in changes in the level of consciousness because of the malfunctioning reticular activating system. The patient lapses into a coma. Then there is slowing of the heart rate, abnormal respiratory efforts, and a terminal drop in blood pressure followed by respiratory failure. Death comes because of the failure of vital centers in the medulla oblongata.

A discussion of trauma to the CNS must include spinal cord injuries. These most unfortunate injuries are common results of motorcycle and diving accidents. Injury to the spinal cord occurs as a result of fractures and dislocations of the vertebrae (Figures 1–16, 2–6). Under normal conditions the spinal canal is large enough to contain the spinal cord adequately, but it does not take much impingement by fractured lamina or by dislocated vertebral bodies to cause spinal cord injury. Cord injury is, of course, variable. There may be only very slight injury or the cord may be severely contused or even completely transected.

Injury to the spinal cord below the neck produces paralysis in both legs (paraplegia), loss of sensation below the level of the injury, and loss of voluntary bladder control. In high neck injuries, all four limbs are paralyzed (quadriplegia), and there is also loss of both sensation and bladder control. Even more disastrous, if that can be imagined, in high cervical cord injuries, the patient is unable to breathe because of paralysis of the diaphragm as well as the muscles of the chest wall. It is obvious that death may occur before a patient can get to the hospital where his or her plight might be recognized.

To be sure, not all spinal cord injuries result in paralysis. The less severely injured may initially have great disability, but significant recovery may occur over the hours, weeks, and months that follow.

Infection

Infection of the CNS and the meninges (dura, arachnoid, and pia mater) results from the invasion of bacteria, viruses, fungi, and parasites. Many types of bacteria invade the CNS and cause disease. The most common are those producing abscesses or suppurative exudates

Figure 2-6 Various Ways Trauma to the Vertebral Column Can Injure the Cord

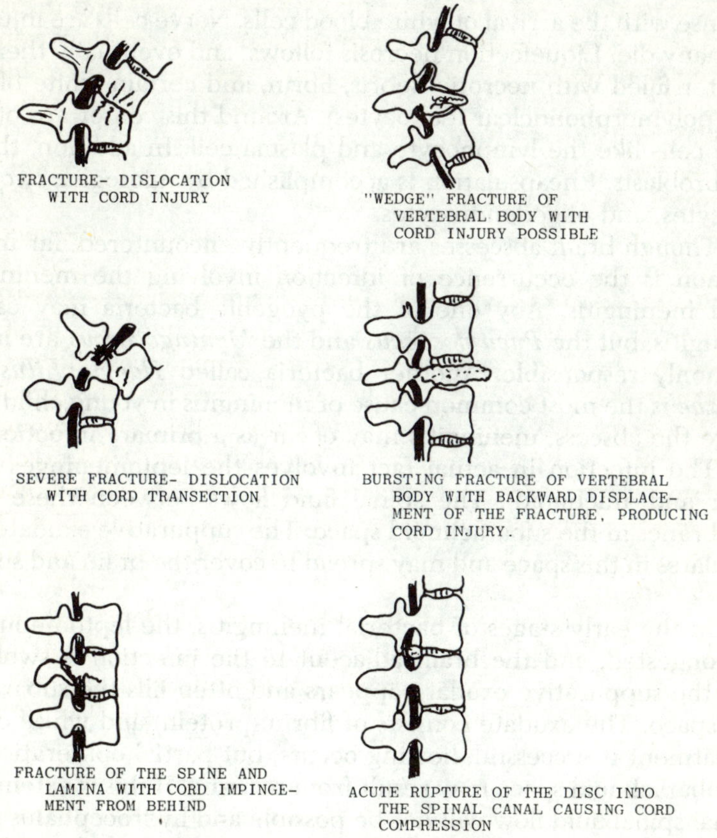

(pus). The common bacteria in this group are the *Staphylococci, Streptococci, Pneumococci, Meningococci,* and *Gonococci*. They gain entrance to the CNS most often from a primary site elsewhere in the body. They may spread by direct extension from infected nasal sinuses, an infected middle ear, mastoid air cells, or a scalp infection. The spread of infection to the brain from distant sites in the body is through the bloodstream. Two very common sites of origin of infected emboli are infected lungs and infected heart valves (bacterial endocarditis).

Abscesses may occur in the epidural space, in the subdural space, or within the brain itself. Brain abscesses are most common in the temporal lobe or in the cerebellum. The formation of an abscess begins with the lodging of an infected embolus in a vessel with a lumen too small for further passage. First, there is an inflammatory response with the arrival of white blood cells. Nerve cells are injured and many die. Liquefaction necrosis follows, and eventually there is a center filled with necrotic debris, fibrin, and certain white blood cells (polymorphonuclear leukocytes). Around this center are other white cells like the lymphocyte and plasma cell. In addition, there are fibroblasts. Encapsulation is accomplished by microglia, swollen astrocytes, and oligodendrocytes.

Though brain abscesses are frequently encountered, far more common is the occurrence of infection involving the meninges, called meningitis. Any one of the pyogenic bacteria may cause meningitis, but the *Pneumococcus* and the *Meningococcus* are most commonly responsible. Another bacteria called *Haemophilus influenzae* is the most common cause of meningitis in young children. Unlike the abscess, meningitis may occur as a primary infection.

The infection in actual fact involves the leptomeninges (pia mater and arachnoid). The spinal fluid flows between these two membranes in the subarachnoid space. The suppurative exudate accumulates in this space and may spread to cover the brain and spinal cord.

In the early stages of bacterial meningitis, the leptomeninges are congested, and the brain adjacent to the infection is swollen. Next the suppurative exudate appears and often fills the subarachnoid space. The exudate consists of fibrin (protein) and white cells. If treatment is successful, healing occurs, but partial obliteration of the subarachnoid space may result from scarring. If this is extensive, normal spinal fluid flow will not be possible and hydrocephalus may develop. The clotting (thrombosis) of veins on the surface of the cerebral cortex is another serious complication of bacterial leptomeningitis.

Nonpyogenic bacteria may cause leptomeningitis. The most common is *tuberculosis;* it almost always is secondary to pulmonary tuberculosis. The exudate produced differs from the exudate seen in pyogenic leptomeningitis. It is located largely at the base of the brain and is gelatinous in character. Healing produces much more scarring than is seen with pyogenic meningitis. Hydrocephalus is a very common complication. The cranial nerves may also be involved by the extensive scarring, producing various cranial nerve palsies.

The bacteria that causes syphilis is another bacteria that may cause meningitis, but far more serious are the processes that occur when the bacteria invades the CNS. Syphilis occurs in three stages:

primary, secondary, and tertiary. The primary lesion is the chancre, which is a single, slightly elevated papule most often on the penis, vulva, or cervix. The chancre may vary in size but within a month or so it is healed. In the primary stage, the syphilis bacteria (spirochetes) spread by way of the lymphatic system and bloodstream. The secondary stage is marked by the appearance of a generalized rash that may involve the mucous membranes. An asymptomatic stage now follows that may last for years. One-third of the infected individuals apparently experience a spontaneous cure and have negative serology tests. One-third have a positive serology test for syphilis but do not develop tertiary lesions. One-third develop recognized tertiary lesions involving the CNS or cardiovascular system.

The cardiovascular lesion in tertiary syphilis is the formation of aortic aneurysms. There are three forms of tertiary syphilis that affect the CNS. One of these forms is meningovascular syphilis, which is characterized by a meningitis occurring at the base of the brain. The healing produces a dense fibrosis, which often seriously obstructs CSF flow. The fibrotic process may also involve certain cranial nerves, and their function can be affected too. The cerebral arteries are involved by a fibrotic process in their walls. The lumen size is thereby diminished, so that ischemia and infarction may occur in the brain.

Tabes dorsalis is another of the tertiary forms of syphilis. In this form, the posterior columns and the dorsal roots of the spinal cord are involved, and there is degeneration of axons and breakdown of myelin. General paresis, or general paresis of the insane, is the third form of tertiary syphilis. Prior to the discovery of antibiotics, GPI was the leading cause of dementia in psychiatric institutions. The pathology takes the form of a progressive loss of brain neurons, especially those in the frontal lobes. At the gross level one sees severe cortical atrophy. Congenital syphilis may occur with passage of the spirochete from the mother to the unborn baby.

Mycotic or fungal infections of the CNS are less common than bacterial infections, but they are by no means rare. The most common fungal infections are cryptococcosis, coccidioidomycosis, and blastomycosis. The disease produced is a basilar meningitis (at base of brain) that very commonly causes hydrocephalus.

Parasitic invasion of the CNS is not common in the United States but very common in other parts of the world, malaria being the most common. These organisms invade the lining of blood vessels. Occlusion of the lumen of the vessel may result. Other diseases caused by parasites that invade the CNS include toxoplasmosis, cysticercosis (pork tapeworm), and hydatid disease (dog tapeworm).

Viral infections of the nervous system are very common. There are many viruses that are pathogenic (cause disease) in humans. Viruses can only multiply within living cells. Almost all contain either DNA (deoxyribonucleic acid) or RNA (ribonucleic acid). The nucleic acid, which carries the genetic code of the virus, is enclosed within a protein shell called a capsid. Viruses appear to cause disease by their ability to modify the metabolic and the reproductive processes of the host cell. Some viruses, however, enter the cell and cause injury or death.

Classification of viruses is complicated and not entirely satisfactory. The classification criteria may include the type of nucleic acid (DNA or RNA), virus particle size, vector of spread (e.g., birds), and type of host cell infected.

Viruses enter the body by several routes. The oral route is most important, with entrance being through the oral or the intestinal mucosa (lining). Mosquito and animal bites may provide the entrance for viruses. Once in the body, viruses multiply within certain cells such as those of muscle, fat, and lymph nodes. The virus, after multiplying, spreads throughout the body in the blood (viremia), and those inclined enter the CNS. Some viruses enter the brain by traveling to it along a peripheral nerve.

If a virus settles in the subarachnoid space, a meningitis occurs with congestion seen in the pia mater and arachnoid. Such meningitis is an aseptic meningitis, meaning that it is not caused by bacteria, which causes septic meningitis. The virus may enter the brain and produce encephalitis, or it may enter the spinal cord and produce myelitis. Often both the brain and cord are invaded, in which case the term encephalomyelitis is used. A patient with aseptic meningitis and encephalitis is said to have meningoencephalitis.

At the microscopic level, in encephalitis there is neuron injury or death with necrosis. There is also an inflammatory response with lymphocytes and polymorphonuclear neutrophils (polys) congregating around the injured neurons and around blood vessels. In some viral infections, particles called inclusion bodies are seen in either the nucleus or the cytoplasm. The Cowdry Type A inclusion is an inclusion seen in the nucleus of the diseased cell. Its presence is fairly specific for viral infections. It stains red with hematoxylin and eosin (H & E) stain. In rabies there is an inclusion called the Negri body in the cytoplasm that stains red with the H & E stain.

When the infection has run its course, the reparative process begins. Dead neurons are removed by phagocytosis. Finally astrocytes become more numerous, producing glial fibers that, in the aggregate, are called glial nodules.

Neoplasms

Neoplasia literally means new growth, but it is not to be used synonymously with cancer, for neoplasm may be either benign or malignant. There are a number of growth abnormalities in addition to cancer. Aplasia is the term used to describe the failure of an organ to develop. If development occurs but ceases without attaining adult size, the word hypoplasia is used. Hyperplasia describes development of an organ beyond average adult size. Metaplasia is the replacing of one adult cell type by another. An example may be seen in lungs in which the constant irritation of cigarette smoking has caused the normal columnar epithelium to change to stratified squamous epithelium. Metaplasia is a reversible process, so that the columnar epithelium will eventually replace the stratified squamous epithelium if smoking is stopped. Dysplasia signifies changes in the characteristics of the adult cells, such as variation in cell size, cell shape, or organization of cells in a specific tissue. Dysplasia may lead to frank anaplasia but not necessarily so. Dysplasia may result from constant irritation, and if the irritant is removed, reversion to the normal adult cells is possible. Anaplasia is irreversible. It may follow dysplasia, but more commonly it is preceded by apparently normal cells.

Neoplasia should be considered as a new growth that consists of an abnormal collection of cells that grow free of control. If the new growth has the characteristics of anaplasia, it is malignant. There are several characteristics that indicate malignancy: There is a great variation in the size of both the cell and the nucleus. The nucleus may occupy most of the cell volume, and there may be an increase in its chromatin. Large nucleoli occur in the nucleus, and there may be more than one in a single nucleus. Often there are very large, bizarre-appearing cells with multiple nuclei. Several cells undergoing mitotic division are seen and many of the mitoses are abnormal. There is invasion and destruction of surrounding normal tissue.

In general, the more closely a malignant neoplasm resembles its adult cell and its tissue of origin, the slower it grows. These neoplasms are considered well differentiated. Extremely anaplastic neoplasms may be so highly undifferentiated that it is not possible to determine the adult cell or tissue of origin.

Benign neoplasms often grow with a capsule surrounding them. The malignant neoplasm may appear to have a capsule, but it is almost never a true capsule. Benign tumors never metastasize (spread). The nomenclature used to designate a benign tumor is derived from its cell origin plus the suffix *oma.* Thus, we have a lipoma (fat cell) or an osteoma (bone cell). The nomenclature of malignancy also considers the cell of origin. If the cell is an epithelial cell, or in other words a cell lining or covering certain structures such as the lining of the lung passages or the skin, the term *carcinoma* is used. Thus, we know that squamous cell carcinoma of the lung arose from dysplasia of the lung epithelium. If the malignant neoplasm arose from muscle, fat, or bone (tissues that do not line body spaces), the term *sarcoma* is applied. A malignant neoplasm arising from fat cells would be called a liposarcoma.

Like normal tissues a neoplasm has a functional cell and a stroma. The functional cell is the rapidly dividing neoplastic cell; the stroma is the supportive connective tissue and blood vessels. In some manner the neoplastic cell stimulates the growth of the stroma. The stromal growth can even surpass that of the functional cell, resulting in a very hard and gritty tumor. If the opposite occurs and the functional cell growth is faster than its stroma, the neoplastic cells outgrow their blood supply and ischemic necrosis occurs.

The growth of malignant neoplasms is quite variable. Some may grow very slowly and, in fact, appear dormant for long periods, only to be reactivated with rapid growth and wide dissemination (metastasis). Other malignant neoplasms metastasize before the primary growth is of any size and long before it becomes symptomatic.

Malignant tumors may spread locally along lines of least resistance. In doing so they erode and destroy normal tissue. It appears that malignant cells have less adhesiveness than normal cells and therefore are more easily broken free, which facilitates their spread.

Widespread metastasis of malignant neoplasms may occur. Blood vessels, especially thin-walled veins, may be penetrated, permitting the tumor cells to go throughout the body. Metastasis to the lungs, liver, and axial bones may occur this way. Spread of tumor cells by the lymphatic system is common, especially for carcinomas. Direct tumor transplants may occur in the peritoneal cavity or the subarachnoid space; tumor cells break loose and implant at points throughout these spaces.

The causes of cancer continue to elude us in spite of great effort and great expense. Certain chemical substances such as hydrocarbons have been shown to cause cancer. These and other substances like cigarette tars are called carcinogens. It has been shown that viruses can cause cancer in laboratory animals. Certain physical agents like excessive X-radiation or atomic radiation can undoubtedly cause cancer. Hormonal influences have been implicated in the cause of cancer, but this has not been proved. Hormonal factors probably create a physiological climate favoring neoplasia. The concept of spontaneous mutation (change in the genetic code) continues to attract proponents.

Brain tumors may be primary or they may be secondary. Primary brain tumors may be malignant or benign. Secondary tumors are those that have metastasized to the brain from primary ones elsewhere in the body. Malignant tumors metastasized to the brain are the most common intracranial tumors. They may constitute as many as 60 percent of all intracranial tumors. Metastatic tumors from the lung are the most common; metastasis from the breast, gastrointestinal tract, and kidney commonly occur. Other malignant tumors may metastasize to the brain but with lesser frequency.

Primary brain tumors, in addition to being classified as either malignant or benign, may be usefully classified as either extracerebral (outside the brain) or intracerebral (inside). Generally those that are extracerebral are benign, whereas those that are intracerebral are malignant (Figure 2-7).

Extracerebral Neoplasms

The meningioma is one of the most common intracranial tumors and one of the most common intraspinal (in the spinal canal) tumors. These tumors arise from nests of arachnoid cells. They may occur over the surface of the brain or underneath the brain next to the brainstem. They grow slowly over long periods of time. The brain can tolerate large tumors because of the slow growth. Those tumors over the surface of the cerebral hemisphere produce indentions in the brain. Those growing at the base of the brain push the brainstem aside, deforming it, involving cranial nerves, and compromising the blood supply. A meningioma growing in the spinal canal slowly impinges upon the spinal cord, eventually causing weakness in the legs (paraparesis) and bladder dysfunction. Most all meningiomas are benign, though they may involve the skull, causing it to thicken and produce a prominent bulge of the scalp.

The neurofibroma and neurilemmoma are tumors, usually benign, that arise from certain cranial nerves and spinal nerves. Intracranially, the eighth cranial (acoustic) nerve is most commonly involved. The tumor grows slowly, pushing aside the brainstem. Clinically the patient becomes deaf, and eventually facial paralysis occurs because the facial nerve lies close to the acoustic nerve. In the spinal canal the neurofibroma is about as common as the meningioma. Like the meningioma the neurofibroma compresses the spinal cord, causing a progressive paraparesis.

The craniopharyngioma is a tumor that occurs in childhood but also in middle age. It arises in the region of the pituitary gland and optic nerves. Clinically the patient has visual impairment, hormone disturbances, and often hydrocephalus. The tumor may be solid or cystic. When cystic, it contains a fluid with cholesterol crystals. Some neuropathologists believe this tumor arises from remnants of Rathke's pouch, a structure seen during a stage of development of the embryo.

The pituitary adenoma is a tumor arising from the anterior lobe of the pituitary gland. In a comprehensive series of reports on brain tumors, the pituitary adenoma accounts for about 8 percent of intracranial neoplasms. An adenoma may arise from any of the three types of functional cells of the anterior pituitary. The chromophobe adenoma is by far the most common. The patient experiences visual impairment, hormonal imbalance, and symptoms of increased intra-

Figure 2-7

B R A I N - T U M O R S

SECONDARY- THOSE THAT METASTASIZE TO THE BRAIN FROM ELSEWHERE. THEREFORE, ALL ARE MALIGNANT

PRIMARY- THOSE THAT ARISE IN AND FROM THE CNS OR IN CLOSE ASSOCIATION WITH IT.

B E N I G N		M A L I G N A N T	
EXTRACEREBRAL	INTRACEREBRAL	EXTRACEREBRAL	INTRACEREBRAL
MENINGIOMA	RARE	RARE	ASTROCYTOMA I-IV
NEUROFIBROMA			OLIGODENDROGLIOMA
CRANIOPHARYNGIOMA			EPENDYMOMA
PITUITARY ADENOMA			MEDULLOBLASTOMA

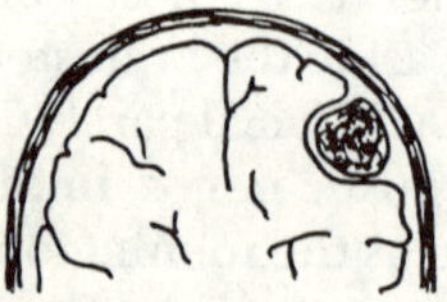
EXTRACEREBRAL BRAIN TUMOR

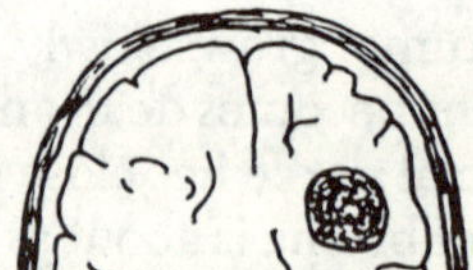
INTRACEREBRAL BRAIN TUMOR

cranial pressure. Patients with eosinophilic adenomas have many of the symptoms of patients with chromophobe adenomas; they also may show features of gigantism or acromegaly because the eosinophil cell produces growth hormone. The basophilic adenoma is the rarest and usually does not attain any great size. The patient with this tumor exhibits Cushing's syndrome because the basophilic cell produces the hormone that stimulates the adrenal gland to produce cortisone and cortisonelike substances.

There are other intracranial and extracerebral tumors, but they are fairly uncommon.

Intracerebral Neoplasms

Most of the intracerebral neoplasms are called gliomas because they arise from the glia. Those few tumors that arise from the neurons are rare by comparison and hence not discussed here. Classification of the gliomas has been a concern of neuropathologists for years. Kernohan's classification is loosely used in the following discussion of them. This classification identifies the cell of origin and then, depending on the degree of anaplasia, grades the tumor I–IV. The grading of the tumor has some prognostic value because it is reasonable to expect longer survival with a Grade I glioma than with a Grade IV glioma.

The astrocytoma is the most common of the gliomas. The cell of origin is the astrocyte. The tumors are graded I through IV, depending on the anaplastic characteristics seen. It is possible that malignant degeneration occurs in astrocytomas. This means that a tumor of lesser grade will, with time, become more anaplastic. In general, the Grade I or Grade II astrocytomas occur more often in children and young adults, whereas more malignant forms are seen in middle life and old age.

At the microscopic level a Grade I astrocytoma has astrocytes that appear normal or near normal. The population of astrocytes is somewhat greater than normal, but one does not see the hemorrhage, necrosis, or vascular proliferation that one sees in the more malignant forms. At the microscopic level the Grade II astrocytoma reveals definite differences in the size and shape of its cell, but mitoses are not seen and hemorrhage and necrosis do not occur.

The astrocytoma Grades III and IV are the most common of all the gliomas. These tumors account for 40–60 percent of all gliomas, and the peak incidence is at approximately 50 years of age. The most common site of occurrence is deep within the cerebral hemisphere invading the basal ganglia and thalamus.

At the microscopic level there is marked variation in the shape and sizes of cells. Large multinucleated giant cells are common. Many cells are seen dividing by mitosis and many of the mitoses are abnormal. There is extensive vascular proliferation; the walls of these vessels are abnormal, for they are thickened often to the degree that the vessel lumen is obliterated. Prominent areas of necrosis and hemorrhage are seen. The vast microscopic variation of these tumors has led to the term glioblastoma multiforme, a name that is probably more commonly used than is Grade III or Grade IV astrocytoma.

A specific form of astrocytoma is seen in the cerebellum of children; it may be solid or cystic. In the cystic form, a small nodule or tumor called a mural nodule is found in the wall of the cyst cavity. Long survivals can be obtained with excision of the cerebellar astrocytoma.

The growth of astrocytomas is progressively invasive; rate of growth is variable, correlating with the anaplastic characteristics of each tumor.

The oligodendroglioma arises from the oligodendrocyte. These tumors account for about 10 percent of all gliomas; they tend to occur rather superficially in the frontal lobes. Unlike most other gliomas, calcification is common in the oligodendroglioma. The calcification can be seen in plain skull X rays. At the microscopic level the oligodendroglioma has a honeycomb appearance. The cell population is dense and their nuclei are small and regular. A clear halo surrounds each nucleus, making diagnosis relatively easy.

The ependymoma is common in children and young adults. These tumors arise from the ependymal cells lining the ventricles and the central canal of the spinal cord. The most common site of occurrence is the fourth ventricle. They also arise from the lateral ventricle, and they are the most common glioma of the spinal cord. There is some variation in their microscopic appearance and in the degree of anaplasia present. Clinically, the ependymoma acts like the various grades of the astrocytoma.

The medulloblastoma competes with the cerebellar astrocytoma for being the most common cerebellar tumor of childhood. The cell of origin is disputed, but these tumors usually arise in the midline of the cerebellum. Obstruction to CSF flow through the fourth ventricle occurs, producing hydrocephalus and symptoms of increased intracranial pressure. At the microscopic level the medulloblastoma has dense sheets of tumor cells that stain darkly. Numerous dividing cells are usually seen in each microscopic field.

Some neuropathologists believe that gliomas may contain cells of differing origin. Thus they may be a composite of the astrocytoma and the oligodendroglioma. Such tumors are designated merely as a malignant glioma.

Although this discussion has been about gliomas in the cerebral hemisphere and cerebellum, it should be stressed that they may occur throughout the CNS. They are seen in the optic nerve, the brainstem, and the spinal cord.

Metastasis of malignant brain tumors beyond the nervous system is rare, but spread within the confines of the CNS is common. The glioblastoma, and particularly the medulloblastoma, may spread in the CSF to implant along the spinal cord and elsewhere in the subarachnoid space.

Demyelination

The presence of myelin is a characteristic unique to the nervous system. Myelin consists of protein and lipid material and acts like an insulator for certain nerve fibers (Figure 1–1). In the brain and spinal cord it is produced by the oligodendrocyte; in the peripheral nerve it is produced by Schwann's cells. Several diseases of the nervous system cause the breakdown of myelin. This breakdown is, in most diseases, a secondary result rather than a direct effect on the myelin itself.

Diseases that specifically attack myelin may be classified into two categories: those in which normal myelin is affected and those in which the myelin is formed or broken down in an abnormal fashion. Multiple sclerosis is the most common demyelinating disease in the first category. Patients with multiple sclerosis experience episodes of acute neurological impairment such as blindness, followed then by improvement. The tendency to exacerbation and remission characterizes multiple sclerosis.

The etiology of multiple sclerosis is not known. Two theories are presently in vogue. The possibility that a virus may cause multiple sclerosis is intriguing. Certainly it is not an acute infection like viral encephalitis, but it may result from a slow virus. It is now recognized that some viruses have very long incubation periods, which on occasion may be several years. The disease called kuru, which occurs in the Fore tribe of New Guinea, is believed to be caused by such a slow virus. This disease causes poor balance (ataxia), slurred speech, and mental deficiency progressing to death.

The other possible cause of multiple sclerosis is that it is some type of an autoimmune process. Recall that the body, in response to certain foreign substances called antigens, produces antibodies; this is how the body gains immunity to certain diseases. It is thought that in multiple sclerosis, antibodies are somehow produced to act against the body's own myelin. It is possible that a slow virus might alter the body's myelin, so that it is indeed a foreign substance that stimulates the formation of antibodies.

At the microscopic level, focuses of demyelination called plaques may be seen to occur randomly throughout the brain, brainstem, and the spinal cord. The optic nerves and optic chiasm are very often involved. The plaques often occur close to blood vessels and are sharply circumscribed. Early in the formation of a plaque, oligodendrocytes assemble. Myelin breaks down and is converted into neutral fat. The axons are naked but they remain intact. In the mature plaque the number of oligodendrocytes decreases. Astrocytes appear and lay down fibers; therefore the term *sclerosis* is applied.

Schilder's disease is another demyelinating disease, a rapidly progressive one occurring in children and one for which there is no treatment.

The leukodystrophies are diseases in which myelin is abnormally formed or abnormally broken down. These diseases are inherited and are basically the result of errors in metabolism. The abnormality in one of these, metachromatic leukodystrophy, results in the accumulation of a substance called cerebroside sulfatide, a substance normally present only in very small amounts.

Degenerative Diseases

Included in degenerative diseases are diseases that are inherited, some that are the result of metabolic errors, and many more that have no identifiable cause. Keep in mind that the etiology of most of the latter will eventually be defined.

The "normal" process of aging is a relentless degenerative process. The brain of an elderly patient shows atrophy with narrow gyri and wide sulci. At the microscopic level there is neuron loss, and glial elements are more prominent. The cause of aging is obscure. Some believe it results from decreased blood flow because of cerebrovascular arteriosclerosis. It is likely that there are several factors probably both intrinsic (within the cell) and extrinsic (outside the cell)—that contribute to the process of aging.

Presenile dementia is defined as dementia that occurs between the ages of 40 and 65 years. The most common disease in this group is Alzheimer's disease. At the gross level the brain shows atrophy. Especially involved are the frontal and the occipital lobes. At the microscopic level there is a severe loss of neurons in the cortex of the brain. Pick's disease is another disease that causes presenile dementia. Like Alzheimer's disease there is prominent cortical atrophy, but it is more localized, especially in the frontal and the temporal lobes.

There are degenerative diseases that involve primarily the basal ganglia. The term *basal ganglia* includes the caudate nucleus, the putamen and the globus pallidus, and the substantia nigra and the red nucleus. Parkinsonism is the most common disease in this class. It may result from infarction in the region of the substantia nigra. It may occur following infection. A number of patients who had encephalitis in the early 1920s have developed parkinsonism. This encephalitis is called von Economo's encephalitis and is thought to be of viral origin. Many cases of parkinsonism occur without any apparent cause and are, therefore, called idiopathic parkinsonism. Finally, certain drugs in high doses can cause Parkinson-like syndromes. These drugs include reserpine, which is an antihypertensive drug, and drugs in the phenothiazine class, which are used as tranquilizers.

The lesion of parkinsonism is in the substantia nigra. At the gross level there is a loss of the normally occurring black pigment (melanin). At the microscopic level the loss of the pigment is observed and there may be some neuronal loss. An inclusion body is common in the cytoplasm of melanin-containing cells.

The biochemical defect in parkinsonism is the depletion of the dopamine in the cells of the substantia nigra. Recently the administration of L-dopa, which is converted by the body to dopamine, has been of great help in the treatment of parkinsonism.

Clinically the patient with parkinsonism has rigidity, bradykinesia (loss of associative movements), and tremor. The tremor occurs especially in the hands. It occurs when the hands are at rest and it appears as though the patient were rolling something between the thumb and fingers (pill rolling).

Huntington's chorea is another degenerative disease of the basal ganglia. The caudate nucleus is most prominently involved, but the cortex also suffers degenerative changes. At the microscopic level there is neuronal loss and fibrosis by astrocytes (gliosis). The disease is inherited and it is manifest by abnormal movements and progressive mental deterioration.

Several degenerative diseases occur that involve primarily the spinal cord. Some involve only motor tracts; others are more diffuse, involving several spinal tracts, the cerebellum, and peripheral nerves.

Amyotrophic lateral sclerosis (ALS) is a degenerative disease that affects the motor system. It involves both upper and lower neurons; thus there is loss of neurons in the motor strip, in the motor nuclei of the cranial nerves, and in the anterior horn of the spinal cord. The cause of amyotrophic lateral sclerosis is not known. It occurs in the fifth to the seventh decade, and it is relentless, with death occurring in approximately 3 years. Patients with this disease have extensive muscular wasting with associated weakness. A common cause of death is aspiration pneumonia because of their inability to swallow.

Friedreich's ataxia is an inherited degenerative disease of the spinal cord. The dorsal columns, the dorsal spinocerebellar tracts, and the lateral corticospinal tracts are involved. At the microscopic level, one sees demyelination and axonal degeneration followed by gliosis. Patients with this disease also have degeneration and fibrosis of the myocardium (heart muscle). Death, caused by thrombosis of the coronary arteries of the heart, is common.

Syringomyelia is a degenerative disease of unknown etiology in which cystic spaces occur in the spinal cord. The space may extend over several cord levels and it may even involve the brainstem. The cavity starts behind the central canal and damages many of the tracts in the cord. The cyst contains fluid and its wall is lined by glial fibers.

There are several rather ill-defined degenerative processes that affect the brainstem and the cerebellum. In olivopontocerebellar degeneration there is atrophy of the pons because of demyelination. The olivary nucleus shows gliosis, and there is demyelination in the cerebellum. In primary cerebellar degeneration there is neuronal loss, especially among the Purkinje cells.

In some instances epilepsy may be a degenerative disease. Seizures may occur in association with known lesions such as tumors, post-traumatic scars, and arteriovenous malformations. There are, however, other instances in which there are no identifiable causes; these are called idiopathic epilepsies. The involved cells, rather than being destroyed, have been rendered irritable, and the manifestation of this irritation is the convulsion. The seizures in idiopathic epilepsy may be of different types.

Grand mal epilepsy is a motor seizure. The seizure may be generalized with movements of all extremities or it may be focal, remaining isolated to a single extremity. The Jacksonian seizure begins with a particular area, like the thumb, being involved first. Next the hand and then the arm join in the jerking. This progression is called a Jacksonian march. It may spread to become a generalized convulsion.

Petit mal epilepsy is characterized by a temporary loss of consciousness that is often associated with head movements. There may be a sudden, short-lived loss of postural tone during which the patient may fall. Sometimes a sudden jerk called myoclonus may be seen with petit mal epilepsy.

Psychomotor epilepsy is a sensory type of seizure that may be accompanied by myoclonic jerks. The patients often experience hallucinations of smell called uncinate fits. There are often temporary emotional disturbances with a clouding of consciousness lasting for brief periods. It is believed that the temporal lobe is the source of psychomotor epilepsy.

It was mentioned that there is no obvious cause for idiopathic epilepsy. In some cases, and especially in psychomotor epilepsy, changes of a degenerative character are seen in the hippocampus lying within the temporal lobe. The particular part involved is called Sommer's sector. At the microscopic level there is neuronal loss, gliosis, and the deposition of material containing iron and calcium.

There is another group of diseases that more rightfully fall under the heading of errors of metabolism than under degenerative diseases. Wilson's disease or hepatolenticular degeneration is a disease in this class that results from a defect in copper metabolism. Copper is deposited in the liver, in the basal ganglia, and in the cornea. There is a deficiency in the blood serum of ceruloplasmin, which may have some function in the binding or transport of copper, but this has not been proved. The microscopic brain lesion is one of diffuse neuronal loss in the basal ganglia followed by necrosis and secondary gliosis.

Phenylketonuria is another disease in which there is a metabolic error. There is a deficiency of the enzyme that converts the amino acid phenylalanine to tyrosine. The phenylalanine accumulation has an adverse effect on the development and myelination of the infant brain.

Intoxications

Many seemingly innoxious substances can be toxic to the body if taken in excess. Their effect on the CNS may not be primary, but none the less the secondary insult to the brain can be lethal.

Cerebral hypoxia (deficient oxygen) may be caused by many toxins. The brain requires as much as 25–30 percent of the oxygen supply to the body, which indicates how metabolically dynamic brain cells are. The oxygen is used to oxidize glucose, which supplies the energy necessary for cellular function. There are two types of hypoxia. The first is a deficiency in the amount of oxygen available to the blood. This occurs in pulmonary diseases like pneumonia where there is a poor exchange of O_2 between the compartments of the lung and the hemoglobin in the blood. Injury to the respiratory centers in the brain from trauma or depressant drugs may decrease the rate of respiration resulting in a deficiency in O_2 availability. Injury to the chest, or diseases affecting the respiratory muscles, such as muscular dystrophy, may make the respiratory effort ineffective. The second type of hypoxia results from inadequacy in the oxygen-carrying ability of the blood. This is seen in the anemia occurring because of excessive destruction of red blood cells or because of defective hemoglobin synthesis. Carbon monoxide, by combining with hemoglobin, drastically reduces the ability of the blood to carry oxygen. This deprives the oxygen of a vehicle of transport to the cells. Serious heart disease, such as congestive failure or fibrillation, affects the dynamics of blood flow adversely and may bring about hypoxia.

Because oxygen is used by the cell to produce energy through the oxidation of glucose, the same end result occurs if there is a deficiency of glucose. This occurs with the excessive administration of insulin or with the presence of an islet-cell tumor of the pancreas (which produces insulin). Cyanide directly affects the enzymatic oxidation of glucose.

It has been shown that, after only 20 seconds of anoxia (total lack of O_2), cortical function ceases. The injury is irreversible if anoxia lasts more than a few minutes. The microscopic features of long-term anoxic states are neuronal death followed by necrosis and eventually gliosis. An additional finding, more specifically the result of anoxia, is the occurrence of multiple, small hemorrhages, called petechiae, throughout the white matter. Certain neurons are consistently injured in hypoxic states; included are those in Layers III and V of the cortex, the basal ganglia, Sommer's sector of the hippocampus, and the Purkinje neurons of the cerebellum.

Some chemical toxins affect both the CNS and the peripheral nerves. Lead is the classic substance in this group. In children it produces severe brain swelling, and in the adult it commonly produces degenerative changes in peripheral nerves. The radial nerve, which is primarily a motor nerve, typically is involved. Arsenic and mercury are two other chemicals that have primary effects on the CNS and peripheral nerves.

Acute ethyl alcohol intoxication produces drunkenness. The major neurological effect, however, is seen in chronic alcoholism. The alcoholic fails to maintain good nutritive intake, and therefore vitamin deficiency results. In this instance thiamine deficiency causes the disease call Wernicke's encephalopathy. The lesion may be hemorrhage or neuronal loss in the gray matter around the third and fourth ventricles.

Vitamin B_{12} deficiency produces combined degeneration of the spinal cord. The effect is primarily demyelination of the posterior columns, the corticospinal tracts, and the peripheral nerves.

Developmental Malformations

There is a multitude of causes of developmental malformations of the central nervous system. Some are inherited; others are the result of infections such as measles. Some medications have been recognized as the cause of developmental abnormalities. Energy sources such as X ray and atomic radiation have been incriminated. There is, however, little doubt that a great number of etiologic factors have not yet been identified.

The embryology of the CNS is rather complicated and is beyond the scope of this book. It seems, however, that many of the causes of malformations of the CNS have their effect at a specific time in the development of the brain and spinal cord. Often there are associated malformations of tissues overlying the malformed nervous tissue. One may see a failure of closure in the bony neural arch of the vertebrae and failure of the skin to close, resulting in direct exposure of neural elements.

Some malformations are incompatible with life, such as total absence of the brain (anencephaly) or spinal cord (amyelia). In some malformations the neurological deficit is overwhelming, but the baby may live for an undetermined length of time. The cerebral hemispheres may fail to form or there may be large cystic cavities, but the brainstem and cerebellum are often present and intact (hydranencephaly).

An encephalocele is a defect that most often occurs in the midline at the back of the head. There is a defect of both skin and bone permitting the meninges and brain to bulge outward. These may be small or very large, containing most of the occipital and parietal lobes of the brain. Surgical closure can be accomplished, but severe neurological deficits may occur because of injury to the brain when it herniates or because of failure of the brain tissue to mature.

Defects similar to the encephalocele occur on the back at various places along the vertebral column. They most commonly occur in the lumbar region, and they appear as a large sac or mass protruding from the back. The mass may be covered by skin, but more often it is covered by thin connective tissue. If only the dura makes up the sac, it is called a meningocele. In this instance surgical closure is done to prevent infection. The baby may have no neurological deficit.

Unfortunately the spinal cord and cauda equina are often an integral part of the mass; such a mass is called a meningomyelocele. These children are usually left with some degree of lower extremity paralysis, and they lack bladder control. Of the children with a meningomyelocele, 80 percent also develop hydrocephalus.

Hydrocephalus may result from certain congenital malformations, but may also be a result of brain tumors or infections. It occurs whenever an obstruction at any point blocks the flow of CSF. CSF continues to be produced, and as a result of the failure of reabsorption, the ventricles become larger at the expense of the surrounding brain. If the site of obstruction is within the ventricular system, obstructive or noncommunicative hydrocephalus occurs. If, however, the block is due to partial obliteration of the subarachnoid space, such as may occur with tuberculous meningitis, a nonobstructive or communicating hydrocephalus occurs.

Most developmental malformations produce obstructive hydrocephalus. The aqueduct of Sylvius is a common site of obstruction. The duct may be incompletely formed, ending in a blind pouch. Sometimes there may be only a thin diaphragm that blocks the aqueduct. An obstruction in the aqueduct often results in marked enlargement of the two lateral ventricles and the third ventricle. The fourth ventricle is normal because it lies beyond the site of obstruction.

The Arnold-Chiari malformation may be associated with obstructive hydrocephalus. This malformation is characterized by displacement of parts of the cerebellum and the medulla oblongata into the upper cervical canal of the spine.

These are just two of the common developmental abnormalities that are associated with hydrocephalus. A tumor in the third or fourth ventricle can also produce hydrocephalus. Infection causing gliosis around the aqueduct may effectively close the duct to normal CSF circulation.

Metabolic Diseases

A survey of metabolic diseases demonstrates the point made earlier —that the CNS does not exist autonomously. Instead, disease in one of the other systems of the body often has a profound effect on the CNS.

The deficiency of thyroid hormone that occurs in hypothyroid states results in mental deficiency in early life. Convulsions and coma may occur in the adult having hypothyroidism, peripheral neuritis, or cranial nerve palsies. Hyperactive thyroid states (thyrotoxicosis) are often associated with eye movement weakness, muscle disease, and myasthenia gravis.

Sudden muscle spasms (tetany) occur in states of low parathyroid function. There may be symptoms of increased intracranial pressure. There is often pathological calcification in the basal ganglia. The deficiency of parathormone causes a low serum calcium level.

Hypoglycemia, which occurs on occasion because of excessive insulin production by the pancreas, may have serious CNS affects. The patients have sweating, pallor, and hunger pangs. In severe hypoglycemia, episodes of confusion may occur as well as convulsions and coma. The lack of glucose at the cellular level is responsible for the symptoms. Recall that oxidation of glucose provides the energy for cell function.

Inappropriate secretion of antidiuretic hormone (ADH) occurs often with trauma as well as with infections and neoplasms. ADH is produced normally by the hypothalamus and is transported to the posterior lobe of the pituitary gland. Normally when a person experiences thirst, ADH is released, which causes the kidney to absorb more water rather than to release it as urine. If there is a deficit of ADH, such as may occur in head injuries, the patient puts out massive amounts of urine and severe dehydration occurs. When this happens, the patient has diabetes insipidus. On the other hand, inappropriate ADH secretion may occur, causing water retention even though the body has no need to conserve it. The fluid spaces of the body increase while sodium is constantly becoming more dilute. These patients have mental confusion, convulsions, and even coma.

Liver disease produces many and varied neurological symptoms. The amount of ammonia correlates reasonably well with the severity of symptoms. In failure, coma may occur and it is aptly called hepatic coma.

Porphyria is a disease that occurs because of excessive production and urinary excretion of porphyrin products. The patient excretes urine that is burgundy red during the acute periods. The patient experiences severe abdominal pains as well as certain neurological symptoms. Neuritis is most profound, with weakness progressing on occasion to total paralysis.

Diseases of the Peripheral Nerves

Turning now to diseases of the peripheral nerves, it is wise to try to categorize these diseases just as was done with CNS disease. Classification is more difficult, but an effort to do so will pay dividends.

Polyneuritis (polyneuropathy) is the term applied when there is widespread disease of the peripheral nerves. Recall that a peripheral nerve is composed of fibers with more than one function. Some of the fibers carry motor impulses, while others carry sensory impulses from the sense organs. Still others go to sweat glands or to blood vessels. Certain diseases of peripheral nerves affect all the fibers; others involve specific fibers within the nerve. At the microscopic level the diseased fibers swell and there is breakdown of myelin. If the disease progresses, the axon cylinders are destroyed and retrograde pathological changes occur in the neurons. If the injurious agent is identified and if treatment is begun, recovery may occur. Incomplete recovery is, however, common.

Malnutrition is a very common cause of peripheral polyneuritis and it is particularly common in the chronic alcoholic. There are some authorities who believe that there may also be a direct toxic effect of alcohol on the nerves. Sensory fibers are especially involved, causing pain and paresthesia. Weakness may follow, beginning in the legs, and paralysis may occur. Korsakoff's psychosis is seen in the alcoholic, and it is a manifestation of CNS effect. The patient is confused, disoriented, and has a loss of memory and the tendency to confabulate. Wernicke's sysdrome also occurs in malnourished states and is primarily due to a deficiency of thiamine. Patients with this syndrome have paralysis of eye movement, staggering gaits, and changes in the level of consciousness.

Lead intoxication is an example of a toxic peripheral neuritis. It involves primarily the motor fibers of the radial nerve. Afflicted patients, usually adults, suffer wristdrop, the inability to extend the wrist and fingers.

The bacterial infection diphtheria may cause a polyneuritis by the production of a toxin. The cranial nerves are often involved, but in severe cases the extremities are affected also.

The infectious polyneuritis of Guillain-Barre's syndrome is a disease of unknown cause that involves both cranial nerves and peripheral nerves. In classic cases the patient has an ascending paralysis beginning in the legs, then involving the trunk, the upper extremities, and often even the face. Respiratory paralysis may require the use of a respirator. Recovery may be complete, but incomplete recovery is more common.

Diabetes mellitus frequently is associated with polyneuritis. Sensory phenomenon with pain and paresthesia is most common, though weakness may be prominent. Better medical control of the diabetes with diet and insulin often lessens the symptoms of the neuritis. On occasion the neuritis involves a single nerve; this is called mononeuritis.

Cancer and especially carcinoma of the lung may produce polyneuritis. The reason is not known but probably it is because of metabolic or toxic factors. Traumatic injuries of the peripheral nerves are common. Crushing injuries or penetrating injuries may severely contuse the nerve or may actually transect it. Recovery from the more extensive injuries is often incomplete. If the nerve is transected and must be surgically reapproximated, the type of nerve injured has much to do with the degree of recovery one might expect. The nerve in which the fibers have one function (e.g., motor) will achieve better recovery than the nerve having fibers of varied function. Thus, recovery of an injured radial nerve will generally exceed the recovery of an injured median nerve.

The major problem, which limits the recovery of a transected nerve, is the inability of the regenerating proximal nerve fiber to grow across the transection and enter its own axon cylinder. It is easily seen how a motor fiber may grow into the axon cylinder that contained a sensory nerve fiber before the injury. Thus the motor fiber would be misdirected and have no chance of reaching the muscle it was intended to innervate. Often the regenerating proximal fiber never finds an axon cylinder, and therefore it grows in an aimless, haphazard manner. Though the two ends of the nerve may appear to have grown together, the nerve is thickened at the point where they join. This widened segment is called a neuroma. Very often no effective nervous impulse will pass through a neuroma.

Another factor that determines the quality of recovery of a sutured nerve is the distance the transection is from the muscle it should supply. A regenerating nerve fiber grows very slowly, often requiring months to reach its destination. A muscle, however, requires constant nervous input to maintain its bulk and tone. Without nervous input the muscle will soon atrophy and be replaced by fat and fibrous tissue. Thus it is often necessary to stimulate the muscle artificially to keep it viable until the arrival of its motor nerve.

The entrapment of peripheral nerves is common in trauma but it occurs in other instances as well. The healing of a fractured bone is accomplished by the formation of new bone, and sometimes a peripheral nerve may become encased in the exuberant bone growth. The radial nerve may be involved in this manner when a fracture of the mid-humerus heals. A fractured elbow may similarly encase or compress the ulnar nerve. Portions of the brachial plexus may be compressed if a fractured clavicle heals with poor alignment.

The carpal tunnel syndrome involves entrapment or compression of the median nerve at the wrist. This may occur from a fractured wrist, from arthritis, or in states where there is soft tissue swelling as seen in pregnancy. Regardless of cause, the common effect of all is to make the tunnel smaller, thereby compressing the median nerve and the flexor tendons as they enter the hand from the forearm. This produces numbness of the thumb, forefinger, and middle finger as well as weakness of the hand grip.

There are diseases of the peripheral nerves that are inherited and that are degenerative in character. Such a disease is peroneal muscular atrophy or Charcot-Marie-Tooth disease. Microscopic degenerative changes occur in the nerves of the leg, especially in the peroneal nerve. There is loss of myelin and degeneration of the axis cylinders. Marked muscular atrophy is a secondary result. The patient's legs appear like stork legs or an inverted wine bottle. Deformity of the feet results, producing clubfeet. The patient experiences pain and paresthesias as well as progressive weakness.

Dejerine-Sottas disease is a rare inherited disease that produces a polyneuritis. The most striking characteristic is the markedly thickened nerves that can be easily seen beneath the skin.

The neurofibroma is the only tumor of note involving the peripheral nerves. These tumors are generally benign, though malignant degeneration may occur in some cases. The neurofibroma may be single or multiple and may occur on any peripheral nerve. When the tumors are multiple they are usually part of the syndrome of neurofibromatosis or von Recklinghausen's disease. In addition to many neurofibromas in the peripheral nerves, these patients may have hundreds of soft polyps on their skin. Light-brown patches of pigment called café-au-lait spots may also occur on their skin. There is an increased incidence of brain and spinal cord tumors in neurofibromatosis. Meningiomas and gliomas are most common. Neurofibromas of the acoustic nerve frequently occur and they may be bilateral. Neurofibromas and meningiomas often occur in the spinal cord.

Muscle Disease

Muscle diseases (myopathies) fall within the domain of the neurologist. Muscle atrophy or wasting may occur in several instances but most often it is not because of intrinsic muscle disease. Atrophy of this type is a secondary effect and should not be confused with muscular dystrophy. Secondary muscular atrophy occurs when a muscle is not used. This happens when a limb is immobilized by a cast for treatment of a fractured bone. Atrophy may occur in poor nutritional states, in trauma, and with infections. If a peripheral nerve is injured, the muscle it supplies begins to atrophy. A muscle requires constant nervous stimulation to maintain its bulk and tone. Pathologically the muscle is a permanent cell with little or no ability to regenerate. Thus if the cause of atrophy is not eliminated, the muscle cell is replaced by fibrous tissue.

Muscular dystrophy is a primary disease of the muscle cell. The cause of muscular dystrophy is not known but most likely it results from an inborn error of metabolism. The various types of muscular dystrophy are inherited and they are characterized by progressive weakness and muscular degeneration. Striated muscles are primarily involved, but in some dystrophies the heart muscle is also affected. The more common muscular dystrophies can be divided into three classes clinically. These are the Duchenne type, the facioscapulohumeral type, and the limb-girdle type.

The Duchenne type occurs only in males, and the onset is in the early years of life. The progression is relentless, with death occurring in the second or third decades. The dystrophy is usually limited to the trunk and extremities. Some of the muscles like the biceps and gastrocnemius appear enlarged, but when tested they are quite weak. Weakness of the pelvic muscles results in a waddling gait. The normal curvature of the lower spine is exaggerated by weakened trunk muscles. Eventually the patient is confined to a wheelchair or bed. Death occurs from pneumonia or because of involvement of the heart muscle.

Facioscapulohumeral dystrophy occurs in either sex and the onset is later than it is in Duchenne dystrophy. The muscles of the face are always affected. The face may become masklike with no expression when laughing. The muscles of the shoulder girdle and upper extremities weaken and degenerate. The progression of the disease is variable, but survival to old age is not uncommon.

Limb-girdle dystrophy occurs in either sex, beginning usually in the first three decades of life. Muscular weakness occurs primarily in the pelvic muscles, but eventually all extremities are involved to one degree or another.

The anatomy of normal striated muscle was reviewed in Chapter 1. In muscular dystrophy, the muscle fibers enlarge (hypertrophy), and some of the muscles split lengthwise. Degeneration of the myoplasm follows, with eventual replacement of the dead muscle cell by fat and fibrous tissue.

The diagnosis of muscular dystrophy is possible by demonstrating microscopically the pathological changes mentioned. There is also an increase of various enzymes in the blood serum, such as creatine phosphokinase (CPK). The electromyogram (EMG) also helps in the diagnosis.

Another group of muscle diseases has in common the characteristics of myotonia, the inability of muscles to relax after a forceful contraction. Myotonia dystrophia is an example of myotonic muscular disease. The myotonia may involve any muscle of the body, but the muscles of the hand are most commonly involved. In addition to the myotonia, the patient with myotonia dystrophia has muscular degeneration similar to muscular dystrophy. Muscles of the face and neck characteristically atrophy. These patients also have early baldness, testicular atrophy, cataracts, and various endocrine (glandular) abnormalities.

There are familial muscle diseases that cause periodic paralysis; these are related to potassium metabolism. The most common is hypokalemic periodic paralysis. During the attack, the serum potassium is lower than 3 milliequivalents per liter. In these diseases there is no impairment of general health, and attacks lessen as the patient grows older.

There are several other primary diseases of muscles. They may be inherited. Some myopathies are limited to specific muscles such as the eye muscles (ocular myopathy); other myopathies are seen in association with endocrine diseases such as hyperthyroidism.

Polymyositis is a common disorder of muscles. It logically should be included in the group of diseases called collagen diseases. The cause of these diseases is not known, but probably it is allergic or autoimmune. Patients with polymyositis very commonly have muscular tenderness. Muscular weakness is seen especially in the girdle musculature and in the muscles of the face. Difficulty in swallowing (dysphagia) is a common complaint. The microscopic changes seen include degeneration of muscle fibers and infiltration of the muscle fibers and spaces around blood vessels by lymphocytes and plasma cells. The course of the disease is quite variable. There may be exacerbations or remissions or the patient may experience only a single acute episode.

Bone Disease Affecting the Nervous System

The CNS lies within the confines of the skull and vertebral column. This armor is largely bony but it is in part made of cartilage and ligaments. Because of this close anatomic relationship, diseases of bone, cartilage, and ligament may affect the CNS secondarily.

Paget's disease causes deformity and thickening of various bones of the body including the skull. Portions of the skull are thickened and may bulge prominently, causing cosmetic problems. More serious though is the encroachment upon neuroforamina (holes in skull) at the base of the skull. The cranial nerves passing through these foramina are trapped and compressed. The eighth cranial (acoustic) nerve is most commonly involved, causing deafness. Fibrous dysplasia is another disease with bone thickening, producing asymmetry of skull contour and foraminal encroachment.

Craniosynostosis (craniostenosis) is the premature fusing of the suture lines of the skull. The brain grows rapidly in early life, so the skull must expand to accommodate this growth. Suture lines are actually the spaces between the various bones of the skull. These sutures remain open until the brain growth slows, and then their closure is accomplished by the formation of bone that bridges the gap between the two adjacent bones. The sagittal suture line is the most common one to fuse prematurely. The coronal and lambdoidal sutures may also fuse, or there may be various combinations of all three that may fuse. If a suture line fuses too soon, those still open must bulge excessively as the brain grows. This results in many strangely shaped skulls, some of which are cosmetic problems if not corrected by surgery early in life. More important is the possibility of restricted brain growth and mental retardation that may result if all or most of the suture lines fuse prematurely.

Several malformations occur at the base of the skull in relation to the upper cervical vertebrae. In certain diseases there is softening of bone which permits the upper cervical spine to protrude into the skull, resulting in brainstem compression. Various malformations of the first two cervical vertebrae (atlas and axis) may occur. There may be incomplete formation of the vertebrae. A potentially serious deformity is the failure of the odontoid process to fuse with the body of C_2 (axis). The stability between C_1 and C_2 is reduced. Relatively minor trauma may cause serious injury to the upper cervical cord.

The ruptured disc is a common cause of spinal cord or nerve root injury. Rupture may occur at any level of the vertebral column. The most common levels of rupture are between cervical vertebrae 5 and 6 (C_{5-6}) and between 6 and 7 (C_{6-7}) and in the lumbar area between lumbar 4 and 5 (L_{4-5}) and 5 and the first sacral level (L_5–S_1)

Picture the disc as a hockey puck lying between the bony bodies of two vertebrae. The circular wall of the disc is composed of dense fibrous tissue called the annulus fibrosis. In the center of the disc is a semigelatinous material called the nucleus pulposus. The disc permits motion of the vertebral column and it also acts as a shock absorber. The disc continues to mature until the fourth decade of life, when degenerative changes begin. The nucleus pulposus loses water and is slowly replaced by fibrous tissue. The annulus begins to weaken and may permit rupture of the nucleus pulposus. The weakest part of the annulus is posterior and lateral.

When rupture occurs the fragment of nucleus pulposus goes into the spinal canal. Because it is laterally placed, it puts pressure on the nerve root that leaves the canal at that level. The patient then experiences pain that radiates along a particular nerve. The ruptured disc in the cervical area causes radiating pain into the arm and hand; in the lumbar area, pain goes into the leg. The patient also has numbness of certain fingers or toes; specific muscles become weak and there can be an absence of reflexes. The radiating pain is called radicular pain, and when present in the leg, the term *sciatica* is commonly used. The herniation of the nucleus pulposus is designated by the abbreviated form, HNP. The lay public commonly uses the term *slipped disc* when talking of an HNP (Figure 2-8).

The herniated nucleus pulposus usually causes compression of the nerve root alone, but if it herniates in the midline, the spinal cord or the cauda equina may be compressed. Recall that the spinal cord ends at about the second lumbar vertebra, and the nerves destined for the lower trunk, bladder, and legs continue in the spinal canal as the cauda equina (horse's tail). Therefore a midline HNP in the lumbar area would compress the cauda equina. In the cervical or thoracic area, a midline HNP could cause spinal cord compression and injury.

The rupture of the nucleus pulposus may occur with trauma. The degenerative changes described may weaken the annulus to the point that a simple sneeze or cough may cause its rupture. Very often, however, radicular pains occur from an HNP with no obvious cause available in the history.

Spondylosis is the term used to describe degenerative changes occurring in the disc and adjacent vertebral bodies. Weakening of the annulus fibrosis may cause it to bulge and initiate calcification. The edges of the vertebrae may also calcify, producing a bony ridge that can encroach upon the spinal canal. The spinal cord may then be injured because the diameter of the canal at the level of the bony ridge may not be adequate for the passage of the cord. Extreme hyperextension of the neck, such as might occur in a rear-end auto accident, may actually pinch the spinal cord at the level of the spondylotic ridge. The bony ridge may extend into the foramen at that level, decreasing the size of the foramen. The nerve root that exits at this level is compressed, and the patient experiences radicular pain. The part of the bony ridge that compresses the nerve in the foramen is often called a spur.

Figure 2-8

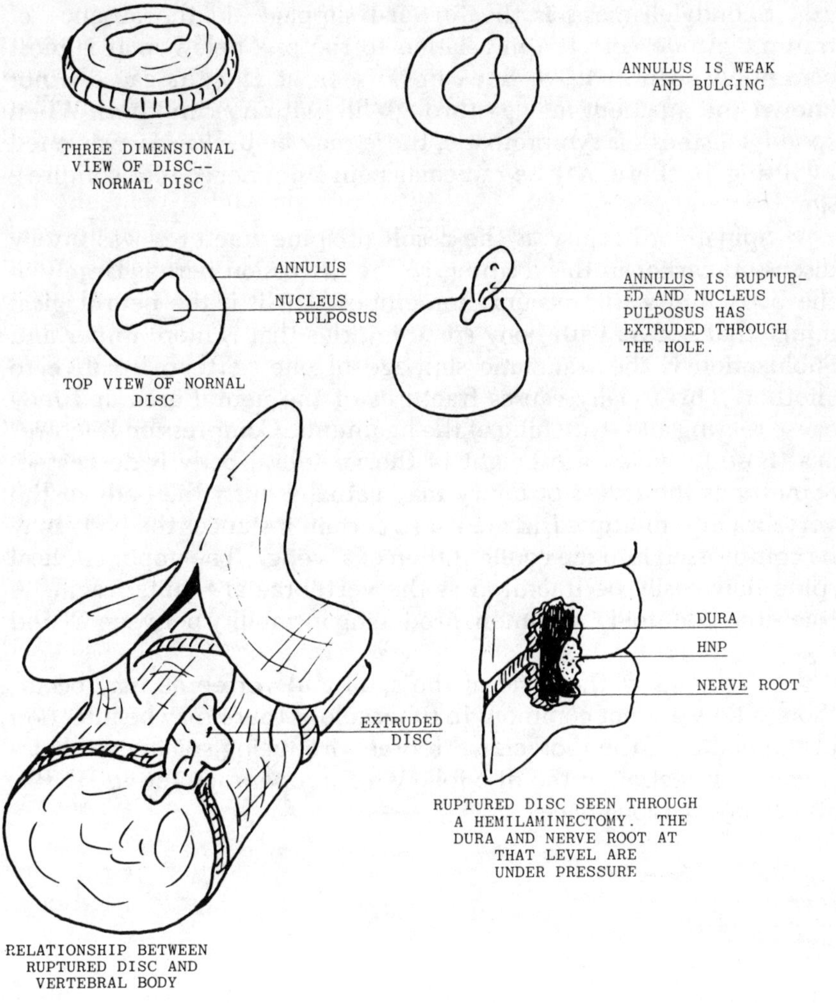

Spondylosis is more commonly symptomatic in the cervical region, but it also occurs in the lumbar spine where it produces cauda equina compression. The changes described also occur in lumbar spondylosis, but in addition there may be prominent thickening of the lamina of the lumbar vertebrae and hypertrophy of the ligamentum flavum. These additional changes cause compression from behind, and when coupled with the anteriorly placed bony ridge, there can be a drastic decrease in the diameter of the spinal canal.

Spondylolisthesis is the forward slippage, in the absence of trauma, of one vertebra in relation to the one below it. It is most commonly seen at L_5–S_1 but can be seen at L_{4-5}. Its cause is not known and a patient may go through life with no symptoms. When spondylolisthesis is symptomatic, there may be backache, worsened by lifting, or there may be radicular pain from nerve root compression.

Spinal cord injury as the result of spine fractures was briefly discussed earlier in this chapter, so the discussion here is largely of the bony injury that occurs. Remember that it is the neurological injury that occurs with bony spine injuries that is more important. Subluxation is the traumatic slippage of one vertebra relative to another. This usually causes fractures of the neural arch and may cause tearing and stretching of the ligaments. Compression fractures are those in which the height of the vertebral body is decreased. Sometimes the forces of injury may actually burst the body of the vertebra into multiple fragments. In certain instances the body may be compressed into the configuration of a wedge. The upper cervical spine may easily be fractured as the vertebrae are quite fragile. A fractured odontoid is common, producing instability between C_1 and C_2.

Infections of the bone of the skull and vertebrae may occur, though they are not common. In tuberculosis there may be infection in the bodies of the thoracic vertebrae, producing spinal cord compression. Infection in the disc following an operation for an HNP is also seen occasionally.

CHAPTER 3

Clinical Evaluation of the Central Nervous System

The evaluation of a patient who is ill should begin with a detailed history and physical examination. Using an orderly approach, one can be complete and detailed without spending an undue amount of time. It should be remembered that physicians who listen to their patients are very often "told" the diagnosis.

Taking a History

The logical place to begin is with the onset of symptoms. Was the onset sudden so that the patient (or relative) can give you the exact day and time, or was it insidious so that only the approximate time can be related? The character of onset is so important because with this information one can often categorize the process with which one will be dealing. Recall the discussions in Chapter 2 of the concept of the injurious agent and of various kinds of injurious agents, including vascular disease, trauma, infection, degenerative processes, metabolic disease, toxins, developmental malformations, and neoplasms.

Figure 3–1 illustrates how knowledge of the type of onset and subsequent course of the disease helps in making the correct diagnosis. In graph 1 of Figure 3-1 patients experience very sudden onset and are immediately the sickest they will be; thereafter they begin to improve. Whether the recovery is complete or incomplete depends on whether or not any irreversible injury was incurred at the

Figure 3-1

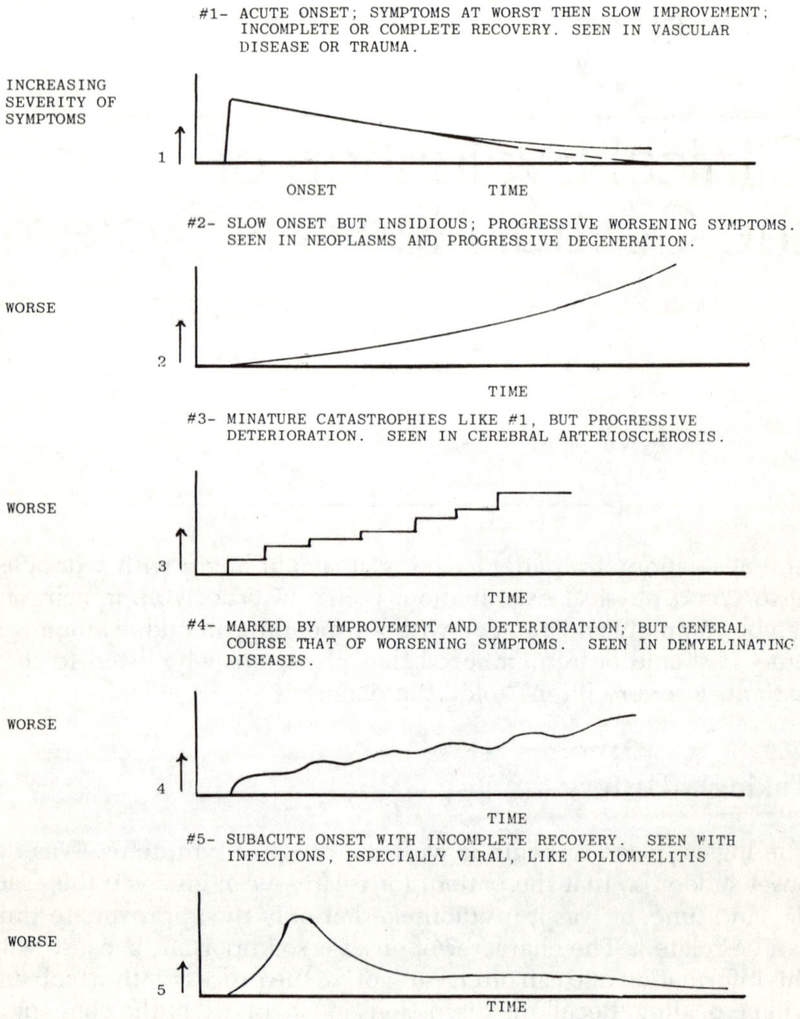

time of onset. In Graph 2 of Figure 3-1 the onset of the disease is so insidious that initially symptoms are vague and are disregarded. With the passage of time (as, for instance, tumor enlarges and invades, causing destruction) it becomes obvious that, whatever the process, it is relentless.

Further information about onset is desirable. Was there an external cause such as a blow to the head or exposure to toxins? Was the patient unconscious? If so, for how long and were there any movements that might suggest a convulsion? If a convulsion did occur, did a specific extremity start jerking first, and were the head and eyes deviated to one side or the other? After the convulsion, was the patient alert or asleep? If the patient was awake, could she or he talk and was there any residual paralysis or weakness? Did the patient have a headache initially and was it associated with dizziness, nausea, or vomiting? Was there any transient numbness, tingling, or weakness on one side of the body or the other? Were there speech difficulties? If so, did the patient know what she or he wanted to say but was unable to, and so forth?

The questions, therefore, are asked so that some concept of the character of onset is obtained. Next, the effort should be to determine the clinical course from its onset to the present moment. Thus, has the patient improved or gotten worse? If worse, in what way? Have the symptoms changed? Is the patient having more pain and what is the pain like? Can the patient do anything to make the pain worse or better? Has numbness or paralysis become worse and is it spreading? If spreading, in what order is it spreading and to what extent? Has the patient taken any medicine on her or his own or from another physician? What medicine was it and what amount was taken? Did it help?

Next the past medical history of the patient should be explored. Remember that most people are not sophisticated medically and may fail to volunteer valuable information. Thus searching questions must be asked.

Has the patient ever had symptoms similar to those presently experienced? If so, when and what happened? Was recovery complete or was there a residual? Had the patient seen a physician? What was the diagnosis? Would medical records be available? What other illnesses has the patient had in her or his lifetime? Were they routine or were there complications? What kinds of surgery has the patient undergone? List them chronologically. Does the patient have any allergies to specific medication? If so this information should be displayed prominently on office and hospital records.

Especially in neurological disorders it is necessary that the history of the patient's birth be reviewed. Were there any prenatal problems such as maternal malnutrition, infection, or threatened abortion? Was the delivery uncomplicated? Was it induced? How long was the labor? Were forcepts required? If a cesarean section was done, was it planned because of a small pelvis or because there was fetal distress? Was the baby premature, and what was the birth weight? Was resuscitation necessary and why? Were there Rh problems, and was an exchange transfusion required because of jaundice? Did the baby sit up, walk, and talk at the expected ages? In school, were there any learning problems?

The family medical history should be examined in detail because many neurological disorders are inherited. Has any member of the patient's family ever had any neurological disease? It is wise, if possible, to get some idea of the symptoms of the diseases that caused the deaths of relatives. Do not be satisfied with old age, palsy, or stroke. The age at the time of death should be noted. If the patient's parents are alive, are they in good health? If not, what is wrong? If they are not living, what was the cause of death and how old were they when they died? Does the patient have any siblings living or dead? Are there any commonly shared medical problems like hypertension, heart attacks, or cerebral vascular disease?

The final part of the patient's history should be the review of systems. In this review the alert physician may uncover symptoms indicating disease in other systems and organs of the body that may affect the nervous system secondarily. Investigate the system of the heart and lungs with questions about chest pain, breathlessness, productive cough, and palpitations. Review the gastrointestinal function by questions about weight gain or loss, food intolerance, vomiting, diarrhea, and abdominal pain. Evaluate the urinary system with questions regarding the ability to control urinary flow versus incontinence, pain with urination, blood in the urine, and flank pain.

The General Physical Examination

The physical examination of a patient with neurological symptoms should include a general examination in addition to the examination of the nervous system. The examination actually begins when the patient comes into the examining room. The observant physician will gather an initial impression of the patient as a whole. Does the patient walk with a limp? If so, is it because of weakness or because of pain? When the patient smiles, does one corner of the mouth seem to droop? Is the speech spontaneous, and are the responses to questions appropriate?

The examination of the head, eyes, ears, nose, and throat is usually performed first. Is the contour of the skull symmetrical or is there a prominent bulge on one side or the other (the tumor meningioma may produce such a bulge)? Are the ears full of wax to explain the patient's complaint of progressive deafness? Are the eyes swollen and is there tearing to suggest an allergic reaction? Auscultation (use of stethoscope) of the head should be done because sometimes one hears a swishing sound when an arteriovenous malformation is present. The swishing sound occurs with each heartbeat as the blood rushes through the malformation. This particular sound is called a bruit.

The neck should be carefully examined. Can you move it freely in all directions or does the patient resist? Stiffness is called nuchal rigidity and occurs with meningitis and subarachnoid hemorrhage. The carotid artery pulse is felt on each side of the neck. Are both carotid pulses present and are they equal? Auscultation is done over the point in the neck where the common carotid artery divides into the external and internal carotid arteries. Arteriosclerosis is very common at this point and deposition of the arteriosclerotic material may significantly narrow the opening in the artery. It is often possible to hear a bruit in such cases as the blood rushes through the narrowed opening.

The lungs are examined by observing the expansion of the chest. Is there good expansion with each breath or is it limited? Tapping with a finger on the chest (percussion) enables the physician to identify variation in lung densities. The presence of fluid in the chest or consolidation of a portion of the lung by pneumonia is identified by a decreased resonance when the chest is percussed. Finally, the lungs are examined by auscultation. With the stethoscope, wheezes can be heard, indicating asthma or chronic lung disease from years of smoking. A fine crackle may be heard, such as might be present in congestive heart failure or early pneumonia.

The heart is examined by both percussion and auscultation. The size of the heart can be determined with percussion. The heart is enlarged by congestive heart failure and long-standing hypertension. The heart sounds are heard with the stethoscope. It is possible to determine whether the heart's rhythm is regular or irregular. An irregular rhythm is called an arrhythmia. Patients with arrhythmias often have neurological symptoms. Blood forms clots in the heart chambers in certain types of arrhythmias, and pieces of the clots may break loose. These pieces, called emboli, then flow with the blood and often go to the brain. They lodge in the small arteries and cause ischemia or infarction of the brain. Heart murmurs can be heard with the stethoscope. Murmurs are often caused when the blood flows through injured heart valves. In rheumatic fever, often the valves are injured and become misshapen and scarred. Bacteria may grow on the diseased valves and in addition, blood clots tend to stick to them. Infected emboli then result and often go to the brain by way of the carotid arteries. When infected emboli lodge in cerebral arteries, brain abscesses or mycotic aneurysms occur.

The abdominal examination is done by feeling (palpating) the abdomen for enlarged organs. An enlarged liver is easily palpated. An abdominal aortic aneurysm presents a large pulsating mass in the midabdomen. Auscultation permits one to hear the bowel sounds. Infection of the peritoneal cavity resulting from a ruptured appendix causes a silent abdomen. Intestinal flu with diarrhea will cause hyperactive bowel sounds. The extremities are examined for focuses of infection or evidence of injury. The arterial pulses are evaluated, and by doing so, the heart's rhythm is checked and some idea of the severity of arteriosclerosis can be gained. Arteries with severe arteriosclerosis are hard, and often the pulse is diminished and even absent. The legs especially should be examined for swelling.

Rectal examinations should be done if at all possible because the greater percentage of rectal cancers are within reach of the examiner's finger. In addition, in males the prostate can be palpated.

If at all indicated in female patients, a pelvic examination is performed. The Pap smear is done to detect cancer of the cervix. The proficient examiner is able to estimate the size, shape, and position of the uterus and ovaries and, therefore, recognize ovarian cysts or other masses in the pelvis.

The Neurological Examination

The neurological examination can be roughly divided into five parts: the motor system, the sensory systems, the reflexes, cerebellar function and the cranial nerves. But first, an appraisal of the patient's conscious state should be made. Is the patient alert? If so, can he or she give you the right calendar date, month, and year? Does the patient know where he or she is? How is the memory for both past and recent events? Can the patient do simple calculations and interpret proverbs?

If the patient is not normally alert, it is best to describe the mental state rather than to use words like *coma,* or *lethargy.* Does the patient respond to verbal commands? If so, is the response appropriate? Does the patient appear preoccupied? Is he or she experiencing hallucinations? Is the patient abusive or hostile?

If the patient is not alert and will not respond to verbal stimuli, describe what he or she looks like. Will pain cause a response? If so, what type of pain and how severe must it be? What is the response made by the patient? Does the patient try to get away from the stimulus or merely assume some pathological position like the decerebrate posture?

A detailed, written description of the initial conscious state of the patient provides a base line for later comparison. Because the patient will be observed by nurses and other physicians, the written description enables others to judge whether the patient is improving or deteriorating.

The Motor System

Examination of the motor system requires that the patient disrobe. Persons of the opposite sex are provided a gown. All muscles should be inspected. Compare the shape and size of specific muscle groups. Are those on the right symmetrical to those on the left? If the patient is right-handed, some allowance should be made, for it is logical that the muscles of the right arm and hand would be larger than those of the left arm. When comparing the muscles of the extremities, it is of value to measure the circumference of the limb at that point. This information can then be objective evidence for future comparison. A muscle that is smaller than normal is said to be atrophic. The phenomenon of decreasing size is called atrophy.

The motor examination also includes the observation and characterization of involuntary movements. The types and causes of involuntary movements are many and varied. Included are the following:

1. *Tremor.* Involuntary and rhythmic movements of the extremities and occasionally the head. Tremors are subdivided as to when they occur:
   a. *Resting tremor.* Seen in parkinsonism, this tremor is present when the limbs are at rest. It is seen especially in the hands as they lie relaxed on the patient's lap.
   b. *Intention tremor.* Occurring in diseases of the cerebellum or its pathways, this tremor occurs as the patient starts to do something, such as reaching with the hand. The tremor becomes increasingly severe as the hand comes near the object.
   c. *Other tremors.* These are seen primarily with activity of the involved limbs. Some tremors have an inherited tendency; others occur with aging; and some occur with hyperthyroid states, alcoholism, etc.
2. *Fasciculations.* Periodic twitches of muscle bundles, these occur when the motor nerve supply to the muscle is injured. Muscles that have fasciculations undergo atrophy.

3. *Myoclonus.* Sudden, nonrhythmic jerks of muscles, these are common just as one is going to sleep and are normal in this instance. They also occur in disease states like encephalitis that affect the neurons of the cortex.
4. *Chorea.* Jerky, irregular, purposeless movements of limbs, body, and face that may occasionally be explosive, these are seen in Huntington's chorea and Saint Vitus's dance (Sydenham's chorea).
5. *Athetosis.* Slow, purposeless, snakelike movements that involve the fingers and toes especially, these are seen with diseases that affect the basal ganglia.
6. *Dystonia.* Involuntary, slow, writhing, twisting movements involving the trunk and proximal extremities primarily, these are seen in disease of the basal ganglia.
7. *Hemiballismus.* Wild, flinging or swinging movements of the extremities, more commonly involving the arms, these occur with disease of the subthalamus.
8. *Spasms or tics.* Various types of twitches occur, very often involving the face, as well as other parts of the body. The majority occur in psychologically unstable individuals.
9. *Convulsions.* Several types occur and are discussed elsewhere.

An estimate of muscle tone is a part of the motor system examination. The muscle examined should be relaxed. The examiner feels each muscle. Are the muscles firm or are they flabby? The normal muscle has some tone so it is firm but not excessively so. The tone of the muscles of an extremity is tested by passively moving the limb through its full range of motion. If there is resistance, there is increased tone. If the resistance is largely in one direction, the limb is said to be spastic; but resistance in all directions of motion is called rigidity. Spasticity occurs in disease of the corticospinal tract, whereas rigidity occurs with disease of the extrapyramidal system. A special kind of rigidity called cogwheel rigidity occurs in parkinsonism; when a joint is passively moved, a ratchetlike resistance is present rather than smooth resistance. There is loss of muscle tone if the motor nerve fibers to a muscle are injured. Decreased tone (hypotonus) also occurs if the sensory nerve from the muscle spindle is injured or diseased. Finally, lesions of the cerebellum cause a degree of hypotonus. Increased tone (hypertonus) occurs with lesions of the pyramidal (corticospinal tract) system and with lesions of the extrapyramidal system.

The final part of the motor examination—the majority of the examination—involves active movement of the muscles by the patient for the evaluation of strength of movement. First, the patient should be asked to perform a series of movements as rapidly as possible. Slowness of movement may be the only evidence of slight weakness. The patient then is asked to do various movements against the examiner's resistance. The muscles of the two sides of the body can therefore be compared. Muscles of the extremities and trunk are tested. The extent of the testing will to a degree be indicated by the history.

The Sensory System

Testing the sensory system requires an alert and cooperative patient. Hysteria, neuroses, and malingering often make the sensory examination of limited value, but with patience a good deal of information can be obtained.

The sensory examination can be divided into superficial, deep, and combined sensation. Testing is most satisfactorily performed by having the patient close his or her eyes. In recording the patient's responses, note the type of stimulus used and if there is anesthesia (complete lack of sensation), hypesthesia (diminished sensation), or hyperesthesia (increased sensation).

Superficial Sensation

1. *Tactile sensation.* This is the evaluation of light touch. A wisp of cotton or a small brush is used.
2. *Superficial pain.* The pin prick is used and it should be firm enough to elicit an unpleasant sensation. Areas of hypesthesia should be demonstrated by a diagram.
3. *Temperature sensation.* Various parts of the body are examined for both heat and cold sensitivity. Symmetrical comparison is important in the examination. Test tubes containing ice and hot water work nicely.
4. *Double simultaneous stimulation.* This is a test of parietal lobe function. Two safety pins are used. With eyes closed, the patient tells the examiner which side of the body is stuck by the pin. Some spot on the extremities works best, but the same general area should be stimulated on each side. After each side has been stuck several times individually, both sides are stuck at the same time. For example, a patient with a left parietal tumor would not feel the pin stick on the right side. This phenomenon is called extinction and occurs only when both sides are stimulated at the same time. When each side is stimulated by itself, the patient feels the pin.

5. *Two-point discrimination.* This is a test of parietal lobe function. Two safety pins are used. This test requires an experienced examiner. The two pins are touched to the patient's skin at variable distances apart. The patient responds by saying whether she or he can perceive two sticks by the pins or just one. The finger tips are able, normally, to distinguish the two pins even though they may be very close together. On the back, however, quite a wide separation is necessary for the two sticks to be perceived as two stimuli. Comparison of one side to the other is important in the use of this test.

6. *Figure writing.* With eyes closed, the patient is asked to identify numerals or letters traced in the palm of her or his hand. This is another parietal lobe test. Both the size of the figure necessary for recognition and comparison of the ability to recognize on each side are required in applying this test. A patient with a left parietal lobe injury or tumor may be totally unable to identify a figure drawn on the right hand though touch and temperature sensation are intact.

7. *Recognition of types of materials.* The patient, again with eyes closed, is asked to tell by touching various objects whether they are rough or smooth, and so forth. Parietal lobe function is evaluated with this test.

Deep Sensation

1. *Joint position sense (kinesthesia).* The patient, with eyes closed, is asked to tell the position of a specific joint as that joint is passively moved. The big toe works well. The patient says the toe is pointing up or down or that it is in between. In diseases of the posterior columns of the spinal cord, the patient will literally have no idea of the position of the toe during the examination. The little finger may be similarly used.

2. *Deep-pressure pain.* The muscles of the forearm, the tendon at the heel, and even the testicles are squeezed to produce pain. This type of pain is very severe when extreme pressures are used. The examiner estimates the amount of pressure that is necessary to produce pain. Is excessive pressure necessary or does the patient seem especially sensitive to the pressure? In tabes dorsalis (syphilis of the spinal cord), this deep pain is commonly absent. In neuritis, hypersensitivity to pain is the rule. Patients in deep coma may only respond to this severe type of pain.

3. *Vibration sensation.* A tuning fork that is vibrating is touched to the prominent bones at the wrist, ankle, and elsewhere on the body. The patient is asked to say when he or she can no longer

feel the vibration. In peripheral neuropathy like that caused by diabetes, vibratory sensation is felt for only a brief period. Diseases of the posterior columns also cause a decreased vibratory sensation because vibration sense travels to the brain by way of the posterior columns.

Combined Sensations

Stereognosis. An object is placed into the hand of the patient, whose eyes are closed. The patient is asked to identify the object or tell the shape. If the patient's primary sensations like touch are intact, the patient's failure at this test indicates disease of the parietal lobe on the opposite side of the body. This failure is called astereognosis.

The Reflexes

A reflex consists of both a sensory and a motor component. The sensory component has a receptor tuned to react to a specific stimulus. In addition there is a sensory nerve that carries information about the stimulation to the brainstem and spinal cord. This information is then evaluated by the cord or brainstem as well as by higher centers of the brain. Appropriate motor neurons are subsequently stimulated and impulses are sent to effector organs like muscles and glands.

Disease or injury to any part of the system described will result in a failure of that system. Therefore a peripheral neuropathy causes absent reflexes because of interruption of either or both motor and sensory transmission. Poliomyelitis attacks the anterior horn cells (motor cells). Therefore the reflex is incomplete because there is no cell to originate the motor impulse. In cases of severe muscle atrophy or disease, the reflex is also incomplete and, therefore, absent, although both the motor and sensory components are functional.

It must be realized that the components of a reflex do not, for the most part, function independently of the rest of the nervous system. Various forces are exerted upon the reflex arc. Some facilitate (tend to increase) the reflex, whereas others act to inhibit it. These forces arise from higher centers like the cerebrum and the cerebellum. They reach the brainstem or spinal cord by way of tracts like the corticospinal tracts. The final effect of these forces is a blend of all forces. It is the character of this resultant force that determines the quantity and quality of the response. To illustrate: A lesion of the corticospinal tract at any point, from its origin in the motor cortex to its termination at the anterior horn cells in the cord, will cause the reflexes to be exaggerated; the functioning corticospinal tract acts to decrease the degree of response. On the other hand, disease of the cerebellum causes a decrease in the reflex; cerebellar function in the normal state tends to increase the response. Other parts of the CNS, like the basal ganglia and vestibular system, also influence the shaping of the resultant force.

The reflexes of the body can be divided into three subdivisions: the deep reflexes, the superficial ones, and the organic ones. The deep reflexes utilize the stretch reflex and are elicited by tapping a tendon or the periosteum (covering of a bone) of one of the bones of the extremities. The common tendon reflexes in this group are those that result when the tendon at the knee, ankle, biceps muscle, and triceps muscle are tapped with a reflex hammer. When the tendon is tapped, there follows a quick jerk of that portion of the extremity. The reflex response is often called a jerk; therefore one may use the terms *knee jerk* or *biceps jerk.* The common periosteal reflex is the radialis periosteal reflex. With a brisk tap on the end of the radius (bone in the forearm), there is a quick flexion at the elbow as the brachioradialis muscle contracts.

The diagnostic value of the deep tendon reflexes is based on the fact that each reflex utilizes a specific nerve root and spinal cord level. The biceps reflex, for example, uses primarily the C_6 (cervical 6) nerve root and spinal cord level for its completion. If the biceps is absent or significantly diminished, the examiner knows the level and location of the disease process. Injury or disease of the corticospinal tract causes the deep tendon reflexes (DTRS) to be hyperactive. Diseases of the cerebellum cause the DTRS to diminish. When the spinal cord is severely injured, causing paralysis, at first the DTRS are totally absent; this is the stage of so-called spinal shock. Later the reflexes return and become very active. In injuries of this type, the reflexes function without the influence of higher centers.

Clonus is a finding seen usually when there has been severe injury (trauma or disease) to the corticospinal tract or to the entire spinal cord. To detect clonus, the examiner grasps the patient's foot and pushes upward under the ball of the foot, maintaining this pressure. If the foot jerks up and down, the patient has clonus. Clonus may last only briefly or it may continue as long as there is pressure upward.

The superficial reflexes are elicited by stroking the skin. The most common reflex in this group is the plantar reflex or, as it is commonly called, the Babinski reflex. This reflex occurs when the sole of the foot is stimulated. An object like a key is used. The examiner starts on the sole of the foot near the heel. The key is then moved along the sole toward the little toe and then across the sole near the base of the big toe. Normally the toes, including the big toe, turn downward. If, however, the Babinski reflex is positive, the big toe extends upward and the other toes flare outward. The positive Babinski or plantar extension response occurs exclusively in disease of the corticospinal tracts.

The abdominal reflexes are another example of superficial reflexes. These reflexes are tested by stroking the skin on one side of the abdomen with a pin while the patient lies on his or her back. The muscles on the same side of the abdomen respond by contracting. The normal abdominal reflex depends on a normal corticospinal tract, so these reflexes are absent in corticospinal tract disease or injury.

There are other superficial reflexes that perform special functions. The corneal reflex is elicited when the cornea is touched by a wisp of cotton. The eye is instantly closed. The gag reflex and the swallowing reflex are other examples of specialized superficial reflexes.

Finally, there is a type of reflex that can be called organic or visceral reflexes. The urinary bladder illustrates the visceral reflex. In the normal state, as the muscular wall of the bladder is stretched, we experience the need to void. We are, however, able to prevent urination (micturition) until an appropriate time. The ability to control urination depends on a normally functioning corticospinal tract. If a disease process injures the corticospinal tract, control is lost. In complete injuries of this tract, the bladder empties automatically as it becomes distended.

The carotid sinus reflex is another example of a visceral reflex. The carotid body is a neural structure found where the common carotid branches into the internal and external carotid arteries. It is very sensitive to pressure. If the blood pressure is excessive or if the carotid body is stimulated by a finger, the heart rate decreases; blood pressure drops and the patient may faint. The carotid sinus reflex is protective but, if overly sensitive, may present problems for the patient and the physician.

Cerebellar Function

The cerebellum functions to coordinate movement and assist in balance. Disease of the cerebellum will result in the following abnormal findings on examination:

1. *Ataxia.* This is clumsy and uncoordinated movements. It can be manifest in several ways:

a. *Adiadochokinesia.* This is an inability to perform rapid, alternating movements. The patients are unable to tap their fingers on a table rapidly.
b. *Dysmetria.* This is an inability to stop a movement at a desired point. When asked to reach for something, patients stop their movement short or overshoot their mark.
c. *Decomposition of movements.* Complex movements lack a normal, smooth-flowing character. They are jerky and seem to be performed in stages.
d. *Disturbances of posture and gait.* Patients walk with a staggering gait. If the lesion is in the vermis or midline of the cerebellum, patients have difficulty sitting upright because the muscles of the trunk are not coordinated. A lesion laterally placed in either cerebellar hemisphere will cause a patient to fall toward that side.
e. *Scanning speech.* Muscles of speech are not coordinated, producing jerky speech with inappropriate pauses and inflection.

2. *Decreased tone.* Normal muscular firmness is absent. Response of tendon reflexes is decreased.
3. *Tremor.* Typically the tremor is one of intention and one that is absent at rest.
4. *Asthenia.* Muscles are weak and move slower than normal.
5. *Nystagmus.* This is a rapid jerking of the eyeball.

The Cranial Nerves

The function of the cranial nerves is complex and includes both motor and sensory components. They should be examined in an orderly fashion because of their complexity. Examination according to their designated number is as good an approach as any:

I. The olfactory nerve provides the sense of smell. Each nostril is tested by alternately closing the other nostril. Familiar odors like peppermint or coffee are tested. Pungent odors like ammonia should not be used. The loss of the sense of smell is called anosmia. Patients with anosmia often complain of a loss of the sense of taste, which illustrates the importance of the sense of smell.

II. The optic nerve is the nerve of sight. Complete evaluation of its function is usually done by the ophthalmologist, but at least gross functional appraisal is possible in the routine neurological examination.

A. Visual acuity is tested by having the patient read test cards. The classic card with letters read from a distance works well.

B. Visual field examination done by asking the patient to cover one eye and look at the examiner's nose with the other. The examiner then brings in various objects from the periphery of the visual field. The patient indicates when she or he sees the object. It is possible to define defects in the visual field if the testing is done carefully. All visual testing must be done with good light.

C. Direct examination of the retina with the ophthalmoscope begins with observation of the color of the retina and any abnormalities such as hemorrhages or infiltrates that are present. Then the optic disc or end of the optic nerve is especially observed. Normally the disc is a pale pink color with numerous arteries and veins coming out of its center and spreading in all directions over the retina. An estimate of the caliber of the arteries and veins is made. Normally the ratio of vein size to artery size is 3:2. In instances of increased intracranial pressure, the veins are engorged and tortuous and the arteries are narrowed. The ratio of vein to artery size may be 3:1 or 4:1. The changes seen in the optic disc with increased intracranial pressure are called papilledema. In addition to the changes in vessel character, the edges of the disc become indistinct and even swollen. When significantly swollen, the disc is elevated compared to the surrounding retina. This requires changing the focus adjustment of the ophthalmoscope a certain degree to see the disc clearly after first looking at the retina. The amount of change needed to get good focus is expressed as a certain number of diopters. This provides a quantitative measure of the degree of swelling; for example, a patient may be said to have two diopters of papilledema. Variable amounts of hemorrhage in and adjacent to the optic disc also occurs with papilledema. If the disc is pale or whitish in color, optic atrophy is present. This occurs following injury or disease of the optic nerve. It is very commonly seen with multiple sclerosis.

III. The oculomotor nerve.

IV. The trochlear nerve.

V. The abducen nerve. These three nerves are examined together because they are all concerned with the eye.

A. Pupil size is closely examined and both pupils are compared for symmetry. The oculomotor nerve carries parasympathetic nerve fibers that go to circular muscle fibers that function to constrict the pupil. The sympathetic fibers that are antagonistic enter the eye by another route and go to muscles that cause the pupil to dilate. Pupillary function is tested by shining a light into one of the patient's eyes. The normal response is for both pupils to constrict. The pathway of this reflex first involves the optic nerve, which carries the impulse that arose from the retina. The impulse is carried to the lateral geniculate body, which lies near the posterior portion of the thalamus. Fibers then go from the lateral geniculate body to the oculomotor nucleus complex. Here parasympathetic fibers arise that run in the third nerve to the circular muscles of the pupil. Therefore if the stimulated optic nerve has been injured, neither pupil will react. If the oculomotor nerve on one or both sides is injured, the pupil(s) will remain widely dilated (owing to the sympathetic effect) and will not react to the light. A judgment is also made about how rapidly each pupil responds to light stimulation. Is the response brisk, sluggish, or is there no response at all? If the pupil of the stimulated eye reacts, that pupil is said to react to direct stimulation. If the opposite pupil is normal, it will also react and is said to react consensually. Therefore the complete and normal pupillary response may be described as equal, briskly active, and reacting to both direct and consensual stimulation. This is why the pupillary function and eye movements are so important when observing a patient following head trauma or after brain surgery. At first there may be just a hint of ptosis and a sluggish pupillary response to light. It is at this point that appropriate measures should be taken to correct the problem. If the neurosurgeon is not notified until a complete third nerve palsy develops, it may be too late to salvage the patient. The phenomenon of accommodation is also tested. The patient is asked to look at a distant object and then to look quickly at an object approximately 20 centimeters away. The normal response is the constriction of the pupil when the patient focuses on the closer object.

B. The upper eyelids are also compared for symmetry. If one seems to droop, it is called ptosis. The oculomotor nerve goes to the levator palpebrae muscle, which is the lifting

Figure 3-2 Third-nerve Compression

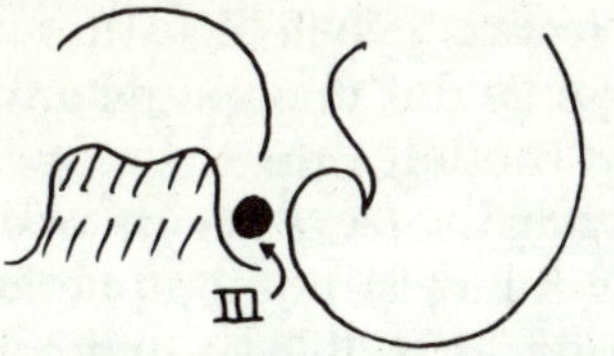

SCHEMATIC DRAWING SHOWING THE NORMAL RELATIONSHIP BETWEEN THE THIRD NERVE AND MEDIAL SIDE OF TEMPORAL LOBE

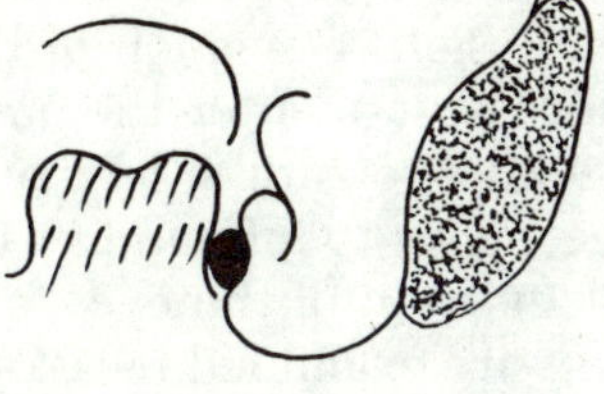

HEMATOMA (STIPPLED) HAS DEVELOPED PUSHING THE TEMPORAL LOBE AGAINST THE THIRD NERVE

muscle in the upper eyelid; so when the third nerve is injured, there is a very definite droop of the upper eyelid on the involved side.

1. Horner's syndrome, a ptosis of mild degree, can be seen with injury to the sympathetic nerves that leave the upper end of the sympathetic chain and go to the head. Injury often occurs with tumors of the chest and neck as well as with trauma. In addition to ptosis, the pupil on the involved side is smaller (miosis) than the opposite pupil, and the eyeball seems somewhat recessed within the orbital cavity. This is called endophthalmous. In addition there is the lack of sweating on the face (anhidrosis) of the involved side.

C. The position of ocular bulbi (eyeballs) is noted. Does the patient seem to look to one side all the time? A patient who has sustained an injury to one of the frontal lobes may very well look constantly toward the side of the injury. On the other hand, a patient having a convulsion will probably have the eyes deviated away from the site of the epileptic focus. The reason for these phenomena is the presence of the frontal eye fields, located in front of the motor strip on each side. For practical purposes the right frontal eye field tries to deviate both eyes to the left, and the left eye field tries to deviate the eyes to the right. Therefore with an injury to the left frontal eye field so that it no longer functions, the right eye field is unopposed and causes the eyes to deviate toward the left side, the side of the injury. On the other hand, when a seizure occurs, one of the eye fields, rather than being injured and nonfunctional, can be considered hyperactive. It is able to overcome the opposite eye field and, therefore, deviates the eyes away from the lesion. Thus it is easily appreciated that the tendency of the eyes to deviate to one side or the other is of help in localizing the site of the lesion. Deviation of the eyes, in most instances, does not last long after the onset of the illness. When occurring with a seizure, it lasts only as long as the seizure. Injury secondary to infarction will on occasion be accompanied by deviation of the eyes for a few days.

D. Ocular movements are examined by asking the patient to follow an object with the eyes. The object is moved throughout the visual field, during which the patient's eye movements are observed. In some instances the inability to move the eyes in a coordinated manner is quite obvious, though often it is rather subtle. These uncoordinated movements cause double vision, which is called diplopia. The patient is asked about the relationship of the two images. Are they side by side? Is one above the other or is one tilted a bit? This information helps to identify the particular muscle and nerve that is not functioning properly. Diplopia can be an annoying problem to the patient because it often causes nausea. It is helpful to patch one eye at a time and then alternate the patch during the day. Figure 3-3 illustrates eye movements. The initials are for the eye muscle and the roman numeral is the cranial nerve that goes to that eye muscle. The arrows indicate the direction the eye will move when a specific muscle contracts. To move the eyes to the left, the patient's left lateral rectus muscle pulls the left eye outward, while the right medial rectus muscle pulls the right eye inward. These muscles are attached to the outside of the eyeball and are, therefore, called extraocular muscles. If one of the muscles fails to function because of direct injury or because of injury to its nerve, the patient has an extraocular palsy. The sixth nerve is the most easily injured of the three nerves. It has the longest intracranial course and it is often injured with increased intracranial pressure. It is common for the pa-

Figure 3-3 Diagram of Extraocular Eye Movements, with Arrows Indicating the Direction a Specific Muscle Will Move the Eye

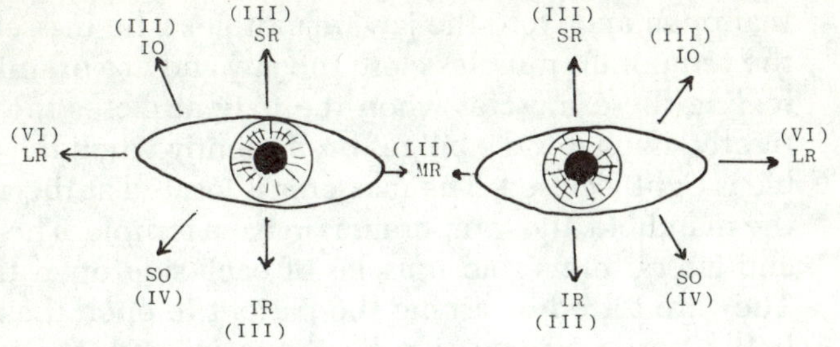

LR- LATERAL RECTUS MUSCLE
MR- MEDIAL RECTUS MUSCLE
SR- SUPERIOR RECTUS MUSCLE
IR- INFERIOR RECTUS MUSCLE
IO- INFERIOR OBLIQUE MUSCLE
SO- SUPERIOR OBLIQUE MUSCLE

tient to experience diplopia because of a lateral rectus palsy. The third nerve is also easily injured, for it is very sensitive to pressure (Figure 3-2). An enlarging or ruptured posterior communicating aneurysm commonly presses on the third nerve. This causes a dilated and unreactive pupil, ptosis of the upper eyelid, and an eye that is constantly looking down and outward. Diabetes mellitus commonly causes a third-nerve palsy, but it is different in one respect. The pupil is not affected. The eyes are also examined for nystagmus, which is a rapid movement of the eyes back and forth. Actually there is a fast movement in one direction and a slower movement back. The nystagmus is characterized by the direction of the fast component. It is further characterized by the plane of movement; horizontal, vertical, or rotary. For example, the patient may have a left horizontal nystagmus, meaning the eye movements are horizontal and the fast component is to the left. Nystagmus has several causes. It is often seen with eye diseases and with cerebellar lesions. It may occur as an inherited characteristic, and it may occur when certain medication is taken in excess. Dilantin intoxication often causes nystagmus and ataxia. Patients who are blind show a certain type of nystagmus.

VI. The trigeminal nerve goes to the face and has both a motor and a sensory component.

A. The motor fibers of the trigeminal nerve go to the muscles that open and close the jaw (mandible). The masseter and the temporalis muscles close the jaw and are examined by feeling these muscles when the patient closes the mouth tightly. Each muscle bulges prominently when the mandible is tightly closed. The masseter is located at the angle of the mandible; the temporalis is in each temple. The medial and lateral pterygoid muscles of each side open the jaw. They are tested by asking the patient to open the mouth. If the nerve on one side has been injured, the jaw will deviate to that side.

B. The sensory nerve fibers give sensation to each side of the face. The nerve divides into three separate nerves before it leaves the intracranial cavity, and each goes to a specific region of the face (Figure 3-4). Their function is tested with a pin sticking each area lightly. The cornea sensation is tested with a wisp of cotton. Many patients find corneal testing difficult. It is reasonably simple if a patient is asked to look to one side and then with the wisp of cotton, approach and touch the cornea from the opposite direction.

VII. The facial nerve, a cranial nerve, has many components with a wide variety of functions. A rather complete discussion is presented in Chapter 1.

Figure 3-4 Divisions of the Trigeminal Nerve

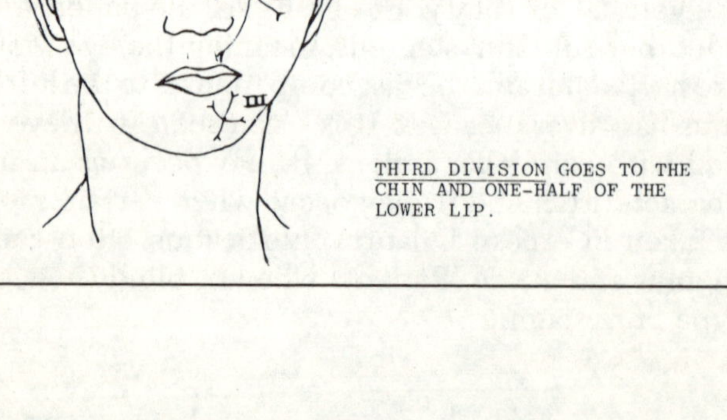

A. This nerve contains motor fibers that go to all the muscles of facial expression. The distinction should be appreciated between the muscles of facial expression and those used in chewing, which are supplied by the trigeminal nerve. The facial nerve is tested by having the patient blow out the cheeks, show the teeth, and whistle or smile. If there is weakness (paresis) or paralysis, the patient cannot show his or her teeth or whistle. The patient will not be able either to close his or her eye on the affected side but will, however, be able to wrinkle the brow if the facial paralysis is central. The distinction between a central facial paralysis and a peripheral facial paralysis was discussed in Chapter 1.

B. The facial nerve also supplies sensory nerves for taste from the anterior two-thirds of the tongue. Taste should be tested when a facial nerve lesion is suspected. The test is performed by placing the test substance on the anterior two-thirds of the tongue. The patient is not to close the mouth, swallow, or in any way manipulate the tongue, because if this is done, the sense of smell comes into play, and the substance dissolves in saliva and may go to taste buds elsewhere. The test substance should be simple—sweet, sour, salt.

C. The facial nerve also sends fibers to some of the salivary glands and to the lacrimal gland (tear gland). To be sure, these functions can be tested, but they are not usually a part of the routine neurological examination. When tearing is affected, the patient may complain of a "scratchy" feeling and the eye is often red.

VIII. The acoustic nerve is divided into the cochlear nerve for hearing and the vestibular nerve for balance.

A. The audiogram is the test used for hearing acuity. It is sophisticated and usually administered by an audiologist. It gives information about the patient's ability to hear the different sound frequencies. A gross indication of hearing is obtained by asking the patient if she or he can hear a watch tick or the snap of a fingernail. The determination of whether there is a difference in hearing ability between the patient's two ears is more important than specific acuity.

1. In the Rinnie test, the base of a vibrating tuning fork is pressed against the mastoid bone, which is located just behind the ear. When the patient can no longer hear it,

the tuning fork is taken off the bone and held close to the ear canal. The patient then listens to the sound and indicates when she or he can no longer hear it. A general impression is gotten about the length of hearing at the two positions. In the first position against the bone, the sound is transmitted by the bone; in the second position the sound is conducted by air. Normally air conduction is better and longer than bone conduction, and this is also true if the disease affecting the hearing involves the receptor organ (cochlea) or the cochlear nerve. However if the hearing loss is due to a canal plugged with wax or from something in the middle ear (interfering with the stapes, incus, and malleus), the bone conduction will be better than air conduction.

2. In the Weber test, the base of a vibrating tuning fork is held against the top of the head in the midline. The patient is asked if he or she hears it better in one ear than the other. Normally the hearing is equal, but if there is middle-ear disease or if the canal is obstructed, the patient will hear the sound better in that ear.

B. The vestibular nerve is closely related to cerebellar function, so the patient may have nystagmus and some of the signs mentioned in the cerebellar examination. A couple of tests should, however, be mentioned.

1. In the Rhomberg test the patient is asked to stand with feet together and eyes closed. It is then noted whether the patient is steady. If not, does he or she tend to lean or fall in a particular direction?

2. In caloric tests, cold or warm water is injected into the patient's auditory canal, which produces nystagmus that varies depending on whether cold or warm water is injected.

IX. The glossopharyngeal nerve has a rather close association with the vagus nerve, but it does have some distinctive function.

A. It provides the sense of taste from the posterior one-third of the tongue. Taste should be tested in the manner described under the facial nerve.

B. It provides sensation to the palate and pharynx. This sensation is best tested by eliciting the gag reflex. The back wall of the pharynx is gently tickled or touched with a dull object, such as a tongue depressor. When the reflex is intact, the patient will retch.

X. The vagus nerve has a very long course. It supplies the muscles of the larynx, pharynx, and palate. It also sends nerve fibers to the heart, lungs, and gastrointestinal tract. From the standpoint of testing, however, swallowing and speech are the most important.
   A. When the vagus nerve itself or its recurrent laryngeal branch is injured, the patient has hoarseness. This occurs because of paralysis of the vocal cord on the affected side. When the patient is hoarse the vocal cords should be examined. Paralysis is readily apparent when the patient attempts to speak.
   B. The patient will have difficulty swallowing because of weakness of muscles of the palate and the pharynx. When attempting to swallow, the patient may regurgitate through the nose.
      1. The patient is asked to open the mouth and say "ah." If one side of the palate is weak or paralyzed, the functioning side will pull the uvula toward it.

XI. The spinal accessory nerve goes to the sternocleidomastoid and trapezius muscles.
   A. The sternocleidomastoid muscle is the large muscle in the neck that runs from the mastoid bone to the medial end of the clavicle. It is tested by putting the examiner's hand against one side of the patient's chin. The patient is asked to push against the hand. The muscle on the side opposite the examiner's hand will become firm and prominent. Both sides are tested and compared.
   B. The trapezius muscle is the large muscle that forms the ridge from the base of the neck to the shoulder on each side. Each muscle is tested by having the patient shrug the shoulder as the examiner's hand presses down on it. The size, tone, and strength of each muscle is appraised and compared with the opposite side.

XII. The hypoglossal nerve is the nerve that goes exclusively to the tongue.
   A. It is tested by having the patient stick out the tongue. If the nerve is injured on one side, the tongue will deviate toward that side. This nerve is like the facial nerve, having a central and peripheral category. When the injury is to the nerve itself, the nerve will atrophy and have visible fasciculations on the involved side. If it is a central lesion, the same deviation may be seen but no atrophy occurs.

CHAPTER 4

Diagnostic Tests

Laboratory tests should never be used in the place of a carefully obtained history and a detailed physical examination. Again, the physician who is willing to listen to the patient is often "told" the correct diagnosis. A few specific tests are then indicated for the sake of confirming the physician's impression. The wholesale use of all the tests in the book is to be condemned, for it results in added expense to the patient and often in needless risk.

Do not forget that an operative permit should always be obtained if a procedure is invasive, that is, if the body is entered by the use of a needle and foreign substances are injected. The patient should be told of the nature of the procedure to be done. A step-by-step description of how the procedure will be performed is often helpful. The patient should also be told why a particular study is needed. Finally, any side effect or complication that might reasonably occur should be discussed with the patient. This is not done to scare the patient but to provide information needed to make an intelligent, informed decision.

Routine Laboratory Studies

Most hospitals require that certain laboratory tests be performed on all patients who are admitted: the complete blood count (CBC), the urinalysis, a serology for syphilis, and a chest X ray. In addition, arterial blood gas determinations are useful for neurological patients.

Complete Blood Count

The CBC includes several determinations performed on the various elements of the blood. A count is made of the number of white cells present. The norm is 5,000–10,000 per cubic millimeter. If the patient has an infection such as a bacterial pneumonia, the white cell count will probably be significantly higher than 10,000 cubic millimeters. Several different cell types are included in the white cell count. The percentage of each type is determined and reported as the differential. The following illustrates the relative occurrence of each type of white blood cells:

Neutrophils (polys)	50–65%
Lymphocytes (lymphs)	25–35%
Monocytes	4–10%
Eosinophils	.5–4%
Basophils	0–2%

The differential count on a patient with a bacterial infection is likely to show a relative increase in the number of polys. If the infection is due to a virus, the lymphocyte count would be increased. A patient with an allergic disease or a disease caused by parasites would have an increase in the eosinophil count.

The CBC includes a determination of the oxygen-carrying capacity of the blood. Oxygen is transported from the lungs to all the body's tissues by hemoglobin, protein in the red blood cell that has a special property that enables it to combine in a reversible manner with molecules of oxygen (0_2). The amount of hemoglobin present in a healthy person ranges from 12 to 16 grams per 100 cubic millimeters. A patient is anemic when the amount of hemoglobin is less than normal. Anemia may occur when malnutrition prevents hemoglobin formation by the body. It may also occur if there is excessive bleeding so that hemoglobin is lost faster than the body can replace it. Another form of anemia occurs when an abnormal hemoglobin molecule is produced by the body, as in sickle cell anemia. Red blood cells with this hemoglobin have a short life-span. Regardless of the cause of anemia, patients with a hemoglobin deficiency are poor risks for general anesthetics and frequently have retarded wound healing.

The CBC also includes the hematocrit, which is the ratio of the total red cell volume to the total blood volume expressed as a percentage with the normal hematocrit being 35–50 percent. The determination of the hematocrit at intervals (every 6 to 8 hours) provides a good index for monitoring internal bleeding that may or may not be occurring. For example, a patient with a ruptured spleen continues to bleed into the abdominal cavity. The initial hematocrit would be normal, but over the next 6 to 8 hours if bleeding continued, the hematocrit would drop. In order to avoid shock (decreasing blood pressure) in this situation, the body must maintain a fairly constant volume of blood. In the short span of several hours, the body can only maintain volume by adding fluid, because red blood cells cannot be produced in sufficient numbers. Thus subsequent hematocrits will indicate a steadily decreasing red blood cell volume if active bleeding continues.

The CBC also includes a platelet count. Platelets are small particles that have an important role in the clotting process. When their number (normal is 200,000–500,000 per cubic millimeter) is diminished, there is an added risk of bleeding with surgery or trauma.

Urinalysis

The urinalysis is a urine analysis with several determinations being made on each specimen. The specimen is collected by having the patient void into a clean container. If an infection is suspected, a sterile container must be used. A portion of the urine is taken for microscopic examination. The technician searches for blood cells, bacteria, and other particles. If several leukocytes (polys) are seen, an infection is probably present even though bacteria are not seen. Red blood cells may be in the urine with infection, but they also occur following trauma or when neoplasms occur in the kidney or the bladder. If the microscopic examination of the urine suggests that an infection is present, some of the urine is cultured in an effort to grow the bacteria and to determine its sensitivity to antibiotics. The routine urinalysis also includes testing the urine for the presence of sugar and protein. The diabetic patient will lose sugar in the urine because of a lack of insulin, which the body needs to metabolize sugar. The loss of protein may occur in patients who have kidney diseases like nephritis.

Serology

The serology, required by most hospitals, is a test to determine whether the patient has syphilis. The routine test has some inherent problems because it may remain positive even though the patient has been properly treated and has no active disease. In most instances when the serology is positive, additional and more specific tests are used to identify those individuals with active syphilis.

Today's technology offers many other tests that in specific diagnostic situations are of great benefit. With a single specimen of blood, several different determinations can be made, and as a result, the cost is quite low. These tests may be used as screening tests to evaluate patients scheduled for surgery, thereby avoiding postsurgical problems caused by previously unsuspected medical illnesses.

Chest X Ray

For admission of a patient to most hospitals, the chest X ray is required for identification of diseases of an infectious nature. It is not uncommon for a routine, admission chest X ray to reveal lung disease in a totally asymptomatic patient. The chest X ray can give other important information. For example, the heart size and its contour may be visualized. An enlarged left ventricle may mean long-standing high blood pressure or it may mean stenosis of the aortic valve resulting from rheumatic heart disease. An enlarged heart with congestion of the lungs may indicate congestive heart failure. An enlarged aortic arch may be consistent with an aortic aneurysm. The chest X ray of a patient who has received trauma may reveal rib fractures, collapsed lungs (pneumothorax), or ruptured diaphragm.

Arterial Blood Gases

The availability of arterial blood gas determinations (CO_2 and O_2 are the gases) has greatly assisted in the care of neurological patients and especially those with increased intracranial pressure. It is known that an increase in the carbon dioxide (CO_2) concentration in the blood causes the blood vessels in the brain to dilate (vasodilation). Because of the great numbers of blood vessels in the brain, significant vasodilation will cause the brain to expand in volume, causing intracranial pressure to increase. If we know the CO_2 concentration, we can make the adjustments necessary to lessen the CO_2 levels and hence the intracranial pressure. Likewise if we know the oxygen concentration in the arterial blood, we can assure that the brain is adequately supplied.

In performing the test, an arterial blood gas sample is drawn with a heparinized syringe (to prevent clotting) from either the radial, brachial, or femoral arteries. The syringe is immediately refrigerated, care being taken that no air bubbles enter. Next the blood specimen is run through a special machine that computes the amounts of carbon dioxide (CO_2), oxygen (O_2), and hydrogen (H^-) contained in it.

Laboratory Studies for Neurological Disease

Skull Series

If the disease process involves the head, a skull series is taken. This X-ray examination includes X rays taken from the side (lateral), the front, and the back of the head. The general contour and shape of the skull is noted. The sinuses are viewed; they may be hazy or opacified by abscess formation, or they may be filled with blood by trauma. In trauma cases the X ray of the bony skull (calvarium) is examined for fractures. Fractures may appear as barely detectable lines or as obvious cracks radiating in every direction. If a fracture is present it is determined if fragments of bone are pressed into the brain. If this has occurred surgery is necessary to remove or elevate these fragments. The direction taken by a fracture is important to note because fractures running in the temple region of the skull may be associated with lacerated dural blood vessels, which would indicate serious trouble: An epidural hematoma is very likely to develop.

In studying the skull series of a patient, certain normally present structures are noted. In many adult patients, the pineal gland contains calcium (it is said to be calcified) and, therefore, it shows up nicely on X ray. The normal position of this gland when viewed from the front is in the midline of the skull. If there is a mass such as a tumor on one side of the brain, the pineal calcification will be pushed toward the opposite side. The thickness of the skull as seen on the X ray is noted. With increased pressure, the skull adjacent to the source of the pressure will be thinner than normal; on the other hand, the tumor called a meningioma may cause the adjacent overlying skull to become thicker than normal. The grooves along the inside of the skull that are formed by the vessels in the dura are examined. They may be more prominent than usual, indicating the presence of an arteriovenous malformation or a meningioma. In patients with prolonged increased intracranial pressure, the bone in the region of the sella turcica (the saddle-shaped structure that contains the pituitary gland) becomes very thin and may appear only as a shadow on an X ray.

The routine skull series may show abnormal calcification within the brain itself. Depending on the density, configuration, and location of the calcification, fairly accurate diagnosis can be made as to the type of calcification seen. Tumors, including the meningioma, the oligodendroglia, and the craniopharyngioma are often calcified. Certain vascular abnormalities like the cerebral aneurysm and arteriovenous malformations are occasionally partially calcified. Infectious processes including cysticercosis and toxoplasmosis may be identified by characteristic calcifications within the brain.

Spine X Rays

X rays of the spine are indicated when the suspected disease process involves the spinal cord, cauda equina, or nerve roots. If trauma is involved one looks for fractures. The fracture may be minor or it may be one of major proportions involving extensive fracture and dislocation of one of the vertebrae. Metastatic carcinoma often spreads to the vertebrae. Where the tumor is growing, the X ray shows areas of decreased density because of demineralization and destruction of bone. In patients with neck or low back pain of no obvious cause, one looks for evidence of arthritis or a ruptured disc.

Lumbar Puncture

The spinal tap is a special procedure performed by the physician when infection or subarachnoid hemorrhage is suspected. This procedure must be done with sterile technique. Patients usually lie on their sides with backs arched outward. The skin is prepared with an antiseptic solution. The physician then anesthetizes the skin with local anesthetic and inserts a spinal needle in the middle line and between the spines of two adjacent vertebrae. The needle is advanced slowly, and the stylet is removed frequently to see if spinal fluid drips out. When the fluid does drip, the point of the needle is in the subarachnoid space, which is the desired location. If the tap is carefully done, clear, free-flowing fluid is usually obtained. In some cases, however, blood will be obtained, which means an epidural vein has been punctured. Occasionally if the blood is allowed to drip, the fluid clears so that grossly normal CSF is obtained. Even then, though, the cell count of the CSF is very likely to reveal numerous RBCs. The physician faces the dilemma of whether to try another tap at another level or wait a few days and try again.

If a satisfactory tap is obtained, the first thing that is done is to record the pressure (normal pressure is 100–150 millimeters of water). This is done with a manometer, which is inserted into the hub of the spinal needle after the stylet is removed. The CSF slowly rises in the manometer, eventually stopping at a certain level, which is the opening pressure (OP) and is recorded as "so many millimeters of water." For an accurate pressure reading to be obtained, a patient must be relaxed; efforts should be made to allay fears of unexpected pain. It is often helpful to have patients stretch out their legs and relax. Straining or pressure on the abdomen will result in an elevated pressure recording.

Most hospitals have disposable lumbar puncture trays that contain the spinal needle, specimen tubes, and syringes as well as sponges and drapes. When the OP is determined, specimens are collected. It is best if three specimen tubes are used, each filled with 3–4 cubic centimeters of CSF. The specimens collected should be taken immediately to the lab and given to the laboratory technician for analysis.

In the laboratory the CSF appearance is noted and recorded. Normal CSF is crystal clear. If hemorrhage has occurred a few days before, the CSF looks yellow-orange, which is termed *xanthochromic.* The color comes from the breakdown products of the red blood cells. If the CSF is cloudy, appearing like ground glass, this is most likely due to the presence of many white blood cells. The patient with meningitis will have CSF of this color.

The spinal fluid specimen is viewed under a microscope by a trained technician. The cells seen, if present, may be polys, lymphocytes, or red blood cells. Each is counted and recorded as a certain number of cells per cubic millimeter. A differential count of the white cells is made, with each cell type recorded as a certain percentage of the total cell population. In bacterial meningitis the predominant cell is the poly (polymorphonuclear leukocyte), whereas the lymphocyte is the dominant cell in cases of aseptic meningitis. If a subarachnoid hemorrhage has occurred, as would happen with a ruptured cerebral aneurysm, the spinal fluid has the appearance of tomato juice. The predominant cell is the RBC, but white cells will be present in the same proportion as in the peripheral blood.

A part of the CSF sent to the laboratory is stained with gram stain (special dye) and viewed under the microscope. Bacteria like the *Staphylococcus* stain purple and are called gram-positive organisms. Other bacteria like the *Pseudomonas* stain pink with gram stain and are called gram-negative organisms. If a fungal infection is suspected, the india ink preparation is made of the microscope slide. This will identify the *Cryptococcus* organism if present. When tuberculous meningitis is considered, the acid-fast stain is used.

Some of the CSF specimen sent to the laboratory is cultured on various media in an attempt to grow the infective organism. When the infective organism is a bacteria, its sensitivity to antibiotics is determined in the following manner: The infected CSF is spread over the surface of a nutritive material on which the bacteria can grow. Blood-agar is the material commonly used for bacterial culture. It is placed in a round, flat dish called a petri dish. Next a paper disc that looks somewhat like a wheel with the spokes gone from the hub is placed over the blood-agar. Around the circumference of the disc, most of the antibiotics available have been impregnated into the paper. Now the dish is covered and placed in an incubator. In several hours bacterial growth can be seen over the blood-agar surface. If one looks along the inner border of the antibiotic dish, there will be areas opposite certain impregnated antibiotics where no bacterial grows, indicating which specific antibiotics have prevented bacterial growth. It may be reasonable therefore to use these antibiotics in treating the patient.

Some of the CSF is analyzed for its sugar and protein content. The sugar value is particularly important if an infection is suspected. In the presence of a bacterial infection, the sugar content will be quite low because the bacteria have metabolized much of it. On the other hand the sugar content will be normal if the infectious agent is a virus. The normal CSF sugar is about half that of the peripheral blood, that is, 45–65 mg%. Normal protein content is 15–45 mg%. The protein concentration will increase in most inflammatory conditions. The concentration of the CSF protein also increases when a block in the subarachnoid space prevents "normal" CSF flow. CSF protein is made up of several different types of protein. In some diseases it is of value to determine the amount of each component, which is done by protein electrophoresis. In multiple sclerosis the amount of gamma globulin is often increased in the spinal fluid.

Multiple lumbar punctures may be done by the physician to evaluate the effectiveness of treatment of certain diseases. For example, successive examination of serial CSF specimens from a patient being adequately treated for bacterial meningitis will reveal decreasing numbers of polys and a return of the sugar content to normal.

Pneumoencephalogram

The pneumoencephalogram (PEG) is a specialized, X-ray examination that is performed by injecting air into the spinal fluid via a lumbar puncture. The air fills the ventricles of the brain and is visible on X ray. The PEG may be done with either general or local anesthetic. In most instances, if the details of the procedure are fully explained to the patient and if an adequate preoperative medication is given, a local anesthetic is well tolerated.

Most hospitals have a special-procedures room adjacent to the operating suite or use the X-ray department for this type of examination. Mechanical chairs designed for the pneumoencephalogram are available. The patient is strapped tightly into the chair to permit rotation in various directions; a somersault may even be done. The back of the chair is open so that a lumbar puncture can be done as previously described. The tap is done with the patient seated upright. Following preparation of the skin by applying an antiseptic solution and after injection of a local anesthetic, a small-gauge spinal needle is inserted into the subarachnoid space. When CSF drips freely from the needle, a few cubic centimeters are collected for laboratory examination. Next a sterile syringe containing filtered air or other gas (such as nitrous oxide) is placed into the hub of the needle. A volume of about 5 cubic centimeters is slowly injected; then 5 cubic centimeters of CSF are permitted to flow back into the syringe. A total of 25–40 cubic centimeters of gas is injected by alternately instilling and removing CSF in 5 cubic centimeter amounts.

It is critical that the head be in proper position during injection of the gas. The chin must be tucked against the front of the neck. In this position, as the air is injected, it rises in the subarachnoid space along the length of the spinal cord. It then collects in the large space called the cisterna magnum, which lies behind the medulla oblongata and just beneath the cerebellum. The gas then enters the fourth ventricle through the foramen of Magendie. It then goes through the aqueduct of Sylvius to the third ventricle and then on to the two lateral ventricles. The gas that is in the ventricles is easily seen on the X ray. Gas, being less dense than either the brain or CSF, appears as a dark shadow whereas the denser substances appear much lighter on the X-ray film. If care is taken in turning or rotating the patient, almost any area of the ventricular system can be outlined by gas.

Sometimes it is helpful to direct the air into the spaces along the brainstem and into the region of the optic nerves and pituitary gland. The presence of air in the subarachnoid space over the surface of the cerebral hemispheres is of value when evaluating cerebral atrophy. When air enters the subarachnoid spaces of the cerebral hemispheres, the patient may experience a rather sudden and a moderately severe headache. If, however, the patient has been told of this eventuality and if adequate premedication has been provided, the patient can tolerate this phase of the study with relative ease.

The indications for use of the pneumoencephalogram are several. First, by placing air in the ventricles, their size and contour is demonstrated. Thus the various forms of hydrocephalus can be evaluated. If a tumor is present in the cerebral hemisphere, it will distort and displace the adjacent ventricular wall. Gas directed to this region of the ventricular system will nicely outline these effects. If a tumor lies in the region of the optic chiasm, gas injected into the basal cisterns can be directed to this area and can outline the actual tumor mass. The size of the tumor can be determined, and some idea of its origin may be provided.

There is one instance when the use of both the pneumoencephalogram and routine lumbar puncture should be avoided or at least done with great care. This is when the patient shows evidence of markedly increased intracranial pressure. The pressence of papilledema (swelling of the end of the optic nerve that can be seen with the ophthalmoscope) should alert one to the possibility of potential trouble. The problem results because of the sudden changes in CSF pressure that might occur with a spinal puncture. When the stylet is removed from the spinal needle in the lumbar subarachnoid space and CSF starts to drip, the immediate effect is the establishment of a relative negative pressure at the tip of the needle. Because the pressure in the head is still high, there is the tendency for the brain to be forced downward through the foramen magnum. If this happens, the medulla oblongata and the cerebellum are forced into the foramen. The effect is like pushing the cerebellum and the medulla through a small napkin ring, and it is ill tolerated. The patient may suddenly die because of failure of many of the vital centers in the medulla.

Another headache, called the spinal headache, is common following a spinal tap. Pressure changes are responsible for this type of headache. When the needle for the lumbar puncture is inserted, first the dura and then the arachnoid are penetrated. When the needle is removed, small holes remain in each membrane through which CSF may continue to leak. Typical of this headache is that the pain is present when the patient is upright and goes away when the patient is flat. When the patient is upright the CSF escapes through the holes to the space outside of the dura. Pressure differences are created, which produce traction on pain-sensitive structures in the head, such as the dura and the major cerebral arteries. When the patient lies flat the pressure in the lumbar region and in the head are equal and the pain goes away. Headaches of this type last from a few hours to several days, until the leakage of the CSF ceases.

Ventriculogram

If the evaluation of a patient requires the instillation of gas into the ventricle and if a pneumoencephalogram is too hazardous, the ventriculogram is used. The classic ventriculogram (ventric) is performed with the patient in the seated position. Like the pneumoencephalogram, the ventriculogram may be done under either a general or a local anesthetic. The procedure should be done in the operating room and with sterile technique. With the patient in the seated position and the head held securely in a mechanical holder, the back of the head is closely shaved and the skin is prepared with an antiseptic solution. A formal draping is performed, after which an incision is made 3–4 centimeters to the right of the midline in the occipital region. In most instances the right side of the brain is used when tapping of the brain ventricles is required. This is because most patients are right-handed and, therefore, the left cerebral hemisphere is dominant. It is advisable to minimize any trauma to the dominant side, even though the trauma is no more than the passage of a brain cannula. When the incision is made in the scalp, a retractor is used to spread the skin edges. A hole is drilled through the skull to expose the dura. A small incision is made in the dura as well as in the pia mater of the brain. A blunt needle of fairly large gauge, called the brain cannula, is then inserted through the brain into the posterior wall (occipital horn) of the right lateral ventricle. When the stylet in the needle is withdrawn, CSF drips freely and a specimen may be collected if needed. A gas (usually filtered air) is then injected to fill the ventricle and displace the CSF. If a more permanent ventricular tap is required, a rubber or polyethylene tube can be placed in the ventricle. In this fashion the skin can be sutured and the flexible tube tied to the skin and incorporated into the bandage. The patient is taken to X ray following the instillation of air and after the application of a sterile bandage. X rays similar to those taken for a pneumoencephalogram are made. The patient may be placed in the pneumoencephalogram chair to facilitate positioning to direct the flow of air to the desired region of the ventricular system.

Variations of the procedure just described may be used. The incision and hole through the skull may be placed to the right of the midline at approximately the coronal suture line, so that the right frontal horn of the lateral ventricle is accessible to the brain cannula or the more permanent flexible tubing. Sometimes a positive-contrast ventriculogram is done. This involves the injection into the ventricle of pantopaque or a similar compound instead of air. Pantopaque is very dense so it shows up clearly on the X-ray film. Because it is a liquid that is heavier than spinal fluid and not water soluble, the two do not mix. It is possible by manipulation of the head to direct the flow of pantopaque to the desired location in the ventricular system.

On some occasions when a pneumoencephalogram alone is not advisable, as with high intracranial pressure, the ventriculogram and the pneumoencephalogram are combined. First the ventricular tap is done, diminishing the elevated intracranial pressure. Then the routine pneumoencephalogram may be done with less worry.

Cerebral Arteriogram

The cerebral arteriogram is one of the most useful diagnostic studies available to the neurosurgeon and neurologist. The basic procedure consists of the injection of a contrast material (liquid that shows up on X rays) into the arteries that go to the brain. The injection is made directly into the blood, and the material circulates with the blood through the brain. During its circulation, X rays are made in very rapid sequence from the front view and the side view of the head. First the large cerebral arteries are visualized; next the smaller ones are seen, followed by the phase when the capillaries are filled. The cerebral veins are seen last, then the contrast material finally fills the large dural sinuses. The contrast material drains from the head via the internal jugular veins, then goes to the kidneys and is rapidly excreted in the urine.

The arteriogram may be done with either a general or a local anesthetic. Pain is experienced both when the needle is inserted into the artery and when the contrast material is circulating through the brain, the latter pain being a hot, burning sensation. In most cases local anesthesia is entirely adequate. Preoperative medication is given but it should not be so great that it depresses respiration. Several cubic centimeters of local anesthetic are injected around the artery before the needle is inserted. A patient who is told of the hot sensation will be able to tolerate it satisfactorily.

Several different arteries may be used for injection of the contrast medium. A direct puncture of the common carotid artery on either or both sides is easily done. Injection of 10–15 cubic centimeters of contrast medium results in swift flow of the material into the internal carotid artery and subsequently into the cerebral arteries. If the cerebral circulation that arises from the vertebral and basilar arteries needs to be visualized, direct cannulation of the vertebral artery is difficult. Even if a satisfactory vertebral artery puncture is made, the dye frequently leaks into the tissue around the artery when the injection is made. Probably the most satisfactory technique for visualization of the vertebrobasilar system is the retrograde femoral technique. The femoral artery in the groin is punctured with a special needle, and the catheter with variable shapes at the tip is inserted through the needle. The catheter is threaded up the aorta to the aortic arch, from which the arteries going to the brain originate. The catheter can be visualized on X ray, making it possible to manipulate its tip so it will enter the artery to be examined. When the catheter tip is in the desired artery, the contrast medium is injected and the sequence of X rays are taken. A similar technique can be used by puncturing the brachial artery in the arm followed by retrograde threading of the catheter. The brachial artery is, however, smaller than the femoral artery, which makes the procedure more difficult.

The cerebral arteriogram can provide a great deal of information to those who have acquired an intimate knowledge of the normal cerebral blood vessel anatomy. If a blood vessel is absent because of occlusion, this will be conspicuous. If the blood vessels are not in their usual position, this will be readily noted. For example, a subdural hematoma forms on the surface of the brain. In doing so it pushes the brain away from the inside of the skull. The X ray will show that the vessels on the brain's surface do not come close to the skull but are separated from it by a void, which is the blood clot. If the patient has a brain tumor or intracerebral hematoma, the normal blood vessels will be pushed out of their usual position. Vessels like the internal cerebral vein, which normally lies in the midline, will be pushed by the mass to the opposite side. Other vessels may be pushed up or down by the pressure effects of the mass. The arteriogram may also reveal blood vessels that are not normally present. The tangle of vessels typical of an arteriovenous malformation is often visualized. Aneurysms and the subsequent arterial spasms that often occur with ruptured aneurysms are seen only with arteriograms. The new vessel growth that occurs in many tumors may be very prominent in the arteriogram. The dye in these vessels frequently produces a very definite, circumscribed glow, which is called a tumor stain.

Serious complications during or following arteriograms are not common but they do occur. The patient should be asked about allergies to local anesthetics and to iodine, which is contained in the contrast material. Sterile technique should be strictly observed with an adequate skin prep, draping, and so forth. Great care must be taken to avoid the injection of air bubbles into the cerebral blood stream. A bubble will act like any foreign body, lodge in a vessel and compromise the circulation beyond that point. Finally, pressure must be maintained at the site of arterial puncture for several minutes after the removal of the needle. Bleeding from the puncture site may be fatal because the accumulating hematoma may compress important, adjacent structures. This is especially true in the neck, where bleeding from the puncture wound in the common carotid may lead to obstruction of the trachea.

Brain Scan

The availability of radioactive isotopes supplies the physician with several valuable diagnostic and therapeutic tools. The brain scan is one such tool, an attractive one because it is easily done, has a wide margin of safety, and affords a high degree of accuracy.

A radioactive isotope is an unstable form of a particular element. Because it is not stable it undergoes decay and changes to another form of the same element. In the process of decay, various atomic particles are emitted: alpha particles, beta particles, or gamma rays. The isotopes used in brain scanning all emit gamma rays. The energy of the gamma rays permits them to pass out of the body, where they can be counted by detection instruments. Several isotopes have been used in brain scanning: iodine^{131}, mercury^{203}, and technetium^{99} (which is most successful). When the isotope is injected into a vein, it has a tendency to concentrate in an area of pathology. There are several reasons for this concentration:

1. Brain tumors usually have more blood vessels than normal brain tissue.
2. The lining of the blood vessels may permit passage of the isotope through its wall, whereas normal vessels would not.
3. The space between cells is probably greater in some pathological states, and so there is more room for the isotope than in normal tissue.
4. The edema that often occurs in the brain adjacent to a diseased area seems to encourage concentration of the isotope.
5. Metabolic factors in tumor cells facilitate entrance of the isotope into the cell itself.

There are two basic detection instruments that intercept the gamma rays and that produce the brain scan: the rectilinear scanner and the gamma camera. The rectilinear scanner requires that the patient be fully cooperative because the scanner passes back and forth over the head, intercepting the gamma rays. Anterior, posterior, and both lateral views of the head are routinely scanned. It takes several minutes to scan one view. The scanner's recorder produces a picture with the head outlined; if a tumor or other lesion is present, it will be conspicuous within the outline.

The second type of detection instrument is the gamma camera or scintillation camera. It is in fact like an ordinary camera, so it is easily used on children and on uncooperative patients. The camera's film is the record. An outline of the head is seen; if disease is present, it is represented as a discrete spot within the head's contour.

The brain scan can be used to diagnose many types of disease. Certain tumors like the meningioma will produce a very positive scan; other types may be less prominent. Brain abscesses are easily demonstrated on scans, but diffuse infections like meningitis are likely to produce a negative brain scan. The brain scan may be of help in evaluating patients who have had head trauma. Subdural hematomas produce a positive scan, but unfortunately, a bruise of the scalp will produce a similarly positive scan. On occasion it is difficult to differentiate between the two, so a cerebral arteriogram is often required. Cerebral infarction will produce a positive brain scan but not for the first week. Thereafter the scan becomes progressively more positive over the next 2 to 4 weeks. The scan thereafter reverts to normal. The changing scan seen with cerebral infarction makes it possible to differentiate between a cerebral infarction and a brain tumor.

On occasion, it is of value to inject a radioisotope into the cerebrospinal fluid. This can be done by a lumbar puncture or by a direct ventricular tap using the technique of a ventriculogram. Iodine^{131} or technetium^{99} are the isotopes commonly used; they must be bound chemically to a large molecule such as a protein. Using a special, commercial, chemical process, human serum albumin is used to bind the isotope and is used for direct CSF instillation.

The CSF circulation may be monitored with this technique by using brain scan every few hours after injection to follow the circulation of the isotope. In communicating hydrocephalus, one sees the isotope moving from the ventricles to the subarachnoid spaces at the base of the brain and then over the surfaces of the cerebral hemispheres. Finally the circulation ceases because the isotope is not absorbed into the cerebrovenous system as it would be in the normal situation.

Injection of protein-bound iodine into the CSF is valuable also in determining the site of leakage in CSF otorrhea or rhinorrhea. CSF otorrhea is the leakage of CSF from the ear because of a skull fracture and a tear in the adjacent dura. CSF rhinorrhea is leakage of CSF through the nose and is also caused by skull fracture and dural tear. If the leakage of CSF continues with no sign of stopping, it is necessary to perform surgery and suture the torn dura. It is, however, often extremely difficult to determine accurately the location of the dural tear. The use of the scanning technique assists in localization by detecting the isotope as it leaks through the torn dura.

Electroencephalogram

The electroencephalogram is one of the oldest but still one of the more valuable tests available to the physician. The EEG is performed by recording very small, rhythmic, electrical potentials produced by the brain. Small electrodes are placed on the clean, dry scalp in a conventional pattern. They are held in position by various glues or pastes. The electrodes are hooked by wires to the electroencephalogram machine, which receives the electrical potentials and greatly amplifies them. Then, by using an ink-writing recorder, it produces a permanent record on paper. Interpretation of an EEG requires very specialized training and is usually done by an electroencephalographer or a neurologist with specialized training.

The normal EEG consists of a number of different waves. By convention, the number of waves per second (frequency) is more important than their height or amplitude. Alpha waves (8–12 per second) are predominate waves in normal adults. Beta waves have a high frequency of 14–60 per second and are intermixed or superimposed on slower waves. Delta waves are slower than 8 per second.

Several factors affect the EEG; some are normal variations; others indicate pathology. Waves in the occipital regions of the brain are slower than those in the frontal and parietal regions. The EEG of an infant has very slow waves of .5–2 per second and fast waves of 20–50 per second. The adult EEG is not seen until an individual reaches 14 to 20 years of age. In sleep or with depressant drugs, the EEG shows a slowing in frequency to 3 waves per second or less. The EEG is distinctive in convulsive disorders. In grand mal epilepsy there is fast activity in the tonic phase and spike-slow wave complexes in the clonic phase. In petit mal epilepsy there is a spike-dome wave of 3 per second. Psychomotor or temporal lobe epilepsy reveals an epileptic focus that originates in the temporal lobe. Focal injury to the cortex that may occur with a brain tumor or trauma produces an EEG that shows a localized, irregular focus of slow waves in the vicinity of the lesion.

Computerized Axial Tomography

Computerized axial tomography or the CAT scan is one of the new diagnostic tools available to the neurological surgeon. It consists of an X-ray tube, detectors, a computer, and data-recording components. With this technique the brain can be studied in layers or tomographic planes. The CAT scan makes detailed pictures of a cross-section of the brain and records them on polaroid film, thus producing a permanent record for detailed study and for future comparison if necessary.

Figure 4-1 illustrates how the CAT scan is performed. The X-ray tube and detector rotate from station to station around the patient's head. In this manner, X rays pass through the head from several angles. In addition, at each station there is linear movement so the X ray passes through the head from one side to the other. As the X-ray beam passes through the various tissues in the head, it is altered. For example, less X ray is able to pass through bone than it

Figure 4-1 How the CAT Scan Works

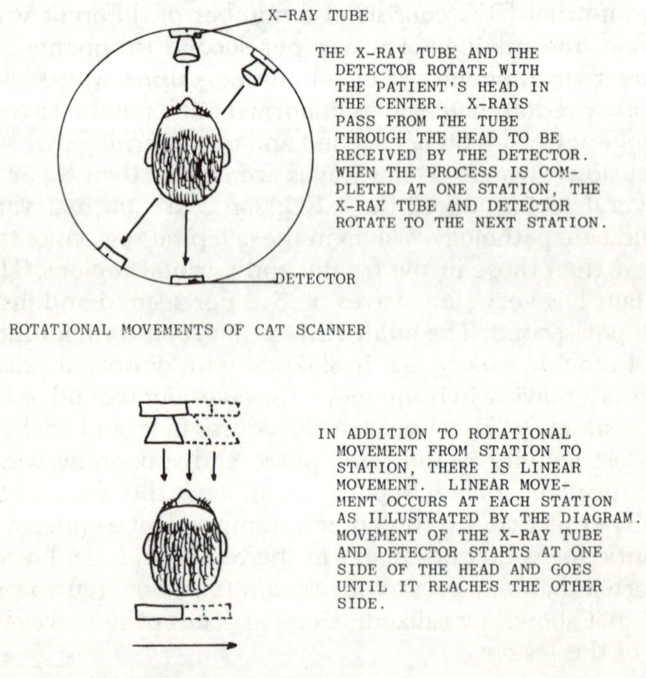

Figure 4-2 Illustration of a CAT Scan Picture with Detail Similar to an Actual CAT Scan

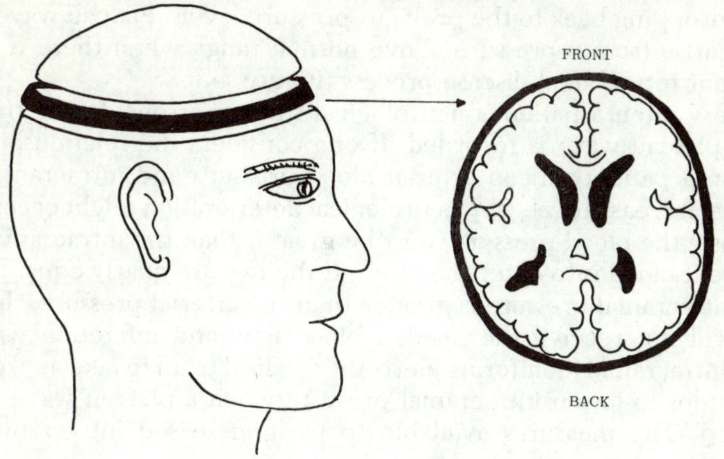

is through brain. This alteration of the X-ray beam is called attenuation. The detectors record the attenuation of the X-ray beam and send this information to the computer. The scanner is calibrated so that, if the degree of attenuation is a certain value, then it is known that the beam passed through a known type of tissue. Thus a brain tumor will attenuate an X-ray beam to a lesser or greater degree than a hematoma. In this manner the CAT scan provides information not only about the size and location but about the nature of the lesion.

The value of the CAT scan is manifold, and it is rapidly becoming the most important neurodiagnostic tool. Newer models accomplish the study quickly so that they can be used on uncooperative and confused patients as well as infants. It is a nonivasive study so that complications do not pose any problem, except for the possibility of allergic reactions to the dye when a contrast medium is injected intravenously as a part of the study. The perfection of the technique is leading to very detailed pictures of high resolution affording more clinically applicable information than is available from other studies (Figure 4-2).

Intracranial Pressure Measurement

The measurement of intracranial pressure provides information that is very useful in the management of neurosurgical patients. The normal intracranial pressure is 0–10 millimeters of mercury with a maximum of 15 millimeters of mercury. Experience has shown that pressure waves called plateau waves (A waves, Lundberg waves) occur when there is an intracranial disease process that causes increased intracranial pressure. Plateau waves indicate a rapid increase in the intracranial pressure, which lasts about 20 minutes before dropping back to the previous pressure levels. Plateau waves usually arise from a pressure above normal range when there is a significant intracranial disease process (Figure 4-3).

Very often a patient's neurological status worsens during the time a plateau wave is recorded. If one considers the relationship between a patient's mean arterial blood pressure and intracranial pressure, it is easy to see why neurological deterioration might occur. Obviously the blood pressure must be greater than the intracranial pressure if blood is to enter the brain. If the two are nearly equal or if the intracranial pressure is greater than the arterial pressure, the brain will not receive the needed blood flow and infarction will occur. Intracranial monitoring alerts the medical team to take appropriate steps to lessen intracranial pressure when a plateau wave is recorded. The measures available to treat increased intracranial pressure are discussed elsewhere.

Intracranial pressure monitoring is not intended to take the place of the neurological vital signs or the clinical observation of the patient. It is a valuable adjunct to be used for the total care of the patient. Of the several different methods that can be used to measure intracranial pressure, each has its advantages and disadvantages.

Intraventricular Pressure Measurement

A small cannula or catheter is inserted into one of the lateral ventricles of the brain through a small, twist-drill hole in the skull. A three-way stopcock is inserted into the other end of this tubing. A manometer inserted into one of the stopcock connections permits direct measurement of the intraventricular pressure and provides a way to calibrate the recording device. A transducer attached to the remaining connection on the stopcock is then attached to the recording module. The recording module provides instantaneous measurements and records the pressure wave forms on an oscilloscope or tape (Figure 4-4). The advantages of the intraventricular technique of measurement are: (1) direct measurement from CSF, and (2) direct access to the CSF if drainage is needed to reduce pressure. The disadvantages are: (1) a definite risk of infection, and (2) potential difficulty inserting the catheter into the ventricle if there is a shift of the ventricle or if it is collapsed because of pressure.

Figure 4-3 Recording Illustrating Plateau Waves

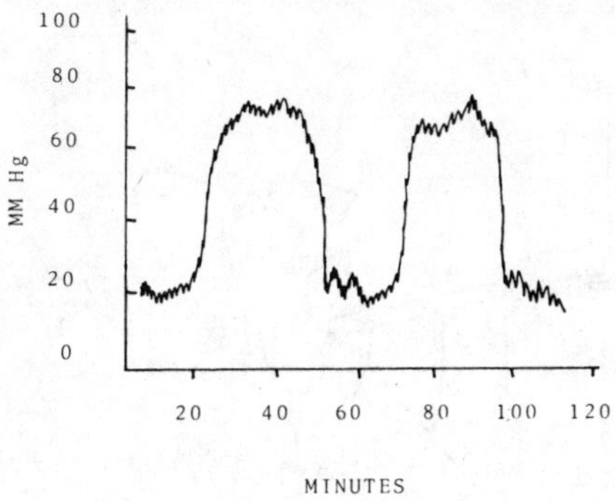

PLATEAU WAVES ARE SHOWN ARISING FROM A BASE PRESSURE OF 20 MM Hg, WHICH IS ABOVE NORMAL. NOTE THE RAPID RISE IN PRESSURE AND THAT IT IS MAINTAINED FOR APPROXIMATELY 20 MINUTES.

Subarachnoid Pressure Measurement

A special screw is inserted into a twist-drill hole in the skull. A hole is made in the dura to permit the tip of the screw to communicate with the subarachnoid space. Then the screw is connected to the transducer and recorder. The advantages and disadvantages are like those for intraventricular measurement, except that the screw is easily inserted, whereas tapping the ventricle may be difficult.

Epidural Pressure Measurement

A device like a balloon, radio transmitter, or fiberoptic transmitter is placed between the dura and the skull. While there is less chance of infection with this technique, there is a question whether the pressure measurements reflect true CSF pressure. In addition CSF cannot be drained to decrease intracranial pressure.

Myelogram

The myelogram is an X-ray study used primarily to study disease in the spinal canal. It is performed in the X-ray department by the radiologist, though some neurologists and neurosurgeons choose to do their own studies.

The myelogram is performed by doing a spinal tap in the manner already described. A large-gauge spinal needle is used because the contrast medium (dye) is a very viscous liquid that will not flow through narrow-gauge needles. When the tap is complete and a specimen of CSF has been taken for laboratory examination, 6–12 cubic centimeters of contrast medium are injected into the subarach-

Figure 4-4 Intraventricular Pressure Measurement

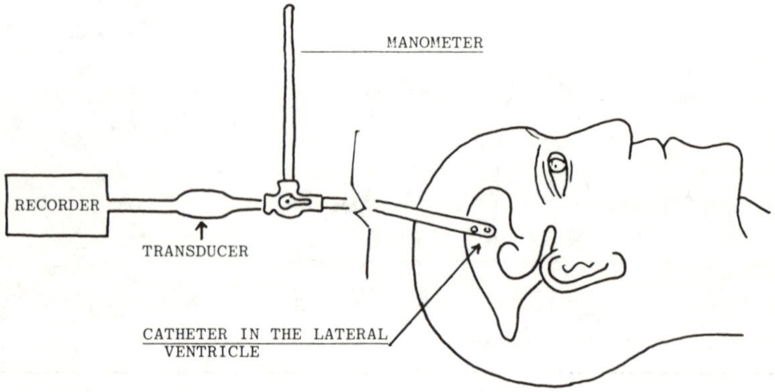

noid space. The dye is not soluble in the CSF, so it remains as a separate entity. The radiologist can, by changing the patient's position, make the dye flow to any point in the spinal canal. When the dye is in the desired location, X rays are taken that show the dye outlining various structures in the spinal canal. Enlargements of the spinal cord caused by a tumor can be detected. Tumors like the meningioma and neurofibroma can be identified and their exact level and size can be determined. A herniated nucleus pulposus in the cervical or lumbar spine can be diagnosed with the myelogram. In some instances the dye can be run into the posterior fossa of the skull to identify tumors or congenital malformations at the junction between the skull and the cervical spine. When the study is completed the dye is returned to the site of the needle and removed as completely as possible. If some remains, there are no serious sequelae.

The myelogram has a bad reputation with the lay public. One will hear fantastic stories about severe pain, paralysis, and even death. Done by a competent examiner it is generally very well tolerated. A low percentage of patients may have a transient spinal headache.

Echoencephalogram

The echoencephalogram or ECHO is a technique that determines the position of brain structures that are normally in the midline: the walls of the third ventricle, the pineal gland, and the large fissure between the two cerebral hemispheres (the interhemispheric fissure). Using a probe that is placed on the patient's temple, beams of pulsating ultrasound are passed into the head. The probe picks up and records returning echoes and transfers this data to a scope that the technician views. Polaroid pictures are made of the scope to provide a permanent record. With the ECHO it is possible to detect shifts of the midline structures. For example, a tumor in the right temporal lobe will shift the midline structures from right to left, a shift easily demonstrated by the ECHO.

In addition to identifying midline structure, a well-trained operator can determine the size of the brain ventricles. This is done by identifying the inner and outer ventricular walls by the reflected ultrasound waves.

Some caution in interpretation of an ECHO is necessary because masses in the posterior temporal, parietal, and occipital regions may attain significant size without producing much of a midline shift.

Electromyogram and Nerve Conduction Studies

The electromyogram (EMG) is a test of muscle and nerve functions. Small, needle electrodes are inserted into the muscles that are to be tested. The electrodes are connected to an oscilloscope, which produces a visual recording that is interpreted by the examiner.

The EMG monitors the motor nerve going to a specific muscle. If the nerve is injured, the muscle will exhibit spontaneous twitches, called fasciculations, which produce characteristic waves that are seen on the oscilloscope. The patient is asked to move the muscle being examined. The EMG reveals whether the number of muscle units that respond is normal, and it gives some information about the function of the myoneural junction. The EMG can also identify and characterize primary muscle diseases like myotonia and muscular dystrophy.

The determination of nerve conduction times evaluates peripheral nerve function. The time required for a nerve stimulus to travel a specific distance is measured. This value is then compared for known values computed for that specific nerve. Tables are available that list the average conduction times for the various nerves of the extremities, such as the median nerve. Peripheral neuropathies characteristically have slowed conduction times.

In certain instances a peripheral nerve can be compressed at different points along its course. For example, the ulnar nerve may be compressed at the elbow or the median nerve at the wrist. The conduction times across these points are usually slowed. Repeated nerve conduction times over a period of time may indicate whether surgical decompression would be of benefit to the patient.

Muscle and Nerve Biopsy

Nerve or muscle biopsies are occasionally of value. In fact, specific peripheral neuropathies or muscular dystrophies can only be identified by biopsy. The sural nerve in the calf of the leg is commonly used when a specimen of peripheral nerve is required.

CHAPTER 5

Nursing Care of the Neurosurgical Patient

By Patricia E. Mahoney

The care of the neurosurgical patient requires a complex interaction of health team skills that vary in type and degree from those needed to care for patients with other disorders. Of the many factors involved in approaching a person who is ill, the professional needs special awareness of the following ones in planning and directing care for neurosurgical patients:

1. Many of the signs and symptoms of these disorders involve subjectivity on the part of patients, significant others, and professionals. Although there has been a great deal of progress in objectifying clinical change, the onset, progression, and improvement in symptomatology is often gradual and may be rationalized by other causative factors. This is especially true of symptoms involving the higher integrative functions, consciousness, and the sensory system. Once the medical professionals have become familiar with their patients, change in the condition of the patients must be evaluated against their underlying personalities, their emotional states, drug effects, and fatigue, all of which increase the difficulty in making clear judgments. Advances in technology have added some clarification but still cannot replace the astuteness of a keen clinical observer.

2. The management of many neurological patients involves long-term follow-up after entry into a complex, multifaceted health

care system. The severe nature of the disorders and their associated chronicity tend to introduce the patients to a large number of health care personnel in the course of treatment. This, in turn, challenges the professionals with complex coordination, goal setting, and communication.

3. Many neurological disorders present patients with moderate to severe loss of control. This may relate to control over themselves and their environment or to a distortion in their perceived and actual abilities. Often crisis intervention is necessary as the impact of illness on patient or family becomes realized.

4. Many neurological disorders still carry a social stigma because they result in obvious insult to cognition, motor function, independence, and appearance. Although society is adjusting its definition of what socially accepted illness is, many neurological problems remain devastating to patient and family.

5. The advance of modern technology has confronted society-at-large with some serious dilemmas relating to coma, the vegetative state, brain death, organ transplantation, therapeutic plans of treatment, and confusion as to who has primary responsibility in the decision-making process. Most of these decisions seem to take on a quality-of-life focus based on the assessment of brain function.

Evaluation of the Patient

Evaluation of the patient begins on initial contact, especially as many verbal and visual cues supplied by the patient on entry into the system can provide valuable baseline information. This provides a basis of comparison for all aspects of future assessment and long-term planning.

Nursing History

A thorough nursing history involves not only direct questioning but special creativity and alertness to more subtle patient cues. Factual content of both subjective symptoms and objective signs is fundamental, but the process of obtaining this information may also provide these other useful indicators (Jones, Dunbar, & Jirovec, 1978):

1. *Appearance and behavior.* These include a general impression of the total patient and may be useful in comparing an initial and

a future impression. They may signal an emotional or organic disorder. Note particularly:

a. *Motor activity and body posture.* These may signal anxiety, denial, decreased attention span, unusual mannerisms, etc.

b. *Dress and hygiene.* Appropriateness of dress and grooming may give clues to dementia, self-image, etc., and should be evaluated according to age, sex, and cultural background.

c. *Body expression.* Body language and nonverbal behavior may signify stress, concentration, lack of concreteness, and movement patterns.

d. *Speech.* This is important in signifying motor dysarthria problems, receptive aphasia, and cognition disorders. Note quality, quantity, and organization.

e. *General manner and ability to relate to the environment.* These may give information as to cognition, affect, mood states, and cooperation.

2. *Mood and affect.* This is best evaluated with a nondirective approach so that the patient is not signaled as to how to respond. Emotional content, completeness of answers, flat affect, and lability should be assessed.

3. *Thought processes and perceptions.* This involves some degree of reality testing and offers information as to the patient's ability to receive, interpret, and respond to environmental cues. Note particularly:

a. *Organization and appropriateness of thought processes.* Assess the composition of the patient's response as well as ideation and interpretation of information.

b. *Thought content.* Note and pursue, if appropriate, any clues to obsessions, hallucinations, delusions, depersonalization, and anxiety.

c. *Perceptions.* Any sensory changes, such as visual or auditory changes, should be especially noted, but also alterations of perceptions of taste, smell, or tactile sense.

4. *Cognitive functions and sensorium.* This area of testing attempts to define objective deficits in higher integrative function and to differentiate between organic and functional disorders. Critical factors such as background, education, culture, memory, and self-perception must be balanced against the cogency of the replies.

a. *Orientation.* This is a basic parameter that implies the degree of the relationship between the patient and his or her environment. Remember that disorientation to time and place may indicate not abnormal function but lack of clarity of environmental cues (especially in strange environments such as intensive care units).

b. *Attention and concentration.* This usually involves testing with serial sevens, repetition of digits, or series of the alphabet.
c. *Memory.* This may indicate organic disease and dementia. Attention should be given both to recent and to remote memory.
d. *Fund of information.* This may indicate the patient's level of intelligence and is evaluated according to knowledge of current events, places, capitals, etc.
e. *Vocabulary.* This again reflects intelligence level but may present problems when the interviewer and patient have different primary languages.
f. *Abstract reasoning.* This is usually tested by asking the meaning of a proverb. It may reveal the use of automatic speech patterns.
g. *Similarities.* Again, this tests concreteness of thought.
h. *Judgment.* Appropriateness of content and consistency with reality may be shown.
i. *Sensory perception and coordination.* This may reflect the patient's sensory, motor, and intellectual skills by asking him or her to copy common figures.

The above list is meant not to be cumbersome but to lend some definition to those qualities of cognitive skills, social and cultural background, and perceptions of reality that a patient may be expressing. Because patients are usually not known personally when they enter the health setting, any information gathered from them about their personality, family relationships, and perceptions of their illness assists all who may care for them. In all stages of contact this information may provide both clues to changes and receptivity to follow-up planning. The family's and the significant others' general response to the patient and the illness is also valuable in assessing their degree of involvement.

The creativity of nurses in making these assessments also extends to their ability to continue to pursue specific avenues of questioning as to such things as other related illnesses, medication routines, bowel patterns, urinary patterns, living patterns, allergies, and expectations of illness. Although hard to accomplish in the busy hospital setting, a complete, knowledgeable nursing history can be vital for every further stage of intervention, especially when inconsistencies are noted.

Physical Assessment

Although the neurological exam is the topic of Chapter 3, some additional points pertinent for the nursing staff in the course of their patient care deserve definition. For example, changes in consciousness and cognition may be noted when patients begin to express interest in their environment, self-image, or seeing family members and significant others or begin to ask about their treatment and prognosis. These are valuable indicators and should not be overlooked.

Motor status can easily be evaluated by observing gait as well as noting difficulty in turning, moving up in bed, or transferring from bed to chair. Postural changes as well as proprioceptive difficulties in maneuvering and walking are significant and have to be evaluated with attention to essential sensory input. For example, a patient may have ambulating difficulties owing to rather sudden blindness rather than to motor dysfunction.

Sensory changes become clear in the course of daily care either from the patient's subjective complaints or from observations of a deficit in a specific modality. For example, the patient who is independent in most of the activities of daily living but who has thermal burns or does not recognize that the bath water is too hot may not only demonstrate a sensory deficit but show implications for teaching. Proprioceptive problems may be seen in ambulating a patient or in assisting a patient to move in bed. In essence the alert nurse can identify information through the constant course of patient care.

Neurodiagnostic Tests

In addition to the indications and descriptions of the neurodiagnostic procedures in Chapter 4, there are certain pre- and postprocedure implications for nursing care that need consideration. Generally, most of these procedures require the informed consent of the patient or a responsible family member to satisfy medical-legal requirements. The nurse's responsibility in participating in this affirmation of consent is to reinforce the information given to the patient, to assess the climate and results of learning, and to deal with the associated anxiety. Specific details about the performance of a procedure and related policies, the place, and other specific orders will vary from facility to facility; and these should be identified in each individual setting.

Because neurodiagnosis is an evolving science, new techniques are replacing older, more formidable procedures. To promote understanding of the need for a complete assessment prior to a set course of therapy, the nurse may have to reinforce the rationale behind a complete battery of procedures as well as the specific implications for the patient of the procedures themselves. This is significant in that many of these procedures still tend to be invasive, painful, and anxiety-provoking—but necessary (Jones et al., 1978).

Noninvasive Techniques

Noninvasive techniques generally involve no specific pre- or post-procedure care, for they are not particularly uncomfortable for the patient. In some instances, contrast substances are used; then the need for the identification of allergies to related dye substances should be explained, and the injection should be described. Otherwise the preparation and aftercare is not complicated. These procedures include:

1. A sleep EEG. A sedative such as chloral hydrate may be administered, which may necessitate explanation and evaluation of post-procedure status for level of consciousness, respiratory patterns, and reactivity.
2. Echoencephalography.
3. CAT scan.
4. Brain scan.

Arteriography

Arteriography is a dangerous yet vital procedure that involves serious attention both preprocedure and postprocedure. Before the procedure the patient and family should be counseled about the serious yet necessary nature of the procedure and about preprocedure protocol: without drink or food (NPO) after midnight, premedication, removal of dentures and rings, and preoperation medication. In addition, what the patient can expect of the procedure (warm flushing during dye injection, salty taste, headache) should be specified without being too suggestive. Postprocedure expectations should be covered as well. The response to this information and the evidence of learning should be documented.

After an arteriogram nursing responsibility centers around the anticipation and notation of any change in general physical status as a result of the procedure as well as specific attention to the injection site. This involves a thorough, frequent neurological check for level of consciousness, pupillary reaction and size, motor and sensory changes, cardiac stability (pulse and blood pressure, including pedal pulses when necessary), and allergic reactions. Care of the site depends on its anatomic location. Bleeding should be checked, and limitations of extremity flexion should be cautioned. If a carotid arteriogram has been done, tracheal-respiratory impairment should be evaluated, and ice bags may be indicated. Edema or bleeding in the tracheal area deserves serious attention. The patient should remain on bed rest until bleeding dangers are passed (usually 12 to 24 hours) but may eat if she or he so desires.

Cerebrospinal Fluid Procedures

The other major category of neurodiagnostic tests involves exploration of the CSF as it circulates through various anatomic spaces (see Chapter 4). In terms of care required, many of these tests involve variations on the same theme.

Lumbar puncture. Special concerns about lumbar puncture include its contraindication in view of markedly increased intracranial pressure, its invasive nature, and the discomfort associated with the procedure and its sequelae. Before the procedure, the specifics of it should be explained and reinforced, such as the position to be assumed (lateral with extreme flexion of head and hips), the possible discomfort of "pressure" as the needle is inserted through the dura (the area will be anesthetized), the possible transient pain and tingling in the legs, and the postprocedure care.

During the procedure the nurse should be alert to the patient's discomfort and tendency to move. Because the nurse will often have direct eye contact, it is often possible to distract and reassure the patient. In addition the nurse should note the opening pressure, the closing pressure, the quality of the CSF, and the specimens obtained.

After the procedure the physical status should be assessed with attention to movement of extremities, local pain, sensory changes, voiding, and CSF leakage. Hydration is encouraged. The nurse should pay attention to headaches and anxiety as well. There is controversy as to the cause of "spinal headaches," and their duration, so strong patient support is needed. The patient should stay in bed with head flat for 4 to 6 hours but may turn from side to side and eat if she or he wishes. Documentation of the patient's response to the procedure is always important.

Cisternal puncture. Similar to lumbar puncture, cisternal puncture is a possible if not an indicated alternative for occasions when CSF needs to be obtained but a lumbar puncture is contraindicated by a subarachnoid block. The implications are similar to those of lumbar puncture except that the procedure is psychologically more traumatic.

Myelography. Also essentially the same procedure as lumbar puncture, myelography differs in the introduction of a dye and its implications, the changes in position during the procedure, and its purpose (to outline the spinal cord and spinal roots on X ray). In preparation for the procedure the same points are taught as for a lumbar puncture. The patient is usually NPO from midnight and premedicated. What the patient can expect after the procedure also needs to be defined.

After the procedure the nurse should observe the patient for the same symptoms as after a lumbar puncture and also for any symptoms of inflammation or infection. Dizziness, nausea, and vomiting; numbness or weakness of an extremity; or an inability to void may also occur. If the dye has not been removed because later films are to be taken, the patient should sit up at a 30 or 40° angle; otherwise flat bed rest should be maintained for 4 to 6 hours.

Pneumoencephalography. In pneumoencephalography the introduction of air into the spinal canal and the rotated positions that the patient may have to assume make both the procedure itself and its sequelae very uncomfortable. This procedure is contraindicated by increased intracranial pressure.

Before the procedure the usual reinforcement of the information given to the patient by the physician is necessary; so is building realistic expectations without introducing undue anxiety. Baseline neurological observations should be obtained. The patient should be instructed about preprocedure orders such as NPO after midnight, removal of dentures and jewelry, and preprocedure medications.

After the procedure the care of the patient should be similar to that following a lumbar puncture plus symptomatic treatment for fever, chills, nausea, and vomiting. Hydration should be encouraged, and the patient should remain on bed rest for a longer period of time (up to 12 hours). Seizures may occur and will have to be treated (see Chapter 12).

Ventriculography. A rather more extensive procedure, ventriculography is similar in concept to a pneumoencephalogram but is preferred in the presence of increased intracranial pressure because it avoids the danger of herniation. The major concern with this procedure is the necessity of making burr holes (an operative procedure) in order to enter the ventricles. This introduces the care associated with anesthesia and the accompanying anxiety.

Before the procedure the patient needs to be prepared physically, psychologically, and educationally. This preparation includes establishing baseline vital signs and explaining to the patient the procedure and its indications, the pain that can be anticipated, the shaving of the head (usually done in the OR), and the usual postoperative care. In addition the patient will be NPO after midnight and premedicated before the procedure.

After the procedure the patient should be carefully watched for signs of increasing intracranial pressure, headache, nausea, vomiting, and changes in vital signs. The head of the bed is usually elevated 10–15° for about 12 hours. Local observation and care of the burr hole is necessary.

Nursing Diagnoses for Specific Nursing Action

To relate systematically the information from patient evaluation to actual nursing care, the next step in the nursing process is to formulate nursing diagnoses. These serve as a classification system and direct nursing action by identifying patient problems or concerns "which are amenable to some intervention which is available in the present or potential scope of nursing practice" (Gebbie & Lavin, 1974, p. 250). These diagnoses are usually accompanied by characteristics that express symptomatology and identify the problem. Although the nursing care of neurological patients is of necessity comprehensive because of their complex and dependent status, it is appropriate to discuss selectively those nursing diagnoses that relate to specific neurological implications.

It must be understood that the following diagnoses and suggested approaches must be adapted to the specific areas of nervous system dysfunction. Generally, however, there are certain principles, aside from basic nursing care, that may pertain in varying degrees to the majority of neurological patients. Although a diagnosis (area of concern) may remain basically the same, a patient often moves on a continuum from an acute, critically ill phase through the various restorative stages. The following, then, are suggested nursing actions for the patient with a neurological or neurosurgical illness; they tend to center around monitoring, maintenance, and directive nursing interventions.

Impairment of Neurological Status

The acutely ill neurological patient presents a variety of signs and symptoms that would be systematically checked in a neurological examination (see Chapter 3). The ongoing observation of neurological vital signs will reflect pertinent elements of the total examination and will yield key information about the patient's status. The frequency of testing should be indicated by the:

1. Acuteness of the patient's condition—ranging from every 15 minutes to every 1 to 2 hours
2. Performance of operative or diagnostic procedures—every 15 minutes for 4 hours, every half hour for 4 hours, every hour for 4 hours, or every 4 hours
3. Performance of any other procedure that may be reflected in an alteration in neurological status—per doctor's orders
4. Need for validation of the stability of the patient—every day or twice a day

Clearly, what evaluations of the patient are necessary depend on both the underlying problem and the nature of the procedure. For example, it is usually not necessary to check pupillary reaction in a patient who has had a myelogram, whereas lower extremity testing and voiding would be most significant.

Level of Consciousness

Changes in level of consciousness may be the most sensitive indicator of change in a patient's condition, so any change should be noted. Generally the use of such categories as semicomatose should be avoided because there may be confusion as to the meaning of the category. Hence it is best to describe the patient's response unless well-defined categories have previously been agreed on. Consciousness should be thought of as including both content and arousal or wakefulness, and both these parameters should be evaluated (Plum & Posner, 1972). For example, a patient who is highly agitated (awake) but is confused in verbalization during an episode of the delirium tremens is easily differentiated from a patient who is very lethargic (degree of wakefulness) but when stimulated will answer questions appropriately, as during increasing intracranial pressure. Generally orientation is assessed by noting orientation to time, place, and person. Remember that the hospital environment itself can induce some forms of disorientation, which must be accounted for. Also drug effect, fatigue, and lack of meaningful stimulation may account for a decrease in orientation, especially to time. Specifically, consciousness can be evaluated by assessing:

1. *Verbal responses.* Check orientation, confused phrases, inappropriate words, incomprehensible sounds, or no sounds. Inability to speak that is of a physical nature, such as that caused by intubation or tracheostomy, must be noted as such.
2. *Eye opening.* Is it to command, spontaneously, to sound, to deep pain, or is their none?
3. *Spontaneous eye movements.* Are they to command, conjugate tracking, or conjugate roving, or are there none? Tracking generally is following a stimulus, whereas roving is not stimulus-directed.

Pupils

Pupils are generally checked for size, regularity, and reactivity (PERLA—pupils equal and reactive to light and accommodation) because these are useful indicators of change for two reasons: The third cranial (oculomotor) nerve is located at the tentorial notch, so its failure to function normally could be an early sign of impending herniation. The nuclei of the third nerves are on the brainstem, and so pupillary reactivity also reflects integrity of the brainstem.

Shape, size, and equality of pupils. Direct pupillary examination without the use of a direct light source reflects brainstem function as well as trauma, surgery, and congenital defects. The best way to record these observations is by noting in millimeters the size of each eye while they share a common, indirect light source. Abnormalities (especially dilation) may reflect herniation, the presence of drugs, or hypoxia.

Reactivity. The most common assessment made is reactivity to a direct light source. It is informative to note if the reaction is brisk or sluggish, but this may lead to some confusion of interpretation.

Motor Status

The evaluation of motor status yields information about both upper motor neuron (brain and spinal cord) function and lower motor neuron (peripheral nerve and local spinal level) function. It can best be evaluated by the following checks:

1. *Best motor response.* This is tested by asking the patient to move on command and noting any inabilities to do so. If the patient is not alert enough for this kind of testing, then motor testing is evaluated by response to pain.
2. *Response to pain.* In deep pain testing (using pressure on a nail bed, preferably on an upper extremity), the significant responses are:
   a. *Localizing.* The contralateral arm is able to approach the stimulus across the midline.
   b. *Nonspecific localizing.* The contralateral limb moves but does not cross the midline.
   c. *Withdrawal.* The patient grimaces or mildly attempts to pull the upper trunk away.
   d. *Abnormal flexion.* Often known as decorticate posturing.
   e. *Abnormal extension.* Often known as decerebrate posturing.
   f. *Other or no movement.*
3. *Leg strength.* On command the patient shows:
   a. Normal strength
   b. Weakness, but patient is able to move against gravity (i.e., raise leg above the bed)
   c. No strength against gravity
   d. No strength
4. *Arm strength.* On command the patient shows:
   a. Normal strength
   b. Weakness, but patient is able to move against gravity (i.e., raise arm above the bed)
   c. No strength against gravity
   d. No strength
5. *Grips.* This last test of motor movement indicates the patient's ability to show a comparison in symmetrical strength. It is evaluated according to:
   a. Normal and equal strength
   b. Weakness
   c. No strength

All of the above involve some degree of potential for change. Responses may differ bilaterally at the same time. Responses may also be stronger or weaker over time. These changes can be noted by using the designations greater than or less than (Bates et al., 1977, p. 211ff).

These vital signs together with blood pressure, pulse, and temperature are significant in demonstrating actual change as well as in noting the potential for danger. The nurse is responsible for recognizing the process of change both from one side of the body to the other (hence the grips test) and from one moment to the next and thus the nurse must be aware of an impending process and report it as the change occurs. With most neurological cases both nurse and patient display a degree of subjectivity. Keeping a record of changes helps to objectify and quantify both patient's and nurse's responses without the need for elaborate keys to response meanings. There are many different versions of neurological vital sign sheets, but the central objective is consistency in the evaluation process.

Aspects of Specific Disorders Requiring Specific Nursing Actions

Patients with field cuts should have their meals, hygiene articles, and other things they need placed within their range of vision. Patients who exhibit any degree of paresis should be assisted by encouraging their use of the functioning side (limb) in the course of activity or by the development of the affected limb in the course of retraining. In patients who have experienced spinal cord trauma, special attention must be paid to perfect vertebral alignment, especially if the trauma has involved the cervical area, which may produce a life-threatening situation (see Chapter 7). A patient who is immobilized in tongs will require careful and monitored support while being turned or moved. It is generally helpful to check with the physician to validate from the X rays what the nature of the damage is and what the exact limitations on movement are. At all times the weights should not touch the ground, and center alignment of the head and body with the weights should be maintained. Lateral flexion of the head while in a lateral position may be as dangerous as anterior or posterior flexion of the neck while in a supine position. Any change in the patient should be evaluated by testing the motor or sensory subjective and objective status of the patient. In conclusion, many of the nursing actions related to an impaired neurological status center around the monitoring aspect of nursing intervention and require careful comparison of the patient to the objective and subjective norms.

Cardiovascular Instability

Patients with neurological and neurosurgical disorders show cardiovascular instability based on several key mechanisms that may be mechanical, chemical, structural, or reflex in nature.

Autoregulation

The ability of the brain to maintain an adequate and constant cerebral blood pressure over a wide range of fluctuation of the systemic blood pressure is called autoregulation. This means that in the normal individual there can be changes in the systolic blood pressure between 70 and 150 millimeters of mercury without significantly affecting the cerebral pressure. The mechanisms underlying this process are thought to be: (1) metabolic (pH, pO_2, pCO_2), (2) neurogenic (neurons in the brainstem), or (3) myogenic (muscle relaxants in the vessel walls).

Cerebral Perfusion Pressure

Generally calculated by subtracting the intracranial pressure from the mean arterial pressure, cerebral perfusion pressure has implications for the control of the systemic arterial pressure in the presence of increased intracranial pressure.

Cushing's Reflex

Cushing's reflex, slowing of the pulse with an increase in the blood pressure when there is impending compromise of the brain's blood supply, is mediated via the vagus nerve and allows for greater contractility and filling of the heart in order to pump more blood into the brain. This reflex is responsible for the characteristic blood pressure and pulse changes in increased intracranial pressure, even though they are late signs in the process.

Structural Integrity of the Cerebral Vascular System

The circle of Willis (see Chapter 1) often allows for continued cerebral perfusion when there is an interruption in the supply of one of its branches. Because it is one of the major anastomotic structures in the brain, it also serves as the site for many congenital abnormalities (aneurysms, for example). Normally there is little mixing of blood between the left and right carotid circulations or between the vertebral and basilar circulations, but this may be altered in the presence of pathology. The major disturbances to circulation may take the form of atherosclerosis, thrombosis, embolisms, inflammation, or compression, the symptoms of which will usually relate to impairment in function of the areas supplied by the offending vessel.

Chemical Factors

The neurotransmitters, especially norephinephrine, epinephrine, serotonin, and the prostaglandins, play an important part in the caliber of the blood vessels. Their release after a subarachnoid hemorrhage is thought to be in part responsible for vasospasm. It is to counteract these substances that many of the drug combinations are now being tried, although their efficacy is questionable. In addition, coagulation factors exert a chemical effect on cerebral blood flow and must be carefully studied when treatment is considered (i.e., surgery may be dangerous for someone on an anticoagulation routine).

Circulating Blood Volume

As in most health problems, changes in the total blood volume are reflected in symptomatology. In neurological patients, where the tendency is to decrease cerebral edema by use of osmotic diuretics, fluid shifts among the vascular, extravascular, and intracellular compartments must be anticipated. Hence complications from shock, for example, when the tendency is to add to fluid volume, may have grave inplications by causing herniation of the brain. Also osmotic changes such as the rebound phenomenon, which could occur 4 to 6 hours after osmotic diuretics have been given, could also produce herniation. This is due to a change in osmotic concentration; the intravascular compartment of the brain begins to pull fluid from the vascular space, which leads to increased intracranial pressure once more. This is usually counteracted by the use of steroids.

Other Related Illnesses

The interaction of all of the above factors may make the treatment of such a syndrome as hypertension a complicated problem. High blood pressure may have contributed to the neurological episode (such as stroke or rupture of an aneurysm), but the continued treatment of the patient may become complicated. For example, in controlling hypertension, consideration must be given to cerebral perfusion pressure so that ambitious therapy to achieve a "normal blood pressure" may not, in fact, produce a strokelike syndrome.

Immobility

The actual state of being immobilized has been shown to add several extra complications to the cardiovascular system, specifically: orthostatic hypotension from loss of muscle tone and disturbance of autonomic reactivity to change in position; increased cardiac work load from redistribution of the blood volume; and pressure against the veins (Olson, 1967, pp. 781, 782).

Nursing Actions

1. Close observation of all neurological vital signs, especially pulse and blood pressure
2. Proper positioning in correct body alignment to prevent obstruction of the jugular venous drainage, which would tend to increase intracranial pressure
3. Frequent turning (every 2 hours) and range-of-motion exercises to prevent thrombus formation
4. Careful monitoring and administration of cardiac drugs and antihypertensive agents
5. Prevention of straining at stool (Valsalva maneuver) by the use of stool softeners
6. Use of antiembolism stockings
7. Careful monitoring of intake and output, especially if osmotic diuretics are in use
8. Early and progressive ambulation with close monitoring of the blood pressure to insure adequate cerebral perfusion pressure, with use of a tilt table perhaps indicated for patients who have been immobilized for prolonged periods
9. Maintenance of a restful environment, which includes adequate stimulation but limits on stress

Respiratory Instability

Because the brain depends on a constant supply of oxygen and will undergo irreparable damage if deprived of an oxygen source for more than just a few minutes, the maintenance of adequate ventilation becomes a necessity. There are several underlying factors that specifically influence neurological and respiratory stability.

Respiratory Patterns

Observation of respiratory rate and pattern may yield some helpful information about the site of neurological damage (Plum & Posner, 1972). For example:

1. *Cheyne-Stokes respiration.* A pattern of breathing in which hyperpnea alternates with apnea, this will usually reflect bilateral

lesions, deep in the cerebral hemispheres and basal ganglia, that damage the internal capsules.

2. *Central neurogenic hyperventilation.* This is sustained regular, rapid, and fairly deep hyperpnea; it may reflect midbrain and pontine dysfunction.
3. *Apneustic breathing.* The pattern is prolonged inspiration alternating with a pause after expiration. It may reflect damage at the pontine level.
4. *Ataxic breathing.* This is a completely irregular pattern of breathing in which shallow and deep breaths occur randomly. It may reflect a lesion in the medulla. (pp. 27–30)

Hence the observation of the respirations may have some value in localizing the neurological problems; the nurse should therefore include this information in assessing the patient.

Reflex Mechanisms

There is a direct relationship between the quality of the blood gases and the caliber of the cerebral blood vessels. An increase in pCO_2 will result in cerebral vasodilation; a decrease in the pCO_2 will cause cerebral vasoconstriction. Neither extreme is desirable, and both have grave implications in the presence of increased intracranial pressure. This makes respiratory management of the neurological patient critical not only for the maintenance of adequate oxygenation but for the maintenance of adequate cerebral perfusion.

Motor Involvement

Clearly, adequate respiration is going to depend on adequate chest excursion and hence on proper movement of the abdominal muscles, the external and internal intercostal muscles, and the diaphragm. Motor impairment usually reflects a neurological disorder, and impending paresis signifies immediate action. Clinical illustrations would be the Guillian-Barre syndrome and spinal cord trauma, especially in the high cervical area. Such conditions often indicate the need for ventilatory assistance with a respirator and involving intubation or a tracheotomy.

Brainstem Instability

Because the brainstem centers (the inspiratory center in the medulla and the pneumotaxic center in the pons) control the rate and rhythmicity of respiration, they may be particularly unstable in many neurological disorders. Also changes in the level of consciousness may be reflected in varying instability of respiration. This becomes even more important in view of drug and metabolic effect.

Immobility

Again, the critically ill patient who is immobilized will tend to be susceptible to decreased respiratory excursion, pooling of secretions, and oxygen–carbon dioxide imbalance (Olson, 1967, pp. 783–784).

Nursing Actions

1. Careful observation and monitoring of (a) respiration—rate, depth, rhythm, and effort—and (b) secretions—consistency, amount, color, and odor.
2. Maintenance of a patent airway, which may involve insertion of an airway by intubation or tracheotomy.
3. Assistance with ventilation as necessary, which may involve total control of ventilation or monitored assistance. Aside from blood gases, the respiratory excursion can also be measured by use of a spirometer, which measures tidal volume and vital capacity.
4. Care of the respiratory tract.

In the immobilized patient, certain nursing functions are critical to maintaining and supporting respiration. Many of these will be described in procedures and policies specific to an individual institution, but they deserve mention here.

Suctioning. Without robbing the patient of an oxygen supply by prolonging the procedure, the respiratory tract must be kept clean and free of secretions. This demands sterile procedure for all aspects of care of patients with tracheotomies and endotracheal tubes. If oral suctioning is done, it should follow tracheal suctioning so that contamination is avoided. Prolonged, extensive suctioning will increase intracranial pressure and should be avoided. Nasopharyngeal suctioning without benefit of intubation or a tracheotomy can be traumatic and can induce vomiting by stimulating of the gag reflex. If secretions tend to be especially tenacious, the insertion of sterile saline into the tracheotomy with immediate suctioning may serve to loosen them.

Tracheotomy and endotracheal tube care. The strings securing the tracheotomy tube should always be tight enough to prevent their being dislodged. They should be tied with knots, and no more than two fingers should be able to fit between the strings and the neck. Care should be taken in changing the strings, and either the change should be done by two people or the new strings should be put on before the old are removed. Tracheotomy care should be done as needed, and only gauze that does not have cotton packing should be used. Patients who have tracheotomies should not use tissues, which tend to shred, but gauze to remove secretions. Endotracheal tubes should be fastened securely, and there are now a number of commercially available fastening products that decrease the trauma to the face that tape often causes. Meticulous oral hygiene should be included in the plan of care, even if an endotracheal tube and airway are in place. The cuffs of tracheal tubes should be periodically deflated, depending on agreed upon procedure. Some of the new low-pressure, high-volume cuffs have eliminated the need for routine deflation. Patients, however, can still aspirate with the cuff inflated.

Humidification. Oxygen or compressed air should never be administered without humidification because secretions will tend to be drier. The various types of oxygen equipment will to some extent limit the kind and amount of humidification used, but warm humidity is preferred. The temperature setting on the humidifier on the ventilator should be checked to make sure that the air is not too hot.

Weaning from the ventilator. The individual condition of the patient will indicate the most appropriate mode of weaning, but several points can be suggested. A weaning procedure should be initiated and carried on during the day and evening hours. While this insures that there are more staff members available for close monitoring of the patient, it is primarily important to insure that the patient receives enough sleep during the night hours. In monitoring the patient during the process, vital signs, color, and respirations should be observed, but blood gas determinations are critical. The blood gas results will only truly reflect the patient's capability if they are taken 20 minutes or more after the process has started. The advent of newer and more sophisticated technology has facilitated the care of patients who need ventilatory assistance, but it never should be forgotten that both the machines and their alarm systems are subject to failure.

Respiratory therapy. Anyone with a compromised respiratory capability or who has undergone anesthesia can benefit from mechanical measures to improve their status. These can vary from routine turning, coughing, and deep breathing as a part of care, to the use of cupping and coughing or intermittent positive pressure breathing (IPPB) and an incentive spirometer. The use of IPPB has to be balanced against the danger of increasing intracranial pressure. These measures should be incorporated into routine nursing care, even when skilled respiratory therapists are available.

Hydration. With an eye to all the various considerations that dictate the fluid balance of a patient, adequate hydration is important to keep secretions from becoming too thick. In addition, any patient who is on a ventilator should be weighed every day to monitor body water. Intake and output should also be recorded.

Problems with Elimination

Patients who have both upper and lower motor neuron disorders may have difficulty with bladder and bowel elimination. As the patient moves from the acute to the rehabilitative phases of illness, the problems of elimination may resolve themselves; but if they remain, as in spinal cord trauma, the psychological impact is major. The eliminatory processes involve sociocultural significance as well as implications for self-image, dignity, privacy, and comfort. Because sexual function in the physical sense is often evaluated along with an assessment of the eliminatory functions, it too is included here; its part in the psychological comfort of the patient is not to be underestimated. Problems associated with neurological disorders can be broken into those affecting urinary function and those affecting bowel function.

Urinary Dysfunction

Neurogenic bladders. Patients who are incontinent may have spastic or flaccid bladders, depending on the integrity of the sacral reflex arcs. With a spastic bladder the reflex arcs causing detrusor muscle contraction are easily stimulated, and small amounts of urine may cause involuntary contraction of the bladder. This may occur after the phase of spinal shock has passed if the sacral nerve roots have been spared. A flaccid bladder involves retention of large amounts of urine with overflow incontinence. Often there has been sacral spinal cord damage in this situation, and the reflex arcs are impaired. Bladder training is most successful when the reflex arcs are retained, but the bladder is able to hold 100–150 cubic centimeters before contracting. Sexual function is controlled by the same spinal cord level as urination, and hence patients with incomplete upper motor and lower motor neuron lesions may be able to have erections, depending on the integrity of sensation, which permits psychogenic stimulation.

Autonomic dysreflexia. A potential danger that exists for patients with spinal cord damage, especially above the midthoracic area, is autonomic dysreflexia. This is due to an interruption of sympathetic nervous system function and may be triggered by a full bladder, a distended rectum, spasticity, or hyperirritability of the skin. These may stimulate vasoconstriction below the lesion level, with a marked increase in systemic blood pressure. As the body attempts to compensate, the sympathetic nervous system above the lesion is stimulated, with superficial vasodilation (flushing of the face) and reflex vagal slowing of the heart. The action is inadequate, however, because of blocking of the impulses at the injury level. A stroke may follow if the stimulus is not relieved or the hypertension is not symptomatically treated with sympathetic ganglionic blocking agents (Taylor, 1974, pp. 717ff).

Antidiuretic hormone. Two common disorders are associated with antidiuretic hormone (ADH). Diabetes insipidus results from too small an amount of ADH being released from the posterior pituitary; inappropriate ADH is usually the result of too much being released. Both conditions can cause marked fluctuations in fluid balance. In diabetes insipidus, as after some head traumas or pituitary surgery, the urinary output is very excessive and the fluid replacement must be matched to the output. If the normal thirst mechanisms are absent, as after anesthesia, then careful records or urinary output serve as the guide. With inappropriate ADH, as following head trauma, oliguria is due not to fluid depletion but to too much fluid retention. Here the situation resembles water intoxication rather than fluid loss. Water and salt are usually restricted.

Immobility. The major urinary problems associated with prolonged bed rest are: (1) pooling of urine in the kidneys, causing a tendency toward stone formation, (2) bladder distention and incontinence, (3) tendency toward infection, and (4) stone formation caused by increased amounts of free calcium, phosphates, and decreased citric acid, the concentrations of which are altered as a result of skeletal-muscle disuse.

Nursing Actions for Urinary System Integrity

1. *Accurate recording of intake and output.* Recording intake and output helps monitor diabetes insipidus and inappropriate ADH,

and indicates general fluid status as well. This is critical in the presence of increased intracranial pressure, especially when osmotic diuretics are used.

2. *Weighting.* Again, daily or routine weightings will reflect fluid status.

3. *Prevention of infection.* Frequent care of the catheter by antiseptic cleansing of it, the meatus, and the perineal area as well as maintenance of a closed urinary system will limit the incidence of infection. Debilitated patients are especially prone to infection because of their immobility, nutritional and fluid imbalances, and incontinence. Very often cross-contamination by health care staff is responsible for infection, and this is a special problem with present and evolving forms of antibiotic-resistant strains.

4. *Routine urine tests.* Aside from periodic urinanalysis and culture and sensitivity testing, neurological patients may need to have both specific gravity and sugar and acetone monitored. The former is important in monitoring diabetes insipidus and fluid balance; the latter is most significant with the large doses of steroids that are commonly used.

5. *Patency of the drainage system.* Kinking of the tubing may lead to bladder distention and autonomic dysreflexia. Of note is the potential for vital sign changes as a result of autonomic discharge when a very full bladder is first catheterized. A way to prevent this form occurring is to drain 500 cubic centimeters, clamp the catheter, and then drain the rest in approximately 1 hour.

6. *Bladder training.* There are several suggested approaches to bladder training. Generally they evolve around drinking regulated amounts of fluid (200–500 cubic centimeters per hour) and making periodic attempts to void, using trigger zone techniques such as tapping the abdomen or thigh or doing push-ups on the toilet. Residual amounts of urine must be checked to determine the progress of the program. Intermittent catheterization is a method that should not be overlooked. It reduces the risks of infection posed by an indwelling catheter, may enhance resumption of good bladder tone, and increases patient independence. Patients with adequate motor function and coordination may incorporate this method into their daily living patterns if properly assessed and taught.

Bowel Dysfunction

Immobility. The major bowel problems associated with staying in bed are related to constipation, which results from diminished expulsive power, loss of the defecation reflex, and lack of exercise. As this process proceeds, dehydration, decreased absorption, and fluid and electrolyte imbalance occur as distention increases (Olson, 1967, pp. 785–786).

Diarrhea. The frequent use of antibiotics may alter the usual bowel flora so that diarrhea and its resultant fluid and electrolyte loss become a major problem. In addition, prepared tube feedings may cause diarrhea.

Steroids. Many neurological patients are treated with steroids, which may produce alterations in electrolyte balance and intestinal bleeding as well. Guaiac testing should be routine.

Nursing Actions for Bowel Function

1. Attempt to establish a regular bowel evacuation routine. This should include recognition of the patient's previous pattern, adequate hydration, adequate diet including foods with fiber and bulk, and stool softeners. A suppository given before the planned time may stimulate the bowel to empty. Enemas on a routine basis should be avoided because they tend to encourage dependency.
2. Observe all stools for color, consistency, amount, and frequency.
3. Prevent constipation through dietary measures.
4. Treat diarrhea by change in diet or medication. Diarrhea may be caused by antibiotic therapy that changes the normal bowel flora. Also tube feedings may be the cause, in which case another type of tube feeding should be tried. Diarrhea may have serious implications because of fluid and electrolyte loss. If diarrhea persists when there is abdominal distention and no record of a recent well-formed stool, impactions should be considered.
5. Because of the frequent use of steroids in neurological conditions, the possibility of intestinal bleeding should always be considered and assessed. Aside from testing the stool itself, the hematocrit and hemoglobin should be checked.

Nutritional Deficiency

The heavy bodily demands placed on patients often immobilized by basic neurological disorders are added to the ongoing needs of the brain for fluid and electrolyte balance and energy supply. The brain is unable to store nutrients and thus must have a constant source of nutrition. A number of factors influence the choice of type and modality of nutritional source.

Presence of a Gag Reflex

Many neurological patients, particularly those who have depressed levels of consciousness, those who have cranial nerve damage, and some of those with upper motor neuron damage, will have a depressed or absent gag reflex. This in turn leads to an inability to take foods or fluids by mouth and to an increased chance of aspiration. Because of this, careful thought must be given to how the patient should be fed—if not by mouth, then what mode is most safe?

Immobility

In an immobilized state, the patient will tend to become catabolic and protein deficient and to show shifts in the utilization of minerals and electrolytes. A diet with a suitable caloric intake must be chosen (there are many commercial brands available), and there are a few other features that must be kept in mind. For example, because of catabolism there must be sufficient protein replacement, which also requires that adequate fluid be given so as not to overload the kidneys. Also the tendency to form kidney stones from free calcium, phosphorus, and other minerals indicates that they should be replaced according to the requirements of bone growth. As previously stated, electrolytes and fluids need to be determined not only with normal maintenance needs in mind but with consideration of special status such as inappropriate ADH and diabetes insipidus.

Nursing Actions

1. Check the gag reflex of any patient who may have questionable function.
2. Select the appropriate feeding tube. Many neurological patients are unable to use their intestinal tract for adequate ingestion, and thus the choice of a feeding tube involves considering the anticipated length of time the tube may be needed, the presence of a gag reflex, possible cardiac sphincter erosion if too hard a tube is used for too long, the possibility of gastric reflux, and the alertness of the patient. Depending on these points, one may consider:
   a. *A nasogastric tube.* This may be of wide lumen and fairly hard plastic, hence leading to sphincter erosion if left in place too long. Also bulk tube feedings will rest in the stomach and, in the presence of a decreased gag reflex, there is the danger of aspiration.
   b. *A gastrostomy tube.* This carries the above dangers but is more suitable for long-term feeding regimens.

c. *A nasojejunostomy tube.* This often is a soft, narrow-lumen tube that extends into the jejunum, thus decreasing the danger of sphincter damage. It empties into an area of the bowel that does not contain a reservoir (i.e., the stomach) and thus decreases the danger of aspiration.

d. *A jejunostomy tube.* Similar to the above, this tube is indicated in long-term tube-feeding situations.

e. *Continuous drip versus bolus feedings.* Both types have advantages and disadvantages. A major deciding factor is safety, because a patient who has a decreased gag reflex or is not totally alert or mobile may be in serious trouble if the clamp on the continuous drip feeding ceases to function while the patient is unobserved. Tube feedings should be considered a serious nursing function.

f. *Hyperalimentation.* Often appropriate for patients who have sustained trauma to their intestinal tract (in addition to their neurological trauma), this is a modern and useful manner of meeting a patient's metabolic needs by an infusion through a central intravenous line. Strict attention should be paid to sepsis and accuracy. Many neurological patients will not need this because they have intact intestinal systems, and the hazard of sepsis is significant.

3. Proceed with the plan of feeding according to accepted procedure.

4. Always feed with the head of the bed elevated and keep it elevated for 45 minutes to prevent aspiration.

5. Inflate the tracheotomy cuff, if applicable, during the feeding.

6. If by-mouth feedings are possible but a patient has dysphagia, test the patient with ice chips or semisolids such as Jello. Ice chips utilize tactile and temperature stimuli to promote swallowing and are not as lethal to the lungs if swallowing is inefficient. Water and liquids tend to be most difficult because they do not properly incorporate the gross motor tongue movements. Remember too that the presence of a trach, even when deflated, may serve as an obstruction to swallowing.

Immobility

The hazards of immobility (Olson, 1967, pp. 785–786) have been outlined as they affect particular nursing problems that have been discussed. In addition, immobility not only affects the psychological status of patients by rendering them dependent but imposes some additional problems by causing further complications.

Interference with Activities of Daily Living

The significance of the limitations imposed on a patient varies according to the severity of the deficit and the acceptability of that deficit to the ego. Hence patients with relatively minor dysfunction may have as difficult a time accepting that deficit as patients who have far greater impairments. From admission, then, the nurse should attempt to set realistic short- and long-term goals and to institute measures aimed at achieving some degree of independence as well as maintaining present function of the musculoskeletal system.

Complications

Preventable sequelae in an immobilized patient include contractures, decubiti, and osteoporosis. Nursing actions should be routinely instituted to guard against these.

Nursing Actions for Complication Prevention

1. The patient should be frequently turned and positioned (at least every 2 hours).
2. Use appropriate splints and supports. It cannot be overstated that the situation should be assessed with the assistance of the occupational and physical therapist. For example, a sling for a flaccid upper extremity may be contraindicated if it will cause shoulder subluxation. Basketball-like sneakers or boots may prevent foot drop more effectively than footboards. Often a soft collar may assist the patient in holding the head up.
3. Active and passive range of motion can easily be incorporated into care during a bath or turning.
4. As soon as possible the patient should be gotten out of bed. The selection of the proper chair is important both for the patient's support and for the nurse's energy. Orthostatic hypotension should be evaluated, and the patient should be encouraged to increase endurance in staying up.
5. Skin care should be constant and thorough and utilize such aids as water and pressure mattresses, padding of extremities, and so forth. It would seem that the most effective measure in the alleviation of decubiti is attention. There are many recommended ways of

treating areas of potential skin breakdown, but nursing attention in the form of keeping the area clean, dry, and unpressured are the most important.

6. Even though it may be time consuming, patients should be allowed to maximize their potential in such activities as dressing, eating, moving, and participating in their own care. Occupational therapy and physical therapy can be most helpful.

Temperature Imbalance

The maintenance of a normal temperature is important for all patients, especially in view of the effects of hyperthermia on metabolic and energy levels, fluid balance, and heart rate. Patients with hypothalamic imbalance may have difficulty maintaining normal temperature, and their course is often characterized by wide fluctuations that have to be symptomatically treated.

Nursing Actions

1. *Hypothermia machine.* These generally provide the easiest means of controlling temperature, but always remember that machines may malfunction. Care must be taken that the patient is not injured by overcooling or overheating.
2. *Alcohol sponge.* This still remains effective for episodic temperature increases.
3. *Medication.* Medications such as aspirin and its derivatives may effectively reduce temperature.
4. *Fluid balance.* If diaphoresis is extensive, additional fluid replacement may be necessary.

Comfort Level

Although generally believed to refer to physical comfort, comfort level necessarily includes psychological comfort as well. Providing an adequate level of comfort involves certain major nursing considerations.

Adequate Rest and Sleep

Hospital environments tend to disrupt normal sleep patterns because they are strange, noisy, and often geared more to the functioning of the staff than to the needs of the patient. In addition, critical care areas usually include care activities that persist around the clock, hence disrupting sleep. The various therapies also tend to exhaust patients. For all these reasons nursing attention should be given to planning regular and consistent rest and sleep patterns. This planning should take into consideration the patient's usual routine. For example, patients who work at night may have a harder time adjusting to a setting in which they are expected to stay awake all day.

Sensory Changes

Altered sensations, whether they be in the form of pain, burning, tingling, or general discomfort, have to be accurately assessed and treated. Changes in sensation may not always reflect decreased sensation but may be paresthesias. Pain medication may not always be the answer; but if used, it should reflect mature nursing judgment.

Medication

Because nursing deals with the whole patient, the evaluation of discomfort must consider the physical as well as psychological state of the person. Patients with chronic pain may have developed a tolerance to their medications so that more may be required. At times, psychological support may accomplish the goal so that medication can be avoided. Prompt postoperative administration of pain medication may break the pain cycle, which can become exacerbated if the pain level is allowed to increase. Fatigue, positional discomfort, and psychological fear and stress may all tend to increase discomfort and require appropriate intervention. Newer and less conventional forms of pain therapy such as biofeedback, acupuncture, and systematic relaxation may all have therapeutic roles.

Safety and Protection

Because of the motor, sensory, and dependency needs of many neurological patients, safety and protective measures need to be incorporated into their plan of care.

Restraining Devices

The policies for using restraints may vary from institution to institution, but generally restraints should not always be negatively regarded. They are a valid part of safety and protection. Patients who are unable to maintain their posture may need to be restrained while sitting. Also patients who have altered levels of consciousness may respond to a noxious stimulus such as an endotracheal tube or a nasogastric tube and may need to have their hands restrained. Restraints should never impair circulation or breathing or contribute to the agitation of the patient. This may mean that the removal of the restraints may be more effective than applying them.

Teaching

Patients with sensory loss—whether it be visual, thermal, tactile, or proprioceptive—will need special instruction and preparation for maneuvering in their environment. This need extends to evaluation of their homes and instruction in how to make them barrier free and to providing advice on home assistance devices.

Psychological Support

The nature of neurological and neurosurgical disorders often lends itself to a need for crisis intervention. This may in part be due to the visible nature of the impairments, the dire nature of the prognoses, the insult to body image and independence, the chronic or life-threatening nature of the diagnoses, and the social stigma that continues to persist in relation to "brain disturbances." In addition, neurological patients may demonstrate changes both in their higher intellectual functions and in their personalities. All of the above comprise a unique challenge to nursing in determining the appropriate intervention for the patient, family, and significant others. When a patient enters the health setting, the nurse should begin to assess not only the patient's coping mechanisms and degree of anxiety but the interactional patterns of the family. A nonjudgmental approach is essential, especially as behavioral changes may reflect a loss of normal inhibitory mechanisms as well as crisis. Total health-team planning that includes the patient and family will usually result in the achievement of common objectives, providing that these objectives are realistically set.

Teaching Needs

Teaching the patient begins when the patient enters the hospital and continues through the entire hospital course. Aside from the formal teaching associated with procedures, surgery, and discharge, informal teaching can relate to all aspects of health care, and it can take place in all contacts with the patient. Some guidelines to remember are:

1. Teaching environments should be selected that contain a minimum of distraction, noise, or movement, especially if memory, concentration, or emotionally potent subjects are to be reviewed. A busy intensive care unit with emergency treatment in progress is hardly the place to teach didactic material or to assess fine coordination skills.

2. Assess the patient's ability to learn. Just as a patient is probably not able to learn while in a state of high anxiety or during the performance of a procedure, so too, teaching should be geared to the patient's ability to receive and process the information. Hence discharge teaching should be initiated far in advance of actual discharge.

3. Audiovisual aides are most helpful in reinforcing teaching and should be used with explanation whenever possible.

4. The results of the teaching-learning process must be evaluated and documented.

Discharge Planning

Discharge planning should begin on admission, should incorporate the total health team, and should cover:

1. The patient's adjustment to the home environment in view of present limitations and predicted prognosis
2. Written instructions for the patient on medications and their action, side effects, dosage, time, and any interactions with other drugs, along with administration times
3. Assistance at home
4. Health care follow-up and further instructions
5. Written patient summaries prepared in advance for patient transfer to another facility

Integration of the Health Team

The care of the neurological patient will often involve a myriad of health care personnel including doctors, nurses, physical therapists, occupational therapists, social workers, speech therapists, home care nurses, and consultants. A major problem in such complex situations is the coordination of all goals, objectives, and activities. This task will often fall to the nurse, as information is transmitted and action is taken. It is most important that good communication exists among the members of the health team so that confusion is prevented and a feeling of trust is encouraged. It must never be forgotten that the patient and family have the primary roles in this planning and should be aware of all components of decisions made.

CHAPTER 6

Craniotomy

The surgical procedure that involves the opening of the skull for brain surgery is generally termed a *craniotomy.* A craniotomy is done for treatment of such conditions as brain tumors, hematomas, and abscesses and for ligation of aneurysms. It is usually described by stating the site of the surgery and naming the reason for it. Thus, an operation for a brain tumor in the right frontal lobe would be called a right frontal craniotomy with excision of a right frontal lobe tumor. If there is a mass in the cerebellum, the resulting craniotomy might be called a posterior fossa craniotomy with exploration and excision of a cerebellar mass lesion.

The decision to perform a craniotomy follows as complete as possible an evaluation of the patient. In certain emergency situations, a surgeon may be forced to proceed under less than ideal circumstances, but even then—by history, examination and the initial diagnostic studies—the surgeon must have a resonable idea about the location of the lesion and a strong suspicion about its character.

General Procedure

The scalp incision used must be planned to provide good exposure, but other factors must also be considered. An effort should be made to minimize exposure of the scar when the hair grows back. In most instances the entire head should be shaved. The bandage (head dressing) stays on better, and the surgeon will not find strands of hair contaminating the sterile surgical field. In some cases, with female patients, limited shaving can be done, but in this day and time with wigs available it is not necessary. In most cases, except with baldness, the incision can be made within the field of hair growth; there is no reason for a scar to be left on the forehead. In posterior fossa craniotomies, a vertical midline incision is usually made that extends to midneck. Female patients have no trouble hiding such a scar with their longer hair. Males, with their generally shorter hair, have minimal scar exposure and it is not unsightly.

The most important consideration in deciding what incision to use is the blood supply of the scalp flap—that portion of the scalp that is turned aside for exposure. Figure 6-1 illustrates some of the incisions that might be used with consideration given to the cosmetic factors and blood supply.

Bleeding is brisk with scalp incisions because of the scalp's blood supply. The bleeding is usually controlled by placing special clips along the edges of the incision or by using the electrocautery forceps. The special clip has a slot into which an applier inserts. When the applier is opened by the surgeon, the clip opens and can be inserted over the edge of the incision. When the applier is removed, the steel or plastic clip compresses any bleeding in the skin edge (Figure 6-2).

When the incision is completed and bleeding has been controlled (hemostasis has been achieved) by the use of the clips, the scalp is easily separated from the underlying bone. The portion of the scalp that is turned aside is called the scalp flap.

The next step in the craniotomy is to turn the bone flap. There are different ways to accomplish this part of the operation. First a hole is drilled in the skull. The classic method was to use a hand drill much the same as that used by a carpenter to drill a hole in wood. Today the hole is drilled with air-driven or electric drills. The basic feature of the drill points is, however, pretty much the same. The hole drilled has slanting sides so that the drill cannot plunge into the brain when the hole is completely through the skull.

In the classic method it is necessary to make several burr holes in the configuration of the bone flap required; the circular bone flap is in actual fact a multisided flap. When the burr holes are completed, a saw guide is inserted into one of the holes and then pushed toward the next hole, separating the dura from the skull (Figure 6-3). A loop on one end of the gigli saw (wire saw) is placed over the hook on the saw guide. The guide is then pulled through the second hole, thereby pulling the wire saw through also. When this is done the wire saw exits each hole. Next handles are placed into the loop on each end

Figure 6-1

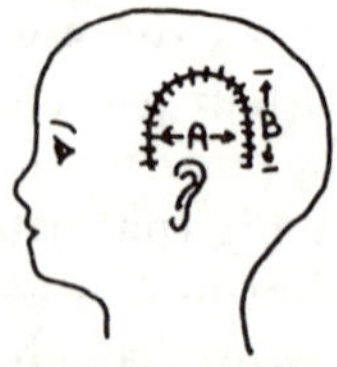

HORSESHOE-SHAPED INCISION

THIS INCISION CAN BE PLACED AT ANY POINT WITHIN THE FIELD OF HAIR GROWTH. THE LOCATION AND AMOUNT OF EXPOSURE NEEDED ARE THE LIMITING FACTORS. THE BLOOD SUPPLY WILL BE ADEQUATE IF THE BASE OF THE FLAP (LINE A) IS AT LEAST ONE-HALF THE LENGTH OF THE FLAP (LINE B).

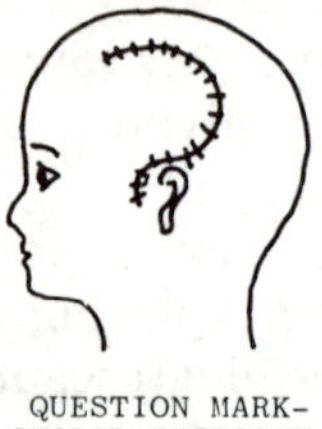

QUESTION MARK-SHAPED INCISION

THIS INCISION PROVIDES EXPOSURE OF THE POSTERIOR HALF OF THE FRONTAL LOBE AND VARIABLE AMOUNTS OF THE TEMPORAL AND PARIETAL LOBES. THE SAME CONSIDERATION OF BLOOD SUPPLY IS NECESSARY HERE AS IT WAS WITH THE HORSESHOE INCISION.

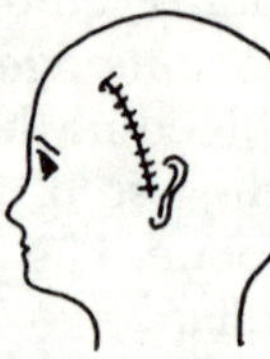

LINEAR INCISION BEHIND HAIRLINE

THIS INCISION PERMITS EXPOSURE OF THE POSTERIOR FRONTAL AND ANTERIOR TEMPORAL LOBES. IT PROVIDES A GOOD APPROACH ALONG THE SPHENOID WING TO THE REGION OF THE OPTIC NERVES AND INTERNAL CAROTID ARTERY. IT IS A GOOD APPROACH FOR POSTERIOR COMMUNICATING ANEURYSMS. THE BLOOD SUPPLY IS NO PROBLEM.

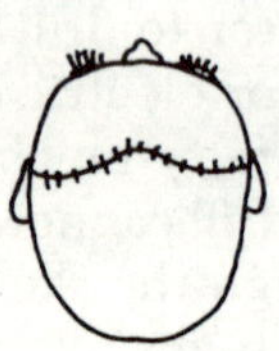

BICORONAL INCISION

THIS INCISION AFFORDS EXPOSURE OF THE FRONTAL LOBES. IT ALSO PERMITS ACCESS TO THE PITUITARY AND OPTIC NERVES. THE SCALP OF THE FOREHEAD IS TURNED FORWARD, EXPOSING THE BONE OF THE FRONT OF THE SKULL TO THE EYEBROWS. BLOOD SUPPLY IS GOOD.

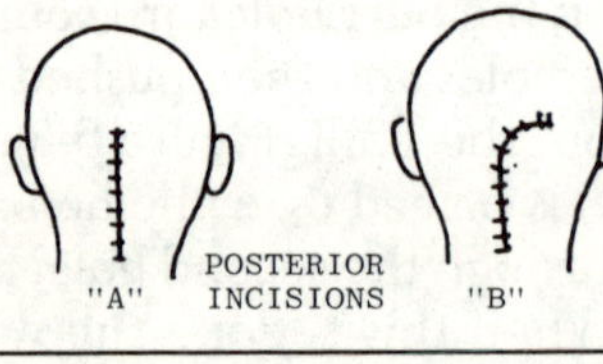

"A" POSTERIOR INCISIONS "B"

THESE INCISIONS ARE USED FOR ACCESS TO THE POSTERIOR FOSSA. "A" IS USED FOR MIDLINE LESIONS WHILE "B" AFFORDS BETTER EXPOSURE TO THE RIGHT SIDE OF THE CEREBELLUM.

Figure 6-2

of the saw, so that the surgeon can now saw through the skull by pulling each end alternately. The saw cut is from the inside of the skull out so that the brain is not cut (Figure 6-3).

Today the availability of electrical or air-driven saws greatly reduces the time required to cut through the skull. These are of great help when the situation dictates the need for speed in getting to the

Figure 6-3

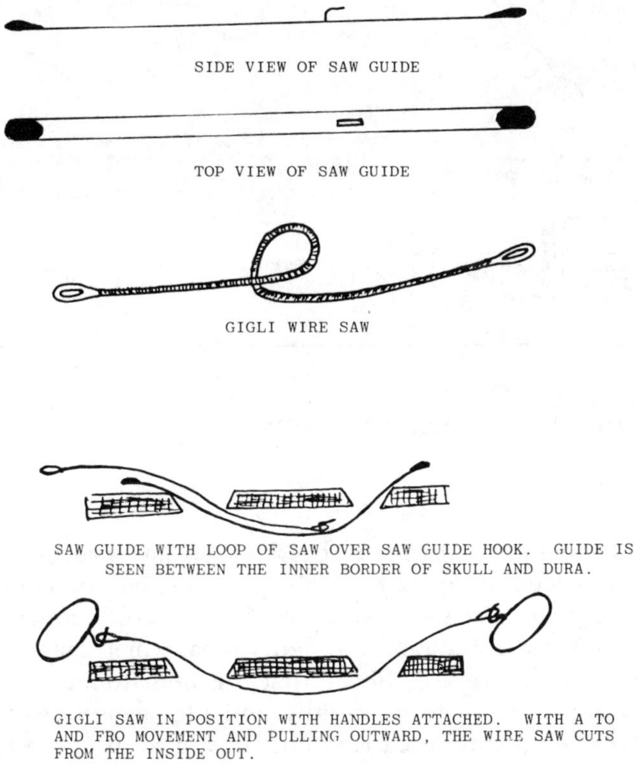

lesion. The mechanical saw and the steps in cutting the skull with it are illustrated in Figures 6-4 and 6-5.

When the craniotomy is done for lesions in the posterior fossa, a bone flap is not turned (Figure 6-6). Instead a burr hole is made and the bone is removed piecemeal, using a bone rongeur. Bone removal usually includes the back wall of the foramen magnum and variable portions of the lamina of C_1 and C_2.

Figure 6-4 Mechanical Saw

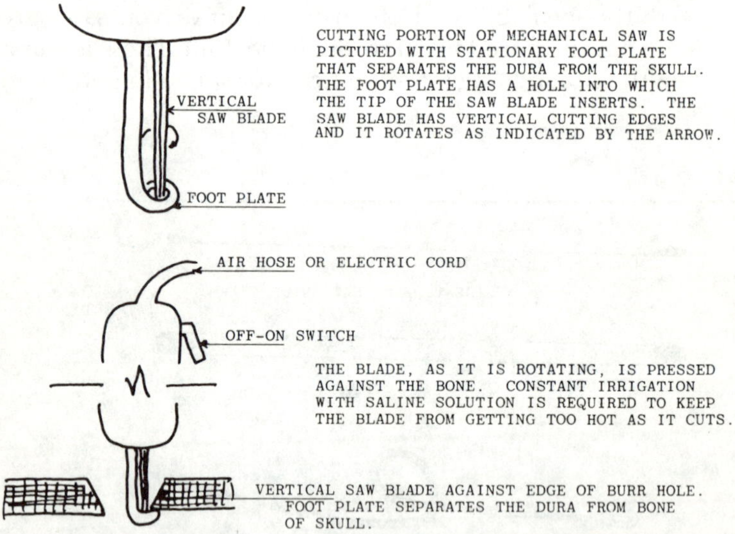

Management of Specific Lesions

Epidural Mass

Turning the bone flap exposes the dura, so any process that has occurred in the epidural (extradural) space will be immediately exposed. Though abscesses can occur, by far the most common lesion to be encountered is the epidural hematoma, which may occur following trauma (Figure 6-7). Recall that this hematoma results from a torn meningeal artery, forms rapidly, and often causes death before surgical treatment can be carried out. In Figure 6-7, the epidural hematoma is pictured lying between the inner table of the skull and

Figure 6-5 Cutting a Bone Flap with a Mechanical Saw

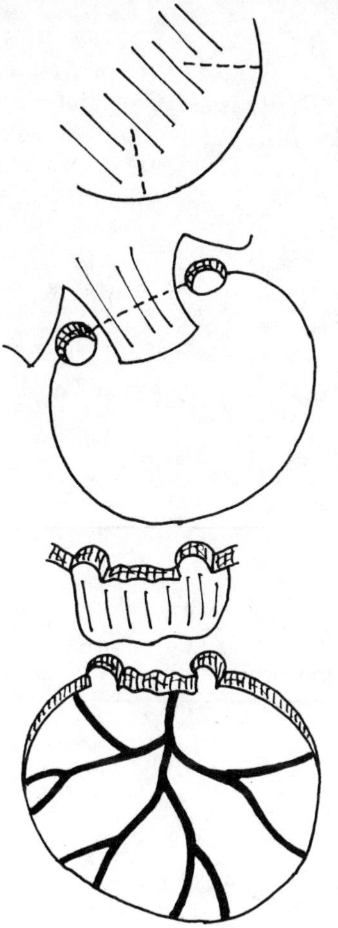

the dura. The brain is indented by this mass. The blood clot is easily removed either by gently scraping it off the dura or by suction. Often the torn meningeal artery can be identified after the blood clot is removed. The bleeding can usually be stopped by cauterizing the bleeding vessel with the electrocautery forceps.

Subdural Mass

If the lesion is a subdural mass; the surgeon is faced with certain considerations when the bone flap has been turned and the dura

Figure 6-6 Removal of Bone Required for a Posterior Fossa Craniotomy

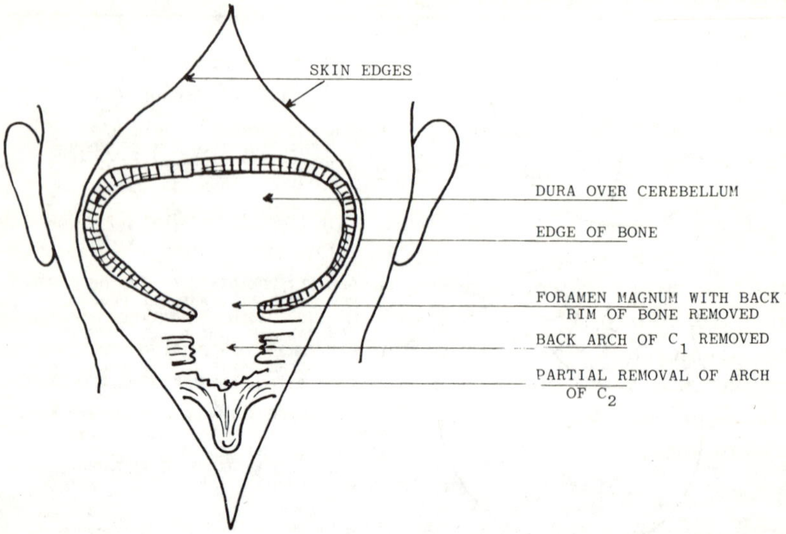

Figure 6-7 Epidural Hematoma

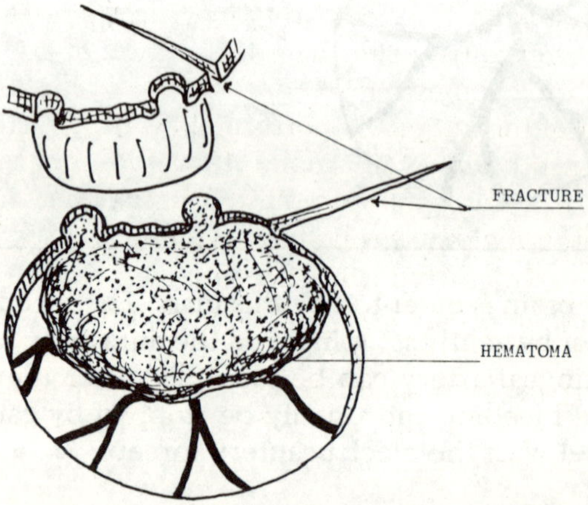

exposed. The opening of the dura, which exposes the brain, should not be done without some planning.

The dural opening should be adequate to accomplish the intended procedure. Poor exposure necessitates compromise on the surgeon's part and prolongs the operating time. On the other hand, wide and unneeded exposure is not good because exposed brain is potentially in danger of injury from instruments and is subject to drying.

If the pressure is high, opening of the dura may permit the brain to herniate through the opening. This can produce local injury to the brain by pressure against the opened dural edge. Rapid herniation may even result in lacerations of the brain. The experienced surgeon can reasonably estimate the pressure by gently touching the dura with the fingertips. If the pressure is judged to be excessive, certain steps can be taken to reduce it: The steps that can be taken are as follows:

1. The anesthesiologist can increase the rate of respiration of the anesthetized patient, which reduces the amount of carbon dioxide in the blood. This causes the blood vessels in the brain to constrict somewhat. The sum total of this effect is to diminish brain volume significantly. Recall that the brain blood vessels are very sensitive to the carbon dioxide levels in the blood: Increased CO_2 causes them to dilate; decreased CO_2 produces constriction.

2. The patient may be given dehydrating agents. These drugs withdraw water from the body's organs, including the brain, and cause it to be excreted as urine. The withdrawal of the water causes the brain to shrink somewhat.

3. The administration of cortisonelike drugs (steroids) often helps to diminish brain swelling and, therefore, helps lessen intracranial pressure. The response to these drugs is usually not manifest rapidly enough to be of great help if given during surgery. If, however, surgery is anticipated, the effect may be very dramatic if the drug is given several hours before the operation.

4. Spinal fluid can be removed. This can be done by tapping the subarachnoid space in the manner described in the lumbar puncture technique in Chapter 4. Removal of the CSF lessens the amount of the fluid in the ventricles and along the base of the brain, thus decreasing the intracranial pressure.

5. The ventricles or the lesion can be tapped with a special brain needle called a brain cannula. If the ventricles are tapped, CSF

can be removed. If the lesion has a fluid component, this can be aspirated through the brain cannula by using a syringe. If the lesion is a tumor with a cyst, it is often possible to aspirate a good deal of the cystic fluid, reducing the pressure. In like fashion, hematomas can be tapped and can be aspirated, but if the hematoma is a solid clot, aspiration is difficult. The cannula is calibrated in centimeters so that, when the lesion is reached, its depth can be determined. When the cannula is in the lesion, the stylet is removed; and in many instances cyst fluid or blood, if present, will come out spontaneously. If nothing comes from the needle, a syringe is attached to the cannula hub and gentle aspiration is applied.

Cannulation of the brain, then, is of significant value. It not only affords a way to decrease intracranial pressure but aids in the location of certain intracerebral lesions. This information is of value when determining how the dura is to be opened. It is usually not necessary to make a wide dural opening when the location of the lesion is known precisely. Sometimes only a short linear incision is all that is needed. The general technique used in opening the dura is illustrated in Figures 6-8 and 6-9.

Intracerebral Mass

A variety of lesions can occur within the substance of the brain. In most instances a brain cannula is passed to the lesion site; this gives the depth and direction to be taken. The brain is then incised, with careful consideration given to the site of the lesion. The surgeon does not electively go into or through the cortex of important areas, such

Figure 6-8 Dura Opened, Exposing the Brain

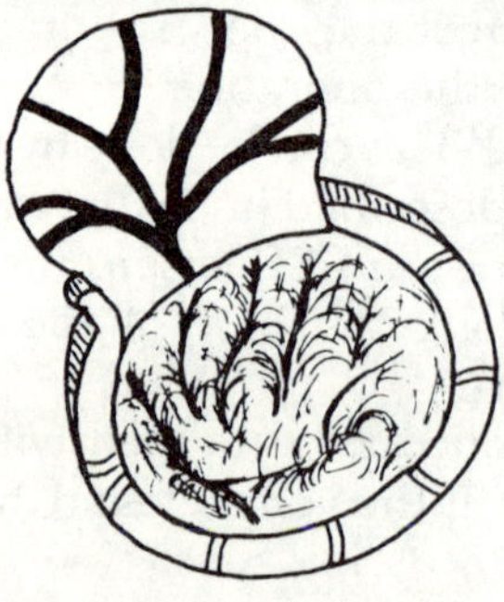

THE DURA IS OPENED BY MAKING A SHORT INCISION IN IT WITH A #11 OR #15 BLADE. SCISSORS ARE THEN USED, TAKING CARE NOT TO INJURE THE BRAIN WITH THE TIPS. EACH CUT SHOULD BE VISUALIZED DIRECTLY SO ONE DOESN'T CUT INTO THE DURAL SINUSES OR CUT VEINS THAT BRIDGE BETWEEN THE DURA AND THE CORTEX.

Figure 6-9 Subdural Mass

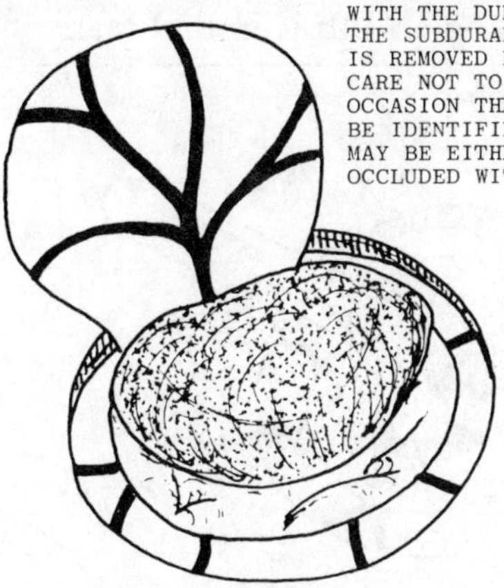

as the speech area or the motor strip. In the effort to help the patient with the operation, one certainly does not want to create further neurological injury. Thus the cortical incision is made where the least chance of injury is likely. It is best if the site has no large arteries or veins that will be sacrificed. The cortex is cauterized and then carefully incised with a Number 15 blade. Now the brain is entered. The surgeon holds a narrow, malleable brain retractor in one hand and a small suction tip in the other. The incision is made deeper with the suction and subsequent gentle retraction. The course into the brain is oriented so that it is the shortest possible route to the lesion. It is often possible to visually follow the track made by the brain cannula. It must be kept constantly in mind that the track made by the suction divides nerve fibers; therefore the surgeon must stay out of the more important areas. Once the lesion is encountered, the operation from that point on depends on the type of lesion present (Figure 6-10).

Tumor

If a tumor is encountered, it is a good idea to take a biopsy of it. Though the surgeon may have a good idea what the tumor is, the pathologist can often be specific and also determine malignancy. Given this information the surgeon must know the prognosis and the best treatment for that certain tumor.

Benign tumor. If, by a frozen section, the pathologist determines that a tumor is benign, an attempt at total gross removal (all tumor

Figure 6-10 Dura Opened and Reflected; Incision in the Brain; Malleable Retractors in Position, Gently Exposing an Intracerebral Mass

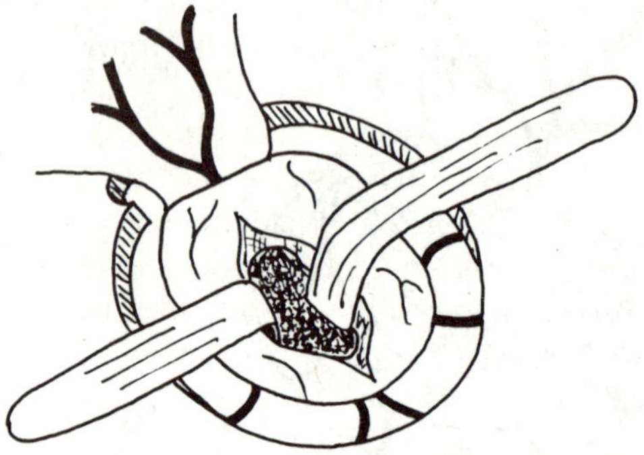

that can be seen) should be considered. Unfortunately this is not common because most intracerebral tumors are malignant. Even though the tumor is benign, it may be difficult to remove it. Thus the surgeon must decide whether an attempt to remove the tumor will cause the patient serious injury; quality of survival is so very important. Sad to say, some benign tumors are in effect malignant because of their location; so much injury is likely from an attempt to remove the tumor that it is best left alone or at least left alone until there is no reasonable alternative.

If removal of the benign tumor is to be attempted, it should usually be done as small pieces rather than as a single mass. The removal in a single mass requires a larger brain incision and greater retraction, and often it is technically more difficult. One situation in which an attempt to remove the tumor as a single mass is better is when bleeding is too great with piecemeal removal. In this case the surgeon works around the outer limits of the tumor, cauterizing and cutting all blood vessels that leave and enter the tumor. It is fortunate that most benign tumors have definite limiting membranes or actual capsules; their limits are much more definite than those of malignant tumors.

When the surgeon is forced to stop resection short of total removal, the tumor will almost definitely recur and again become symptomatic. Fortunately many of the benign tumors grow slowly so the patient may live several years before symptoms occur again. It is possible that a benign tumor that is not totally removed can be reoperated on several times. But because of scarring, each reoperation becomes more difficult.

Primary malignant tumor. If a tumor is malignant it must be decided if an attempt for total removal should be made. The surgeon is aware that a total gross removal does not mean the patient will be cured for it is most likely that the tumor will recur and go on to cause the patient's death. The surgeon can, however, remove a sizable portion of the tumor, thereby relieving the high intracranial pressure and lessening local pressure on adjacent nerve pathways. Clinically the patient should be relieved of headache and might experience some improvement in neurological symptoms. The surgeon's mission, then, is to improve the patient's symptoms at least for awhile, knowing that ultimately he or she will fail. An additional period of life in comfort and relatively free of handicap is worth a good deal.

It is best, if the patient will not be injured further, to attempt removal, thereby relieving the increased intracranial pressure. This treatment can then be supplemented with X-ray therapy and chemotherapy. If removal is attempted, the principle is to work within the tumor, removing it with suction or forceps. By working from inside outward, injury to adjacent normal cells and fiber tracts can be minimized. The limits of some tumors are difficult to determine. There is often an insidious change from obviously malignant tissue to relatively normal-appearing white matter. In fact uninvolved white matter next to the tumor often does not appear normal because of edema. The surgeon must make a judgment about when to stop removal. Primary brain tumors, and especially the astrocytoma, often have very ill-defined borders, whereas metastatic tumors in the brain may have very definite borders and "shell out" quite easily. Following the removal of the tumor, bleeding is stopped using the electrocautery forceps and gelfoam (Figure 6-11).

The failure of surgery to cure malignant brain tumors necessitates the consideration of the use of radiation therapy and chemotherapy. The employment of these modes of therapy requires knowledge of certain principles and clinical concepts.

Radiation therapy kills cells that are actively dividing. Because tumor growth is accomplished by rapid division of malignant cells, it is logical that radiation therapy would be helpful in cancer treatment. There was for some time a question, however, whether in actual practice radiation therapy was effective in the treatment of malignant brain tumors; there is now no doubt about its usefulness.

Figure 6-11 Methods for Stopping Bleeding in Neurosurgery

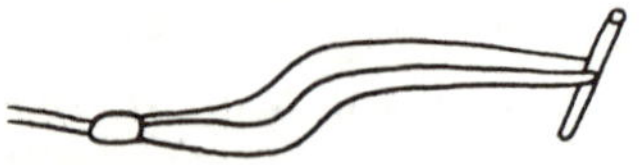

ELECTROCAUTERY FORCEPS

1. ELECTROCAUTERY FORCEPS- THE BLOOD VESSEL IS GRASPED BY THE FORCEPS. THE SURGEON STEPS ON A FOOT PEDAL THAT CAUSES THE TIPS OF THE FORCEPS TO GET HOT AND COAGULATE THE VESSEL.

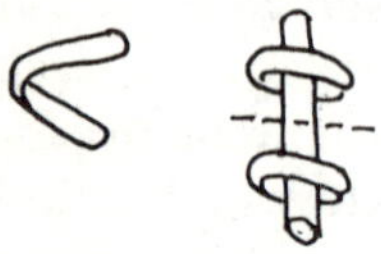

VASCULAR CLIPS

2. VASCULAR CLIPS- THE LITTLE METALIC CLIP IS HELD BY A HAND-HELD APPLIER. IT IS CRIMPED ACROSS THE BLOOD VESSEL. IF A VESSEL NEEDS TO BE CUT, TWO CLIPS ARE APPLIED AND THE VESSEL IS CUT BETWEEN THEM WITH SCISSORS.

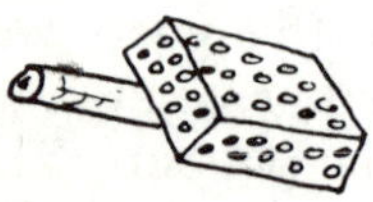

GELFOAM

3. GELFOAM- GELATIN SPONGES ARE USED AND MAY BE CUT TO ANY SIZE: USUALLY ABOUT ONE-HALF TO ONE-FOURTH THE SIZE OF A POSTAGE STAMP. THEY ARE SOAKED IN SALINE OR THROMBIN SOLUTION OR MAY BE USED DRY. THEY ARE PLACED ON A BLEEDING VESSEL AND PRESSED GENTLY TO IT. THE GELFOAM STICKS FIRMLY. IT WORKS WELL FOR BLEEDING VEINS AND SMALL ARTERIES. CAUTERY OR CLIPS ARE NEEDED FOR LARGER ARTERIES. THESE GELFOAM PADDIES ARE LEFT IN PLACE.

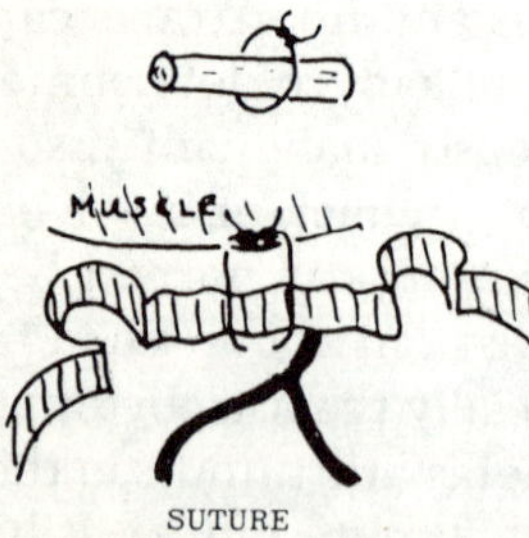

SUTURE

4. SUTURE- BLEEDING VESSELS CAN BE TIED WITH SUTURE BUT IT IS NOT OFTEN NEEDED IN NEUROSURGERY.

"TACK UP" SUTURES ARE COMMONLY USED TO STOP BLEEDING THAT COMES FROM THE EPIDURAL SPACE. THE SUTURE PULLS THE DURA TIGHTLY AGAINST THE INSIDE OF THE SKULL, WHICH HELPS TO DISCOURAGE BLEEDING. WHEN A CRANIOTOMY IS CLOSED THESE STITCHES ARE COMMONLY USED ROUTINELY TO PREVENT THE FORMATION OF EPIDURAL HEMATOMAS POST-OPERATIVELY.

It has been observed that a patient's length of survival is significantly prolonged when radiation therapy is given following surgery. Thus the combination of surgery and radiation therapy is more effective as treatment than is surgery alone or radiation therapy alone.

The optimal amount of radiation therapy is 5,000–6,000 rads. Usually the entire head is irradiated with approximately 4,500 rads, and the remainder is restricted to the vicinity of the tumor.

Patients receiving radiation therapy to the head usually lose their hair. In some cases it will grow back later but it is rarely ever normal. The scalp is usually red and has the tendency to become dry and scaly during the period of radiation treatment. Much of the discomfort experienced, such as itching and scaling, can be minimized with the use of moisturizing body lotion or creams.

Chemical substances are also used to treat malignant tumors of virtually every organ of the body. Their use in the treatment of leukemia in childhood is very effective. Although they are minimally effective in treating malignant brain tumors, research continues toward developing more effective substances.

Chemotherapeutic agents act to kill rapidly dividing cells, which is why they are useful in treating malignancies. It was initially believed that, because of the blood-brain barrier, chemical substances would be relatively ineffective for the treatment of malignant tumors of the brain. Evidence indicates, however, that within the substance of the tumor the blood-brain barrier is altered so most substances pass freely between the vascular space and the tumor cells.

The most effective chemotherapeutic agents in the treatment of malignant brain tumors are the nitrosoureas. BCNU is the designation of the member of this group most commonly used. It is given intravenously in short courses and is repeated every 6 to 8 weeks.

There are many adverse side effects from the use of most chemotherapy agents because their effects are not limited to tumor cells. Bone marrow, which like tumor cells has rapid cell division, is also affected. Therefore the patient receiving chemotherapy may develop a low white blood cell count, decreased platelets, and anemia.

Clinical studies indicate that, if chemotherapy (BCNU) is given following surgery to a patient with a malignant brain tumor, there is a significant prolongation of life. When it is given along with radiation therapy after surgery, the length of survival is even greater. Therefore available evidence indicates that, if possible, a patient should have a full course of radiation following surgery and should be placed on a chemotherapy program.

Metastatic tumors. Metastatic brain tumors such as those from lung or breast may also be treated with radiation and chemotherapy. There are, however, some differences to consider between the management of metastatic brain tumors and that of primary malignant brain tumors.

Recall that craniotomy is indicated if a primary malignant brain tumor is suspected and if it can be done without undue risk and without producing severe neurological deficit. If, however, the tumor is likely to be metastatic (if there is a known malignancy elsewhere in the body), it should be realized that the patient probably has more than one brain metastasis. In the case of multiple brain metastases, a craniotomy would probably be of little benefit to the patient. If the metastasis is shown by computerized axial tomography (CAT scan) to be solitary, and if it is an immediate threat to life, surgery may be considered. However, the neurosurgeon should never, in the latter case, forget to consider the patient as a whole. For example, to remove a solitary metastasis from the brain would be foolish were the patient soon to die anyway from widespread metastasis to other organs of the body.

Radiation therapy is useful for metastatic brain tumors as well as primary malignant ones, although clinically it is probably of more benefit with primary malignant tumors. On the other hand, radiation therapy may be the only thing to offer the patient with cerebral metastasis. This is especially true of the patient with multiple metastases. So far chemotheraputic agents have little to offer the patient with cerebral metastasis. Certainly there is no strong statistical evidence to support their value.

The value of corticosteroids (cortisone) has been discussed. They are particularly valuable in reducing brain swelling, which occurs with both primary malignant and metastatic brain tumors. For some reason metastatic tumors especially cause swelling of the brain that surrounds them. The patient with headache and nausea caused by such swelling is often dramatically improved in a short time after cortisone is given. When a patient is given radiation therapy, the malignant cells often swell initially. Corticosteroids may be needed to lessen this reactive swelling until the cells die and undergo necrosis.

Hematoma

The diagnosis of an intracerebral hematoma is usually made by history and confirmed by cannulation with a brain cannula. It is difficult to remove the entire clot by aspiration through a cannula. This is especially true when the hematoma is relatively new. It is, therefore, necessary to remove it under direct vision through a cortical incision. The hematoma is easily removed with a small suction tip. Gentle irrigation with saline will wash out portions of the clot in many cases. When removal is accomplished, the hematoma cavity should be searched for actively bleeding vessels. Usually the original bleeder has stopped bleeding long before surgery because of the local pressure effect of the hematoma itself. If indeed this does not occur, the patient usually dies before getting to the hospital. When the surgeon is satisfied that no active bleeding is occurring, the craniotomy is closed in the usual manner.

Brain Abscess

The treatment of brain abscesses is never clear-cut. In some cases there is disagreement whether surgery is even indicated. Certainly the timing in the use of surgery is of paramount importance. The early stages of abscess formation are by nature largely local inflammation with brain swelling. There is at this point no pus present, so surgery would be of no help and could even be hazardous. It is best to wait until the abscess is well-formed with a strong capsule surrounding the collection of necrotic material before doing surgery. Antibiotics are used during the phase of inflammation and early capsule formation. The choice of antibiotics depends on the suspected bacteria and its sensitivity to antibiotics as determined by culture. The bacteria is identified by a search elsewhere for a primary source of infection, such as infected sinuses, ears, or scalp lesion.

Brain abscesses may occur secondary to lung infections or infections that begin on scarred heart valves. If the patient shows signs of increased intracranial pressure during the early stages of abscess formation, dehydrating agents and even cortisonelike drugs can be tried in addition to antibiotics. The effort is to buy time, giving the body a chance, with the help of antibiotics, to recover from the inflammation or to form a thick wall around the central collection of pus. In some instances, in spite of these stopgap efforts, the surgeon's hand is forced because the patient's status begins to deteriorate from the results of increased pressure. When this occurs a craniotomy must be done. The skin incision and bone flap turned depend on the location of the abscess. A decision is then necessary on whether the lesion should be tapped by a brain cannula. Cannulation will tell the depth and direction of the abscess. On the other hand if the capsules are very thin and are penetrated by the cannula, infection can spread along the cannula tract, or pus may spill onto the brain and dura when the stylet is removed.

If antibiotic administration has been long enough, the abscess may be sterile; but the surgeon cannot count on it. If spillage does occur, the surgeon must decide how to manage the situation. One choice is to aspirate as much pus as possible through the cannula and then irrigate the cavity with saline or antibiotic solution. (Not all antibiotics can be used in irrigation solution used in the brain. They are often toxic; and when they are used, it is at a lesser concentration in most instances). Some type of tubing (catheter) may be threaded along the cannula tract, terminating in the abscess cavity. The other end could exit the wound and be incorporated into the dressing. This method would provide a way for frequent irrigation and antibiotic installation.

The surgeon may, as an alternative, choose to enter the cavity directly through a brain incision. Then she or he could probably drain the cavity better and could irrigate with an antibiotic solution more effectively than through the catheter. The wound could then be closed, the intracranial pressure having been lessened. The patient would contine to receive the appropriate antibiotics.

If the index of suspicion of a brain abscess is high, the surgeon could decline use of the cannula, certainly avoiding penetration of the capsule, and make an attempt to remove the abscess intact, thereby avoiding contamination of the surgical field. The problem with this attempt would be the requirement for a larger cortical incision and, very likely, greater retraction. Again the surgeon must keep in mind the possibility of causing greater neurological injury.

The last option is to avoid surgery at all costs. Certainly with adequate antibiotic coverage, abscesses may heal. They have been shown to lessen in size, and eventually only a small, wrinkled scar remains.

Arteriovenous Malformations

A craniotomy done for removal of an arteriovenous malformation (AVM) presents some special problems. Recall from Chapter 2 that an AVM consists of a tangle of abnormal blood vessels occurring within brain tissue. AVMs occur in the cerebral hemispheres, cerebellum, brainstem, and even the spinal cord. The AVM is fed by arteries that make direct connections with veins that subsequently drain the malformation. Thus there are no capillaries, which normally occur between arteries and veins. Because of the absence of capillaries, adjacent brain tissue is not provided with an adequate oxygen supply. It is at the capillary level that the exchange of oxygen and carbon dioxide normally occurs. Consequently neurons adjacent to the AVM function abnormally or at least poorly. Seizures are commonly associated with AVM and are a manifestation of abnormal function of neurons. In addition to the absence of capillaries in an AVM, the vessels present are often thin-walled and commonly rupture. Their rupture causes the formation of a spontaneous intracerebral hematoma. When a spontaneous intracerebral hematoma forms, it is necessary to perform a craniotomy to remove the hematoma. The patient deteriorates because of the increased intracranial pressure produced by the enlarging hematoma.

Actual removal of an AVM is possible in some cases, but consideration of several factors is required before this is attempted. Many AVMs simply are inoperable because of their size and location. It is not uncommon to find an AVM that occupies a good share of one cerebral hemisphere. It gets its blood supply from several vessels and often from cerebral vessels on both sides of the brain. The draining veins are usually multiple, and they are often deep within the brain. In the case of these massive AVMs and those located in important areas, nothing can be done to remove them that would not be likely to be disastrous to the patient.

When the AVM is small and not in the more important areas of the brain, removal is commonly attempted. The surgeon studies the cerebral arteriograms carefully, often making diagrams of certain parts of the AVM. The basic effort is to shut off the blood supply to the AVM. Thus the major feeding arteries are identified, isolated, and then divided. The arteries are occluded by applying metallic clips or by using the electrocautery forceps. The surgery is usually done with an operating microscope. This provides not only magnification but also a good light. The surgeon works around the entire AVM, identifying and dividing all feeding arteries. When veins are encountered, they are left alone. If a major vein is occluded and divided before the majority of the arteries are divided, the AVM will burst and bleed profusely. When all of the arteries are divided, the AVM shrinks in size dramatically. Finally the few remaining veins can be divided, and the entire AVM can be lifted out of the brain.

Aneurysms

No problem in neurological surgery is more ticklish than taking care of a patient with a ruptured intracranial aneurysm. The onset of this illness is as sudden as if the patient were hit in the head with an ax. The rupture of the aneurysm often occurs during times of exertion, such as during a bowel movement. A sudden and terrific headache occurs because the blood that goes into the subarachnoid space is very irritating. The patient has marked stiffness of the neck, which is called nuchal rigidity. It too is a manifestation of this irritation.

When an aneurysm ruptures, the survival of the patient depends on whether the bleeding stops or not. If it does not, death is usually swift, and many such patients die before reaching the hospital. Those who survive, because the bleeding stops, show a great variability in neurological status. Some are normal, complaining only of headache, whereas others are deeply comatose, showing signs of severe and probably irreversible brainstem injury. There are several causes for severe neurological injury when an aneurysm ruptures. Large hematomas occur in addition to the blood that mixes with the CSF (subarachnoid hemorrhage). The hematomas may occur outside of the brain, or the pressure of the jet of blood coming out of the bleeding aneurysm can lacerate the brain, permitting the formation of an intracerebral hematoma. Regardless of the site, the hematoma causes markedly increased intracranial pressure.

Acute hydrocephalus is another complication that can occur. The blood in the CSF spaces along the base of the brain causes obstruction of the subarachnoid space and halts CSF circulation, creating another potential source of increased intracranial pressure. Still another complication is arterial spasm, and unfortunately it happens quite often. Why spasm occurs is not really known, but it is probably a response to certain substances in the blood, specifically in the red blood cells. Spasm is not always present initially but it may appear at any time following the bleed. It may occur in a patient who initially had no neurological findings. The problem produced by the spasm is that it may be so severe that the amount of blood that can flow through the spastic vessels is inadequate. The brain is then ischemic, and massive infarction with severe neurological deficit or even death can occur.

The diagnosis of a ruptured aneurysm can usually be made by history. A lumbar puncture confirms the diagnosis when bloody spinal fluid is obtained. A cerebral arteriogram is then done to locate the aneurysm and to identify any associated hematoma or spasm.

If a hematoma is present and the patient is deteriorating, a craniotomy is done to remove it. It is probably best to leave the aneurysm alone at that time and plan to go back after it when the patient has had a few days to stabilize.

If significant spasm is present on the arteriogram, nothing should be done surgically. Surgery to ligate an aneurysm when severe spasm is present is almost always a disaster for the patient. It is best to wait, supporting the patient, until the spasm resolves. It may be necessary to repeat the cerebral arteriogram every 4 to 5 days until this study shows no significant spasm.

The initial stages of a craniotomy to approach a ruptured aneurysm are the same as in any craniotomy. A skin flap and bone flap are turned in the manner already described. The intracranial pressure is often increased, so it may be necessary to take steps to lessen the pressure before opening the dura. When the dura is opened, the final approach toward the aneurysm is achieved by gentle retraction.

Several different approaches may be made depending on the location of the aneurysm. The initial effort is to reach the artery from which the aneurysm arises and to reach it before the "takeoff site" of the aneurysm. This permits proximal control that may be needed if the aneurysm ruptures. If it should rupture prematurely, a temporary clip may be placed across the artery for a brief period until control is achieved. For example, for either anterior or posterior communicating aneurysms, the internal carotid artery is first exposed. Using malleable brain retractors, the surgeon then follows the course of this vessel by very careful and gentle retraction of the brain. If a posterior communicating aneurysm is present, it will soon be encountered because it arises directly from the internal carotid artery (Figure 6–12).

On the other hand if there is an anterior communicating aneurysm, the surgeon continues to follow the internal carotid artery until it branches into the anterior and middle cerebral arteries, then follows the anterior cerebral artery to the origin of the aneurysm. In like fashion the middle cerebral artery is followed if a middle cerebral artery aneurysm is present. Aneurysms also occur in the posterior fossa, but surgery to approach them is basically the same except that a posterior fossa approach is used.

By reviewing the pictures of the aneurysm on the cerebral arteriogram, the surgeon knows the best way to handle the aneurysm when it is exposed. Without a doubt the best way is to ligate the base of the aneurysm. This can be done if the neck of the aneurysm is narrow enough. Ligation may be done by simply tying a ligature

Figure 6-12 Exposure of a Cerebral Aneurysm

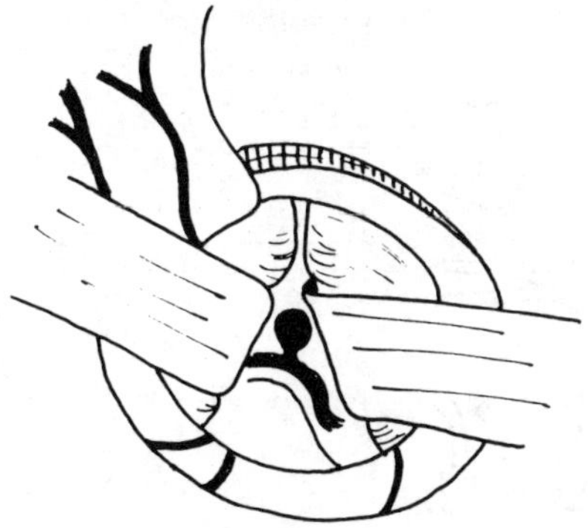

around the neck. This, however, may be difficult because of poor exposure. Consequently various types of metal clips have been developed. The best are small, delicate, spring-loaded clips that look something like a clothespin. They are placed in position with a handheld applier, which the surgeon uses to open the clip and to place it over the neck of the aneurysm. When the clip is released, it closes and stops blood flow into the aneurysm.

Unfortunately the aneurysm may have a configuration that makes clip application impossible, as when the neck of the aneurysm is too broad. Often, important vessels come off the side of the aneurysm so that clipping the neck would stop blood flow through these vessels. In this instance, sometimes by using curved or angled clips, just a portion of the aneurysm sac can be clipped, perserving blood flow through the vessels. This may be quite adequate because the fundus or dome of the aneurysm is usually the site of rupture (Figure 6–13).

Figure 6-13

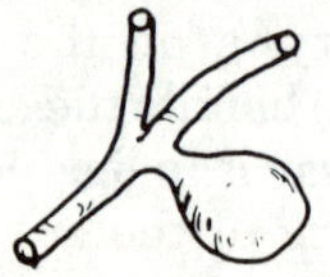

THIS ANEURYSM HAS A NARROW NECK. IT IS IDEAL FOR DIRECT CLIPPING.

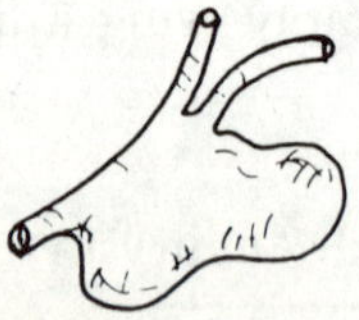

THIS ANEURYSM HAS TOO BROAD A BASE FOR CLIPPING. IT WOULD BE NECESSARY TO STRENGTHEN THE WALLS WITH METHYL-METHACRYLATE OR SOME OTHER SUBSTANCE.

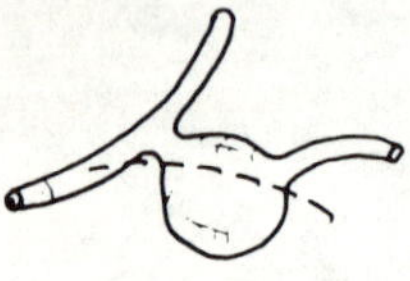

AN IMPORTANT VESSEL ARISES FROM THE WALL OF THE ANEURYSM. DIRECT CLIPPING OF THE NECK WOULD NOT BE WISE. A CURVED CLIP ALONG THE DOTTED LINE MIGHT WORK. IF NOT, THE ENTIRE ANEURYSM AND ARTERIES COULD POSSIBLY BE ENCASED.

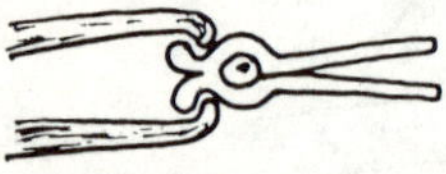

SIDE VIEW OF AN ANEURYSM CLIP WITH THE TIP OF THE HAND-HELD APPLIER SHOWN HOLDING THE CLIP.

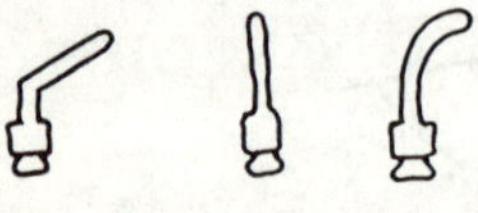

TOP VIEW OF THREE CLIPS, ILLUSTRATING SOME OF THE SHAPES AVAILABLE.

When clipping an aneurysm is considered ill advised, some other form of treatment must be used. The basic effort in most of the alternative approaches is to reinforce the aneurysm. Many materials have been used, including muscle and muslin. These substances are packed around the aneurysm sac, with the hope that, with some scarring of the wall of the aneurysm, it will become stronger. These attempts have been largely unsatisfactory because it is usually impossible to surround the entire aneurysm. If an attempt is made to expose the aneurysm completely, bleeding will occur in many cases.

Certain agents like methyl methacrylate have been developed to surround the aneurysm. These agents are prepared at the time of the operation. Initially they are liquid and can be squirted through a syringe or poured around the aneurysm. Within a few minutes the liquid becomes more viscous, and soon it solidifies into a hard material. If the entire aneurysm is thoroughly encased, there is little chance of rebleeding; but total encasement is often difficult at best. Some surgeons have found it helpful to put a few drops of this material around a clip that has been placed at the base of an aneurysm. This holds the clip in place, for it is possible for a clip to work its way off the neck.

Extracerebral Tumors

Some tumors occur inside the dura (intradural) but outside of the brain (extracerebral). The meningioma is a common tumor in this group. It occurs over the surface of the cerebral hemisphere as well as in the posterior fossa and along the brainstem. Because it is usually a benign tumor, total removal should always be attempted; if any of the tumor remains, it will recur. Judgment is, however, required because it is senseless to injure the patient when attempting complete removal; it could be better to risk recurrence and plan to reoperate later if necessary.

In operating on meningiomas that occur over the surface of the cerebral hemisphere, the dura is opened in a circular manner around the site of tumor origin. Because meningiomas arise from dura, the involved dura must be removed along with the tumor. Meningiomas grow very slowly and progressively embed themselves into the brain. In removing them, after the dura is incised, the surgeon works around the sides of the tumor, cauterizing and dividing all entering vessels. Gentle traction on sutures that are placed in the dura and attached to the tumor slowly lifts the tumor out of its bed. Great care is taken to protect the brain in the tumor bed because it is easily injured. In many cases it is eventually possible to remove the tumor as a single entity, along with the attached dura (Figure 6–14).

When the meningioma is in the posterior fossa and adjacent to the brainstem, total removal may not be practical. The capsule of the tumor may adhere densely to the brainstem and cranial nerves. Even using the operating microscope it may be impossible to remove all vestiges of tumor without seriously injuring the patient. In these cases the surgeon opens the tumor capsule and guts the tumor, then tries to remove as much capsule as possible, leaving behind those portions that are adhering densely to the brainstem and cranial nerves.

The other more common extracerebral tumors, such as the acoustic neuroma, the pituitary adenoma, and the craniopharyngioma, are handled like the meningioma. The capsule is opened and the tumor is gutted. Although removal of the entire capsule is desirable, often small attachments must be left. When removal has been completed, bleeding is controlled by cautery and plegettes of gelfoam.

Figure 6-14 Craniotomy Showing a Meningioma (Stippled) Embedded in the Surface of the Brain, with Two Retraction Sutures in the Edge of the Dura Pulling the Tumor Upward (the Portion of the Dura Attached to the Tumor Is to Be Removed with It because the Tumor Arises from the Dura)

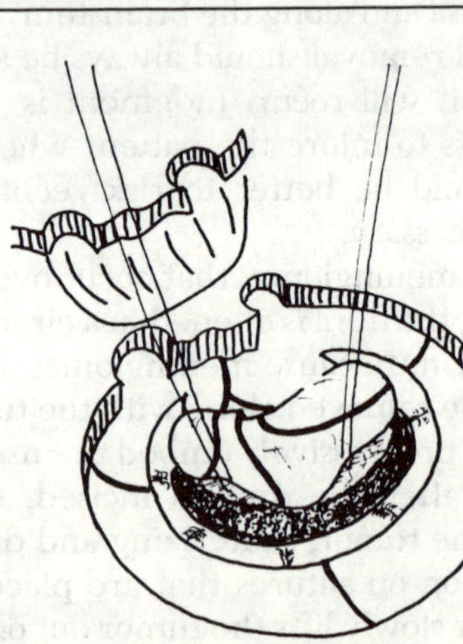

Closure of a Craniotomy

A craniotomy is never closed until all bleeding has stopped. It is a good idea to observe the brain for several minutes to be assured that no bleeding is occurring.

The dura should always be closed in a watertight manner. If CSF leaks from a craniotomy wound, the chance of meningitis developing is quite good. The dura can be closed by closely spaced, interrupted stitches or by a continuous running stitch. When a portion of dura is missing, as when a meningioma has been excised or when the dura is severely shredded in trauma, it may be necessary to sew in a graft. This piece of free tissue may be obtained from the fascia lata of the thigh or from the temporalis fascia if this is exposed by the scalp incision. Fascia is strong tissue that forms the compartments in which muscles work. It is cut to the desired size and configuration and then sewn into the dural defect.

The bone flap is then put into its normal position and tied or wired securely. A hole is drilled through the bone on each side of the saw cut. The suture or wire is passed through the holes and then tied. The scalp is then closed. Classically this is done in two layers with the galeal stitch being inverted. The galeal stitches are interrupted, whereas the skin stitch may be interrupted or continuous.

Finally a sterile bandage is applied to protect the wound from contamination. It should be tight enough to discourage bleeding under the flap but not so tight that it is uncomfortable.

Preoperative Care

I. A complete history and physical examination should be on the chart for quick referral by the anesthesiologist or other members of the medical team.
   A. This pertinent information should include not only the present illness and physical findings but also:
      1. Past medical illnesses
      2. Allergies
      3. Medication regularly taken by the patient, such as heart medications, insulin, etc.

II. The routine laboratory studies should be posted appropriately on the chart.
   A. Special studies that might be indicated should also be available. This would perhaps include pulmonary function studies, coagulation studies, etc.

B. Medical clearance should be obtained by an internist if the patient has significant medical illnesses such as diabetes mellitus and cardiac disease.

III. The X rays should be available in the operating room for quick referral if needed.

A. A chest X ray should be done on all patients undergoing general anesthesia.

B. Special studies like cerebral angiograms, brain scans, CAT scans, etc., should be available and they should be preselected for quick referral if required.

IV. Blood should be drawn, typed, and cross matched, and a sufficient supply should be available in case it should be needed during surgery.

A. If any special blood components, such as packed cells or split packs, will be required, arrangements should be made for this to be done ahead of time.

V. An electrocardiogram should be obtained on all patients over 35 years of age if a general anesthesia is to be given. If the patient has any history of cardiac disease, an EKG should be done regardless of the patient's age.

VI. An indwelling catheter should be placed in the bladder if a long procedure is likely and especially if dehydrating agents will be given.

VII. Elastic stockings or elastic wraps should be applied to the legs and should extend from the tip of the toes to the groin.

A. The stockings or wraps are used to prevent pooling of blood in superficial veins. If a seated position is used in surgery, elastic stockings or wraps are especially necessary.

B. The wraps are also valuable in the postoperative period to lessen the chance of thrombophlebitis.

VIII. Hair should be washed with hexachlorophene or an iodine soap preparation the night prior to surgery.

A. Care should be made that the patient is not chilled.

B. IMPORTANT: Shaving should not be done the night before surgery for the following reasons:

1. Close shaving with a razor is painful.
2. Scratches or nicks may be made that harbor bacteria.
3. The surgical procedure may be postponed or canceled for some reason.
4. Shaving adds to the anxiety and apprehension the patient experiences.

IX. Ideally, preoperative rounds are performed by the anesthesiologist who will administer the anesthesia. In doing so, he or she can greatly assist the surgeon as well as the patient by:

A. Reviewing the chart and noting the need for any preoperative studies that might have been overlooked.
B. Answering questions the patient may have; discussing starting the IV (the induction of anesthesia) and forewarning the patient of a possible sore throat from the endotracheal tube, or other matters of importance.
C. Writing the orders for the preoperative medication to be given. After seeing the patient and after reviewing the chart, it is possible to prescribe a more ideal premedication.
D. In writing the preoperative medication, it must be remembered that some patients take cardiac medications, insulin, and other drugs. These should be included in the preoperative orders if indicated.

X. An operative permit should be signed and witnessed in the presence of the surgeon, if at all possible.
A. In getting informed consent the patient should be told of the various alternatives of treatment available. The advantages and disadvantages of each type of treatment should be discussed. All reasonable complications should be mentioned. These complications should include those of anesthesia as well as of surgery. In other words the patient must be presented with all pertinent information with which to make an intelligent decision regarding the course of treatment to be followed.
B. It is wise to discuss the alternative treatments in front of all members of the immediate family or responsible individuals. This is particularly important if the patient for one reason or another is unable to assume an active role in the decision.

Care in the Operating Room

I. The patient should be transported to the OR suite by a stretcher or in his or her bed. The side rails should be up. The patient should be appropriately covered and should be transferred on elevators and by routes not utilized by the general public.

II. On arrival in the OR, the patient should not be left unattended.
A. There may be unexpected reactions to the preoperative medications or there may be respiratory depression, vomiting, etc.

B. The patient should not be put in the hall outside of the OR where he or she may see things that are not understood.

III. When the patient is taken into the OR, it should be quiet with all personnel working in an efficient and orderly manner.

A. Loud music or laughter will do little to bolster the patient's confidence.

B. During the induction of anesthesia, it is especially important that absolute quiet exist.

IV. The IV should be started with a large-gauge needle so that blood or other medication can be given rapidly if required. For the patient's comfort, it is helpful if local anesthesia is injected into the skin before the large-bore needle is inserted into the vein.

V. When the patient is placed on the OR table, be sure the indwelling catheter is draining and that the tubing is NOT kinked.

VI. When the patient is asleep and placed in the desired position, check to be sure there is not undue pressure over bony prominences. Also see that all pulses are present and that there is no compression of peripheral nerves.

VII. The ground for the electrocautery should be well placed and NOT in contact with the genitalia or located over bony prominences.

VIII. The eyes should have ointment applied, and they should be taped shut. This is particularly important when a craniotomy is done because prep solutions may get into the eyes.

IX. When the endotracheal tube has been inserted and securely taped, care should be taken not to move the head from side to side excessively during the positioning and the shaving of the head.

A. Excessive movement can irritate the vocal cords and the mucosa of the trachea. This causes possible laryngeal spasm or tracheal edema postoperatively. This is especially true with infants and young children.

X. EKG leads must be properly placed and secured.

A. After draping, it may be difficult to replace the leads.

XI. A nasogastric tube may be required, particularly in cases of trauma where the patient may have eaten or drunk something just before the accident.

A. It is wise to ask the patient, before putting him or her to sleep, if he or she has taken anything orally. The patient may not realize the importance of strict avoidance of food or liquids prior to surgery.

XII. The insertion of a rectal temperature probe will be needed if the surgical procedure will be a long one.
   A. This should always be done with infants and small children because they lose body heat more rapidly than adults.
   B. If hypothermia is to be used, a probe for constant temperature monitoring is mandatory.

XIII. The decision about how much hair should be shaved will depend on the incision and the exposure required.
   A. Enough should be shaved to prevent hair from contaminating the wound and to permit extension of the incision if necessary during the operation.
   B. Close shaving with a razor should be done after the patient is asleep because it is painful.
   C. Take care not to contaminate adjacent sterile equipment during the shaving procedure. If the shaving is done dry, airborne, particulate matter may result. It is probably best to moisten the area to be shaved with soapy water or shaving cream. The use of a depilatory is preferred by some surgeons.
   D. Remember to save the hair if any significant amount is shaved. It should be given to the family.

XIV. The particular position on the operating table will be dictated by the intended surgical procedure.
   A. Be sure the position is secure.
   B. Look for constrictive straps, tape, or clothing that may compromise blood supply.
   C. Avoid excessive flexion of the neck, which might kink the endotracheal tube.

XV. The preparation of the skin must be done by a member of the surgical team who understands and practices strict sterile techniques.
   A. There are several acceptable prep solutions available.
   B. Always check the patient's chart for allergies when selecting a prep solution. Sensitivity to iodine is common.
   C. Be careful not to let the prep solution run into the eyes. Careful preparation should be done of the ear, not letting the solution run into the canal. It is a good practice to plug the canal with a sterile cotton ball.

XVI. Remember the anesthesiologist when draping the patient and when positioning surgical tables and mayo stands. The anesthesiologist should have easy access to the patient during the entire surgical procedure.

Postoperative Care

I. After the closure of the wound is completed, a sterile dressing is applied.
   A. The entire head should be wrapped with the dressing. It should be fairly tight to minimize bleeding and to prevent its coming off easily, thereby contaminating the wound.
   B. If at all possible, the ears should not be included in the dressing because they will become sore from the constant pressure. If they must be incorporated in the dressing, it will help if a folded sponge is placed behind each ear to reduce the pressure.
   C. If bleeding appears on the dressing in the immediate postoperative period, the bandage should merely be reinforced. If bleeding is excessive, the surgeon should be called, for it might be necessary to put in an additional skin stitch to stop the bleeding. In most cases bleeding of this type is from a small bleeding vessel in the edge of the incision. If the dressing must be totally changed, it should be done with strict sterile technique.

II. The surgeon should write an operative note in the progress notes. This provides vital information used by the rest of the team caring for the patient.
   A. It gives the type of anesthesia and mode of administration; for example, endotracheal tube, mask, etc.
   B. The position of the patient during the procedure, such as seated or prone, should be mentioned.
   C. The procedure performed should be named and defined, with pertinent findings listed.
   D. A list of the surgeon(s) and assistants should be given.
   E. An estimate of the blood loss is made, and a list of the fluid, blood, etc., that was given during the operation is noted.
   F. Mention should be made of any drains used or remaining in the incision. Any other pertinent information about the wound or dressing should be included.
   G. If possible, potential problems that might occur postoperatively should be mentioned.

III. The surgeon should accompany the patient from the OR to the recovery area or the neurosurgical intensive care unit. There the surgeon can relay to the members of the team who will be recovering the patient:
   A. The postoperative status of the patient; for example, comatose, hemiplegic, or one pupil dilated and nonreactive.

B. What should reasonably occur as the patient recovers from the anesthesia. If the patient was comatose before surgery, it is likely that he or she will be comatose after surgery. If he or she was weak on the right side, the right side is likely to be weak on recovery.

C. Potential hazards or problems that might occur.

IV. The surgeon then writes the postoperative orders. They must be complete, providing for all the immediate needs as well as anticipating problems or complications that might occur. The following points discussed are a part of the usual postoperative orders:

A. Vital signs, including both routine and neurological ones. Initially these are monitored every 15 minutes; but if, as the patient is observed, the vital signs are stable, they may be taken less frequently.

1. At first they should be taken every 15 minutes for 2 to 4 hours; next, every 30 to 60 minutes until the surgeon changes the orders.
2. The usual craniotomy patient should be checked every hour during the first 24 to 48 hours. Then, depending on the clinical state of the patient, the vital signs can be taken every 2 to 4 hours.
3. The surgeon should recall how frequently she or he has asked that the vital signs be taken. Initially the patient must be watched closely. However, on the third or fourth day if the patient is doing well, it serves no purpose to awaken the patient during the night to take the vital signs or to take them too frequently.

B. Fluid intake and output (I&O) must be recorded, and one cannot overemphasize the need for accuracy.

1. The patient should be without drink or food (NPO) the first 12 to 24 hours. This helps prevent vomiting and assures an empty stomach if the patient has to be taken back to surgery for one reason or another.
2. Classically the neurological surgeon tends to keep patients dry, but this should not be overdone. It is better to keep the patient adequately hydrated. This is possible only if an accurate I&O record is maintained. Efforts should be made to avoid overhydration.
3. The average-sized adult patient should receive 3,000 cubic centimeters of fluid per 24 hours. This will provide good hydration and an adequate urinary output. If the patient is losing fluids through a nasogastric tube and by

ventricular drainage, these volumes of replacement fluid must be increased. In addition, significant amounts of fluid may be lost if the patient has a high fever or a rapid respiratory rate.

4. If the urinary output is excessive, it is wise to determine the output of urine hourly. This occurs with diabetes insipidus, where vast amounts of urine may be produced in a very short period of time. When this occurs, the IV rate must be increased to compensate.
5. A close watch must be kept on the serum electrolytes in the postoperative period. They should be obtained every 24 hours or more frequently if diabetes insipidus occurs or if dehydrating agents are used.
6. When the patient is alert and without nausea, fluids may be given orally and the diet may be advanced as tolerated.

C. Airway maintenance is mandatory in the postoperative care of the craniotomy patient. There are few things that can happen to cause a patient to deteriorate as fast as an inadequate airway.

1. Initially when the patient arrives in the intensive care area, the endotracheal tube may still be in place. As the patient recovers from the anesthesia, he or she may not be able to tolerate the tube, so it must be removed. It is in most cases highly undesirable to have a patient in the immediate postoperative period do a lot of violent bucking or coughing on the endotracheal tube.
2. In certain cases it may be of benefit to give intermittent positive pressure breathing (IPPB) treatments postoperatively. The effort is to prevent pulmonary complications such as atelectasis and pneumonia. IPPB should never be used, however, as a substitute for good tracheobronchial nursing care. Good care includes:
   a. Suctioning as needed
   b. Deep breathing
   c. Coughing
   d. Postural drainage by frequent changes in position
   e. Humidification of inspired air
3. There are, however, major contraindications to the use of IPPB. The following list should be kept in mind when considering its use:
   a. Patients with significant pulmonary hemorrhage should probably not receive IPPB. This is because

air might be forced into the pulmonary blood vessels. The air then may travel to the brain as emboli, causing ischemia or infarction.

b. Patients with a pneumothorax (collapsed lung) should not get IPPB until a chest tube has been inserted. This is because the pneumothorax will enlarge as the positive pressure forces air through the lacerated lung into the pleural space. Thus a patient who has a pneumothorax should probably not undergo general anesthesia either until a chest tube has been inserted.

c. Patients with bullous emphysema (thin-walled blisters on the lung) may develop a pneumothorax with IPPB because the positive pressure can rupture these air-containing blebs.

d. The comatose patient may have air forced into the stomach when a mask is used to give IPPB. This elevates the diaphragm and limits its excursion. The patient will then experience difficulty breathing after the IPPB treatment is discontinued. Belching and vomiting are also likely with gastric distention.

e. IPPB increases intracranial pressure during the phase of positive pressure.

D. An indwelling urinary catheter must be used with care to prevent a urinary tract infection.

1. Be sure the catheter or drainage tube does not become kinked, preventing drainage.
2. Unexplained restlessness on the part of a patient with altered level of consciousness may occur if the bladder is distended.
3. See Chapter 5 for care of the catheter.

E. Prophylactic measures must be taken against increased intracranial pressure.

1. Constant intracranial pressure monitoring may be done.
2. Vital signs should be taken to clinically recognize potentially serious, increasing intracranial pressure.
3. See below "Postoperative Problems and Complications."
4. As a part of the postoperative care, prophylactic treatment for increasing intracranial pressure may be accomplished by:
   a. Ventricular drainage
   b. Dehydrating agents

c. Steroids (dexamethasone)
d. Assuring no pulmonary problems

F. For management of fever see below, "Postoperative Problems and Complications."
   1. Constant monitoring of the temperature via rectal probe is advisable.
   2. Prophylactic treatment to prevent pulmonary infection may be accomplished by:
      a. Frequent airway suctioning
      b. IPPB
      c. Position change for pulmonary drainage
   3. Contingency plans if fever becomes excessive could include:
      a. Aspirin rectally or Tylenol orally.
      b. Alcohol baths as needed.
      c. Ice baths as needed.
      d. Hypothermia blanket if the temperature cannot be reduced by other methods. Care should be taken to watch for cardiac arrhythmias when the temperature of the body is decreased.

G. Medications to be given postoperatively must be ordered.
   1. Pain medication may be needed, although craniotomies are for the most part not very painful.
      a. The scalp and dura are pain-sensitive structures; the bone is not.
      b. Subarachnoid blood may cause headache postoperatively and may require some analgesia.
      c. If the patient complains of an increasingly severe headache, consider as causes increased intracranial pressure or infection.
      d. An excessively tight head bandage may cause pain.
      e. The treatment of pain in the postoperative craniotomy patient should, if at all possible, avoid narcotics, for they may alter the level of consciousness, depress respirations, and affect pupillary reactivity.
   2. For use of anticonvulsants, see below "Postoperative Problems and Complications."
   3. Other medications, such as cardiac medication, insulin, etc., that are routinely taken by the patient must be ordered.

H. Nasogastric suction may be required and should be done routinely with a trauma patient.

I. Orders for specific positions, etc., may be required.
   1. The patient should be turned from side to side frequently to promote pulmonary drainage and to protect the skin.
   2. The head of the bed should be elevated 30° if the vital signs are stable. This facilitates venous drainage and tends to lessen intracranial pressure.
   3. Avoid flexion of the neck by a pillow if the patient has an altered level of consciousness. Acute flexion of the neck tends to obstruct the airway.
   4. Provide for measures to prevent skin breakdown and for other requirements of body hygiene.

J. Orders for rehabilitation should be given.
   1. Dangle the patient; mobilize as soon as possible.
   2. Active and passive exercises should be done as indicated.

Postoperative Problems and Complications

I. Increased intracranial pressure.
   A. Changes indicative of increased intracranial pressure are:
      1. A change in the level of consciousness; the patient responds less well to verbal commands.
      2. Focal signs develop such as progressive weakness.
      3. Pupillary changes occur; for example, a sluggish pupil or an enlarging, unreactive pupil.
      4. Intracranial monitoring will show the appearance of plateau waves.
   B. Causes:
      1. Postoperative hematoma—bleeding at the site of surgery—may occur even though there was no apparent bleeding at the time of closure.
         a. Prevention:
            i. In preparation, the clotting mechanisms of the patient should be checked; this is especially true in cases of severe trauma.
         b. Treatment:
            i. Evacuation of hematoma by reoperation
            ii. Correction of clotting defects, etc., as indicated
      2. Cerebral edema occurs maximally at 36 to 72 hours following surgery and may be bothersome and difficult to manage.

a. Causes:
   i. Excessive retraction on the brain during surgery.
   ii. Partially resected tumors, such as the gliomas, may swell severely postoperatively.
   iii. Diffuse swelling of the brain may occur following trauma.
   iv. Carbon dioxide retention, secondary to respiratory problems, can cause increased intracranial pressure.

b. Treatment:
   i. Correct the basic cause of the swelling, such as an inadequate airway and hyperventilation.
   ii. Administer corticosteroids (dexamethasone) during the stages of swelling.
   iii. Use dehydrating agents such as mannitol, urea, or oral glycerol.
   iv. Establish ventricular drainage.
   v. A decompression procedure, such as a lobectomy, etc., can be done, but only in extreme situations.
   vi. Hypothermia by the use of hypothermia blanket.

3. Acute hydrocephalus may occur either if there is significant bleeding during the operation, filling the basal cisterns, or after surgery, in the posterior fossa.
   a. Treatment:
      i. Ventricular drainage
      ii. Definitive, permanent shunting procedures such as brain-to-cardiac or brain-to-peritoneal shunts

II. Fever.

A. The general treatment of fever is:
   1. Aspirin or Tylenol given by rectal suppository or orally. Care must be given when giving aspirin when the patient is getting steroids because of the possibility of gastrointestinal bleeding.
   2. Ice or alcohol baths.
   3. Hypothermia blanket.

B. Causes:
   1. Pulmonary problems. Fever in the first 12 to 24 hours is probably due to atelectasis.

a. Pneumonia may develop rapidly in the postoperative period, especially if there has been aspiration of stomach contents or aspiration of blood.
b. Treatment:
    i. Care of airway with frequent suctioning
    ii. IPPB
    iii. Antibiotics as indicated

2. Thrombophlebitis, common in neurosurgical patients, is the forming of a blood clot in a vein secondary to inflammation in the wall of the vessel.
    a. Signs and symptoms:
        i. The patient may have generalized fever or locally increased temperature.
        ii. There is local tenderness, swelling, and often redness.
        iii. Unfortunately thrombophlebitis may occur in the deep veins of the legs and pelvis and be totally asymptomatic.
    b. The major concern, if thrombophlebitis is present, is the possibility of pulmonary embolism.
        i. This occurs when the blood clots break loose and go to the lungs.
        ii. If the clots are large enough, sudden death can occur.
    c. Causes:
        i. Injury to the lining of the vein is common with trauma, if intravenous needles are left in place for extended periods, and if certain medications are given intravenously.
        ii. In trauma, alterations in the plasma proteins may produce an increased coagulability of the blood, which may encourage clot formation.
        iii. Obstruction of blood flow in an extremity imposed by prolonged bed rest or constrictive clothing may cause thrombophlebitis.
    d. Prophylactic treatment:
        i. Get the patient up as soon as possible after surgery.
        ii. Use elastic stockings, which collapse the superficial veins of the legs. If elastic bandages are used, check frequently to be sure they are properly applied.

iii. Change IV sites frequently, especially if there are any signs of inflammation occurring. This is especially important when intravenous medications are given that are known to irritate the lining of the veins.
iv. Moist, warm soaks should be applied to the area of inflammation.
v. Elevate the involved extremity.
vi. Give antibiotics if indicated.
vii. Use anticoagulation if permissable.
viii. Use vena caval ligation if embolization continues to occur in spite of therapy.

3. Infections of a craniotomy wound may occur under the scalp flap in the epidural or subdural spaces or as a brain abscess. Fever usually does not occur from the wound infection for 5 to 6 days after the craniotomy, although a particularly virulent organism may produce fever sooner.
   a. Treatment:
      i. Antibiotics as indicated by culture and sensitivities
      ii. Debridement, incision, and drainage of the infection if a mass such as an abscess is present and if the antibiotics fail to eradicate the infection
4. Meningitis may occur secondary to contamination at the time of the craniotomy. Always keep in mind the possibility of meningitis occurring secondary to trauma because of the CSF rhinorrhea; the injured patient lies supine or on one side so that the spinal fluid leaks into the pharynx and is, therefore, not detected.
   a. Treatment:
      i. Antibiotics as indicated by the culture and sensitivity of the spinal fluid
5. Genito-urinary infections are most commonly caused by gram-negative organisms, and gram-negative shock may occur.
   a. Prevention:
      i. Conscientious catheter care and irrigation
   b. Treatment:
      i. Antibiotics as needed
      ii. Steroids if gram-negative shock occurs

6. General sepsis—infection elsewhere in the body—is especially likely in trauma, where soft tissue infection may occur.
7. Hyperthermia of central origin (hypothalamic). Although both hypothermia and hyperthermia may occur because of hypothalamic dysfunction following a craniotomy, a fever should be considered to be due to an infection until proved otherwise. Disturbances of hypothalamic temperature control may occur from head injury, hydrocephalus, or tumors in the region of the hypothalamus.
   a. The signs and symptoms of postoperative hyperthermia include:
      i. Fever. The shape of the curve should be plotted to differentiate between sepsis and central fever. The curve tends to remain high and unrelenting in fevers of hypothalamic origin, rather than spiking periodically as in infection.
      ii. There may be a depressed or altered level of consciousness.
      iii. There may be accentuation of neurological deficits or the development of new ones.
      iv. There is an increased heart rate, increased respiratory rate, and diaphoresis.
      v. Shock is possible if gram-negative organisms are present.
      vi. Often there is evidence of other hypothalamic dysfunction, such as diabetes insipidus.
8. Subarachnoid hemorrhage—blood in the subarachnoid space—may cause low-grade fever with the temperature elevation typically no more than a degree or so.

III. Postoperative seizures can be a major problem in the postoperative period. As a part of the informed consent and operative permit, the patient should be appraised of the possibility of postoperative seizures.

   A. Causes:
      1. Electrolyte imbalance
      2. Hyperthermia
      3. Anoxia

4. Retraction or invasion of the brain as necessitated by the surgical procedure

B. Prophylactic treatment:

1. Some neurosurgeons routinely include anticonvulsants as a part of their routine orders. If this is done the patient should continue to take them for several months. If no seizures occur, then they may be slowly withdrawn over a period of time.

IV. Cerebrospinal fluid fistula—the drainage of CSF from a craniotomy wound—is a serious complication because of the possiblity of infection. It occurs because of the failure to get a watertight closure of the dura. This is common when the dura is badly shredded by trauma or when a segment of dura is removed because it was intimately involved by the pathological process. The surgeon must make great effort to close the dura either primarily or by suturing a graft in the dural defect.

A. Treatment:

1. If a dural closure is not possible, the scalp must be closed in a watertight manner, and a snug head dressing should be applied. The head dressing will prevent the accumulation of spinal fluid under the scalp flap. The dressing should be left on long enough, though changed periodically, to permit the wound to heal completely. If CSF leaks through the incision, in spite of all efforts, it may be necessary to put a stitch in the incision at the site of drainage. Prophylactic antibiotics should be given while active leakage of spinal fluid is occurring or if there is a likelihood that it will occur.
2. The leakage of spinal fluid through the nose is a common complication when surgery is done in the region of the pituitary gland. This is especially true when the approach to the pituitary is through the sphenoid sinus. In this approach, the nose is packed postoperatively, and it is when the packing is removed that the CSF leakage will occur if a fistula persists.
   a. The patient is warned not to blow the nose or cough, and to try to avoid sneezing.
   b. A sterile drip pad is taped to the nose when spinal fluid leakage is occurring. The nursing personnel must observe how often it is necessary to change the pad, and they should also note changes in the character of the drainage.

V. Gastrointestinal bleeding may occur in two instances in patients who have a cerebral lesion or who have suffered a head injury.

A. Causes:

1. Dr. Harvey Cushing noted the relationship between cerebral lesions and the occurrence of gastric and duodenal ulcers. It has been shown that there is a direct correlation between gastric acidity and hypothalamic function. Bleeding may be severe, with shock and even death occurring before surgical treatment can be provided.
2. Peptic ulceration with hemorrhage or perforation is a common complication of corticosteroid therapy. The efficacy of the use of steroids to treat cerebral edema make it imperative that the nursing team watch for signs or evidence of gastrointestinal bleeding.
   a. Nasogastric aspiration is wise on occasion in the postoperative period. The aspirate will reveal bright red blood when the bleeding is active.
   b. The patient's bowel movements may appear tar-like in color and consistency, indicating gastrointestinal bleeding. In the postoperative period it is wise to check the stool for occult blood periodically even though no gross bleeding is occurring.
   c. If there is any suggestion of active bleeding, periodic monitoring of the hemoglobin and hematocrit should be done.

B. Treatment:

1. Fluid administration and blood transfusion as required.
2. Nasogastric suction with periodic gastric irrigation with iced saline.
3. Administration of antacids via the nasogastric tube as indicated.
4. Avoid aspirin.
5. If possible, decrease or stop corticosteroids.
6. Maintain a ready supply of blood, typed and cross matched, for adminstration if needed.
7. Obtain a general surgical consultation early.

VI. Electrolyte imbalance of a serious nature may develop in spite of diligent efforts to maintain a satisfactory intake and output. The following conditions may occur and tax the expertise of the medical team:

A. Diabetes insipidus occurs following surgery in the region of the third ventricle and after some head injuries. There is a relative deficiency of ADH (antidiurectic hormone), which acts to regulate the volume of urine produced by the kidneys.
   1. Signs and symptoms:
      a. Clinically, in addition to the large urinary output, the alert patient will crave water.
      b. Patients with a lowered level of consciousness will quickly become dehydrated and shocky if treatment is not begun.
      c. If diabetes insipidus is suspected, the medical team should begin to check the hourly urinary output. If the output is more than 150–200 cubic centimeters an hour, the surgeon should be notified.
      d. The urine specific gravity should be checked and will range between 1.001 and 1.004 if diabetes insipidus occurs.
   2. Treatment:
      a. Administer vasopressin, which is available in an aqueous form or as vasopressin tannate in oil. The aqueous form may be given intravenously, subcutaneously, or intramuscularly. If given intravenously, the effect is very short-lived, although its effectiveness lasts only a few hours when given subcutaneously or intramuscularly. Vasopressin tannate in oil, given intramuscularly, will remain effective for 24 hours or longer.
         i. Vasopressin should not be given to a patient with significant coronary artery disease.
      b. After vasopressin is given, care must be taken not to give excessive amounts of fluid intravenously. At the onset of diabetes insipidus large volumes of fluid may be needed intravenously to replace the urine lost, but after giving vasopressin, watch the I&O closely and avoid water intoxication.
      c. If the problem remains chronic, vasopressin can be given as a nasal spray. In addition, the use of thiazide diuretics may assist in lessening the urine output.

B. Inappropriate ADH secretion occurs in several pathological states, among which are brain tumors, head trauma, tuberculous meningitis, and carcinoma of the lung.
   1. Signs and symptoms:

a. Clinically there is fluid retention with dilution of all body-fluid spaces. This leads to dilution of the serum sodium and chloride.
b. There is also the loss of sodium in the urine. Therefore, the patient develops hyponatremia (low serum sodium), which may cause changes in the level of consciousness, seizures, and even death.

2. Treatment:
   a. Restrict the fluid intake.
   b. If the patient is in coma, it may be necessary to give hypertonic saline.

VII. Fat embolism. In cases of extensive soft-tissue trauma and long-bone fractures, globules of fat may be forced into the general blood circulation.
A. Signs and symptoms:
1. Initially the fat globules go to the lungs and obstruct many of its capillaries. This is manifest on the first or second day after injury. The patient becomes short of breath, breathes rapidly, and may become cyanotic.
2. Many of the globules pass from the lungs and go to other organs of the body, including the brain, kidneys, and skin. In the brain, smaller caliber vessels are occluded, producing hypoxia, manifest clinically by restlessness, seizures, and coma.
3. Petechial hemorrhages are seen in the skin.
4. Fat globules appear in the urine.

B. Treatment:
1. There is no specific treatment.
2. Efforts are directed toward minimizing hypoxia by administrating oxygen.

VIII. Problems and complications involving other systems of the body. The medical team must be constantly aware of these. Treat the whole patient.

Special Considerations Determined by Specific Lesions

Aneurysms and Arteriovenous Malformations

I. Preoperative. The major efforts include prevention of rebleeding and stabilization of the patient in preparation for surgery.

A. Quiet environment. Many of these patients are in extreme pain with headache and stiff necks. A quiet, private room without the noise of a television, telephone, and bothersome visitors is mandatory. The environment should be restful and suited to the individual.
B. Dark room. Blood in the subarachnoid space causes marked sensitivity to light (photophobia). Window curtains should be drawn closed. The members of the medical team should never turn on a light at the bedside or overhead without first warning the patient.
C. Pain and sedation. The headache and neck stiffness, secondary to a subarachnoid hemorrhage, are very painful. The patient needs adequate medication for relief. Mild sedation is in order if the patient is restless. There is, of course, some risk that subtle or early signs of deterioration will be masked by the analgesics and sedation. Judgment and close observation are needed.
D. Avoidance of sudden rises in intracranial vascular pressure.
   1. Coughing. The patient should be cautioned against coughing, and cough medication may be needed. Prevention of smoking by the patient or visitors is absolutely necessary.
   2. Avoidance of constipation. Stool softeners should be used routinely. No medications should be given rectally. Temperatures should only be taken orally.
E. Avoidance of hot or extremely cold fluids or food.
   1. There are potential, adverse effects if hot liquid or food is taken orally when a patient is not expecting it.
   2. Patients may spill hot fluids such as coffee in the bed or on themselves.
F. Supervision of daily care. The medical team alone should bathe the patient. Their skill in giving the bath, dressing the patient, and changing the linen lessens physical exertion and emotional stress.
   1. Avoid chilling during the bath.
   2. Avoid embarrassment.
   3. Instruct the patient regarding the plan of action.
G. Management of vessel spasm. As discussed elsewhere, the presence of blood in the spinal fluid may cause cerebral vessels to go into spasm. As a result, there is a marked decrease in the amount of blood that can flow through the vessels. Severe ischemia and brain infarction often occur.

Present treatment is not wholly successful but seems to help in some instances.

1. Intravenous isoproterenol may help to lessen spasm. The patient must be closely watched because cardiac arrhythmias may occur that require a lidocaine drip.
2. Low molecular-weight dextran and corticosteroids are often used, but their effect on spasm is debatable.
3. In most instances all that can be done is to wait until the vasospasm lessens, giving good supportive care in the interim.

H. Antifibrinolytic efforts. The rationale in the use of antifibrinolytic agents is the concept that a blood clot forms around the aneurysm when it ruptures. The clot, therefore, lends some strength to the aneurysm wall or in some way helps to lessen the likelihood of rebleeding.

1. Aminocaproic acid is given intravenously, which helps to retard the breakdown of fibrin in the blood clot. In this manner the patient may, ideally, be readied for definitive surgery with less chance of rebleeding. In the past it has been recognized that rebleeding was most common approximately 7 to 9 days after the initial bleeding occurred; this correlates with the time of clot breakdown. The patient is begun on the drug with a loading dose of 4–5 grams of aminocaproic acid intravenously and then receives 1 gram intravenously every hour. This should never be given intravenously in an undiluted form.

I. Signs of increasing intracranial pressure. Any time in the preoperative period a patient who has suffered a subarachnoid hemorrhage may deteriorate because of increased intracranial pressure. A number of different processes may cause the increased pressure.

1. Rebleeding can occur at any time, and as the hematoma accumulates, intracranial pressure rises. If this happens and the bleeding continues, the patient will die before he or she can be taken to surgery.
2. Hydrocephalus commonly develops after subarachnoid hemorrhage because the CSF pathways are blocked. This is managed by performing frequent spinal taps, by removing spinal fluid, or by ventricular drainage. It may be necessary to perform some type of a permanent shunting procedure.

3. Brain swelling, secondary to anoxia and infarction, is common when vascular spasm occurs. The treatment consists of efforts to lessen spasm, minimize anoxia, and counter the brain swelling with corticosteroids and dehydrating agents.

J. Management of hypertension. Patients who have had a subarachnoid hemorrhage usually have an elevated blood pressure, and often it is quite high. While it is advisable to lower the blood pressure, caution must be taken in doing so. Remember the intracranial pressure is likely to be above normal; therefore a greater blood pressure is needed so sufficient blood can flow into the brain. Obviously, this is critical. If the blood pressure falls below the intracranial pressure, blood flow into the brain will cease. In addition, spasm of the cerebral arteries will necessitate higher-than-normal blood pressures.

1. The neurosurgeon should watch that a well-meaning medical consultant does not order antihypertensive drugs that will drop the blood pressure excessively.

II. During surgery on aneurysms.

A. Induced hypotension. As the surgeon gets close to the aneurysm, the chances of rupture increase because of retraction and manipulation. It is, therefore, logical that, if the blood pressure is dropped, there will be less chance that the aneurysm will rupture.

1. The anesthesiologist can give agents intravenously to drop the blood pressure. It is wise that the pressure not remain low for an excessive period of time, but it can be tolerated for 30 minutes or a bit longer. The pressure is usually dropped to 60 or 70 millimeters of mercury.

B. Hypothermia. Sometimes the surgeon will find it necessary, especially if the aneurysm ruptures during surgery, to put temporary clips on the parent artery. When this is done, bleeding stops or decreases, giving the surgeon a chance to put a clip on the aneurysm itself. The temporary clip can only be left in place a short time because the brain, dependent on the blood flow through that artery, will quickly become anoxic and infarction will occur. If, however, the body temperature is dropped by using cooling blankets, the metabolic rate of the brain cells decreases. This makes it safe for the surgeon to leave the temporary clip in position for longer periods of time. Hypothermia also causes the brain to shrink a bit, which facilitates exposure during surgery.

1. At the lower body temperatures, cardiac arrhythmias occur; therefore, close cardiac monitoring is necessary.

III. Postoperative. All the problems and complications discussed following a craniotomy apply to craniotomies for aneurysms and arteriovenous malformations as well. In addition:

A. Vascular spasm continues to be a problem in the postoperative period. The patient may awaken with no neurological deficit, only to deteriorate hours or a few days later. Just why the spasm is delayed is not clear. When the patient deteriorates, arteriograms should be done to rule out a postoperative hematoma and to substantiate the suspicion of vasospasm. Many neurosurgeons routinely do arteriograms postoperatively to be sure the aneurysm has been properly clipped and that the clip has not slipped off. The author routinely puts a drop or two of methyl methacrylate on the spring mechanism of the clip to prevent its opening and slipping.

Brain Tumors

I. Preoperative. Patients are prepared as for any craniotomy, but there are a few points that should be mentioned.

A. If the intracranial pressure has been significantly elevated for several days or weeks, efforts should be made to reduce it prior to surgery. This is accomplished by corticosteroids and dehydrating agents like mannitol or urea.

B. If the tumor is in the posterior fossa, producing hydrocephalus, ventricular drainage should be established 2 to 3 days prior to surgery. This gives a period of time during which stabilization can occur.

C. If the tumor is metastatic to the brain, an effort must be made to be sure that there is a single metastasis and that there are not widespread metastases throughout the body. If these two criteria are not met, the craniotomy is probably not indicated.

II. Postoperative. The considerations listed for the routine craniotomy apply in the postoperative period. In addition:

A. If the tumor is a primary malignant glioma, such as a glioblastoma multiforme, and if the surgical excision was subtotal or if only a biopsy was taken, postoperative swelling of the remaining tumor will be severe.

1. Vigorous efforts are required immediately with high doses of corticosteroids and dehydrating agents.

B. If the tumor removed was a meningioma, the adjacent brain will swell dramatically following the removal of the tumor. The patient will show signs of increased intracranial pressure with a decreased level of consciousness. Also focal signs such as hemiplegia may develop.
   1. Vigorous efforts to counter the swelling are needed, using corticosteroids and dehydrating agents.
   2. When this clinical picture occurs, the possibility of a postoperative hematoma being present must not be forgotten.

Spontaneous Intracerebral Hematomas

I. Preoperative. Usually there is only time for quick appraisal, cerebral arteriograms, and surgery if indicated. The decision whether to operate requires sound judgment considering the following points:
   A. Surgery should not be done if the patient shows signs of irreversible brainstem injury and pending death.
   B. A poor surgical result is probable if the hemorrhage occurs deep within the basal ganglia and especially if it ruptures into the ventricles.
   C. The patient's age and general health status should be considered.
   D. Patients with long-standing hypertension are poor surgical candidates.
   E. The *quality* of survival must be considered. If the hemorrhage is in the dominant hemisphere, hemiplegia and aphasia will probably remain.

II. Postoperative. The usual postoperative orders and considerations apply.

Infection and Abscesses

I. Preoperative. The preoperative period is essentially one of expectancy. Efforts are made to postpone surgery as long as possible or to obviate it entirely.
   A. Antibiotics are given in high doses. If the treatment is begun during the stage of cerebritis, cure may be achieved without an abscess forming.
   B. If an abscess forms, antibiotics permit the postponement of surgery until a thick capsule can form around the abscess.
   C. Surgery is indicated if:

1. The mass of the abscess causes unmanageable increased intracranial pressure or progressive focal lesions.
2. Hydrocephalus occurs because of obliteration of the CSF pathways. A shunting procedure may be necessary.

D. Brain swelling may be significant, especially during the stage of cerebritis, and it may require treatment.
   1. Corticosteroids and dehydrating agents are used. Corticosteroids are used in spite of the fact that theoretically they may adversely affect the body's response to infection.

E. There are two complications that may occur, causing the patient to rapidly deteriorate:
   1. The rupture of the abscess with spilling of its contents into the ventricles or subarachnoid space.
   2. Thrombosis of the dural sinuses or cortical veins, with infections of the central nervous system. The patient usually develops seizures, various focal deficits, and an altered level of consciousness. Infections on the face in the region of the nose may lead to thrombosis of the cavernous sinus, which is a life-threatening complication.

II. Postoperative. The usual postoperative orders apply.
   A. If the capsule of the abscess is broken during its removal, infected material will contaminate the wound. This requires close observation of the surgical wound and appropriate steps if signs of infection occur.

Head Trauma

Every patient who sustains a head injury should be considered a potential surgical candidate. Therefore, much of the management should be considered preoperative.

I. Preoperative. The major responsibility is continued close observation of the patient to detect early clinical changes indicative of a progressive intracranial process. If this occurs, appropriate diagnostic procedures should be performed immediately. If a surgical lesion such as a subdural hematoma is identified, the patient is made ready for surgery as outlined for any craniotomy.

II. Postoperative. The postoperative management of a head injury is similar to that for any craniotomy.
   A. Continue to observe for CSF rhinorrhea and evidence of infection.

CHAPTER 7

Laminectomy

The basic operation performed when spinal surgery is done is called a laminectomy. A review of the anatomy of the vertebral column and of a single vertebra will facilitate the understanding of terms used in describing a laminectomy.

The vertebral column consists of seven cervical, twelve thoracic, five lumbar, and five sacral vertebrae. The first two cervical vertebrae, called the atlas and the axis, are specialized in their function and differ in their configuration from the other vertebrae. The five sacral vertebrae are usually fused into a solid, bony mass called the sacrum.

Figure 7-1 is a diagrammatic representation of an "average vertebra." There is a single spine that projects backward. At the base of the spine, two laminae flare to each side, forming the roof or neural arch over the spinal canal. The neural arch is supported on each side by a pedicle.

The pedicles arise from the body of the vertebra. It is the vertebral body that supports our body weight. The intervertebral disc lies between two adjacent vertebral bodies. The disc functions by absorbing shock and by permitting motion. Broad ligaments span the gap between adjacent spines and laminae. The interspinous ligament connects the spines; the ligamentum flavum or yellow ligament connects adjacent lamina. On each side, at the point where the lamina and pedicles meet, are the facets. These are actually joints by which the vertebra articulates with the vertebra below it (inferior facet) and the one above it (superior facet). The facets, along with the interspinous ligament, ligamentum flavum, and intervertebral discs, permit movement between adjoining vertebrae.

Figure 7-1 The Vertebra

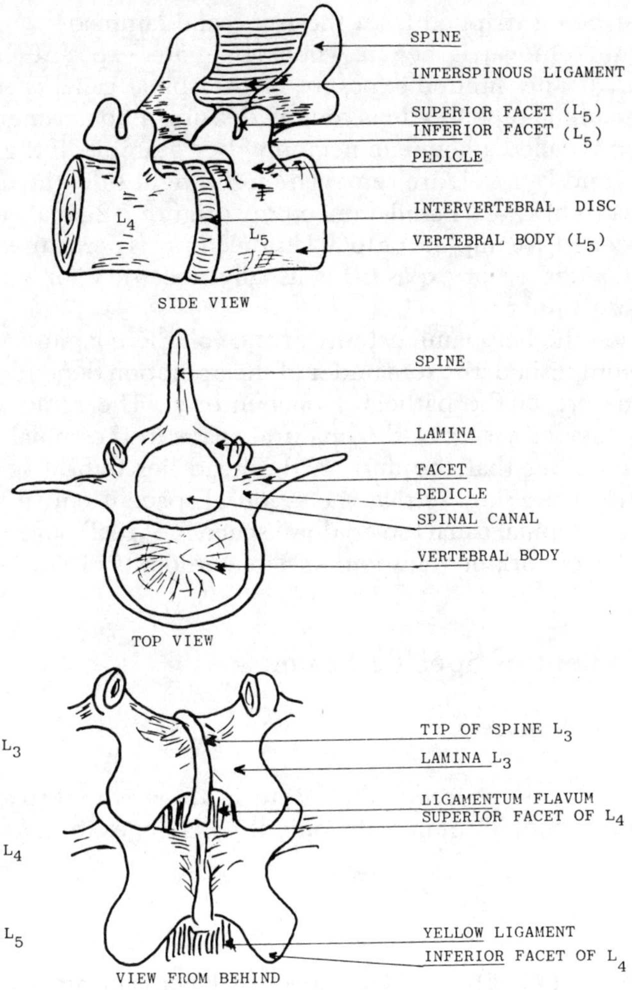

General Procedure

In order to gain access to the spinal canal, the surgeon first makes a vertical, midline incision on the back or neck at the appropriate vertebral level. The incision goes through a layer of fat of variable thickness until the tips of the spines are exposed. Next, the paraspinous muscles are stripped away from the spine and lamina, using a periosteal elevator. Depending on the nature of the surgical procedure to be performed, the surgeon may expose one or both lamina. The muscles are held away from the midline by mechanical retractors after being stripped from the spine and laminae.

Bone removal is begun when adequate exposure has been achieved. If only limited exposure of the spinal canal is sufficient, only the lamina on one side is removed, using a bone rongeur. This operation is called a hemilaminectomy. For example, if the laminae of the L_4 and L_5 levels are removed on the right side, the operation is called a right L_4–L_5 hemilaminectomy (Figure 7-2). If a wide exposure is needed, a complete or total laminectomy is performed (Figure 7-2). This degree of exposure is usually necessary for surgery on spinal cord tumors.

When the hemilaminectomy or the complete laminectomy has been accomplished, the remainder of the operation depends entirely on the nature of the pathology encountered. The removal of the lamina provides access to the epidural space in the spinal canal.

Remember that the dura in the head lies tightly against the inner side of the skull so that the epidural space is only a potential space. In the spinal canal the epidural space is a "real" space containing a rich network of veins and variable amounts of fat.

Management of Specific Lesions

The Epidural Space

The many disease processes that occur in the epidural space of the spinal canal include trauma, degenerative changes, tumors, and infection.

Trauma

The involvement of the epidural space by trauma occurs when there are fractures of the vertebrae. Fragments of fractured bone may be displaced, and often they impinge upon the epidural space. In some instances the fragments press against the spinal cord. The various types of vertebral fractures that may occur have been discussed in Chapter 2 (see Figure 2-6).

If the spinal cord is compressed by fragments of a broken vertebra, the surgeon must decide if surgery should be done to relieve the pressure. If the fragments of displaced bone are from a fractured lamina forced into the spinal canal, the surgical approach is from the

Figure 7-2

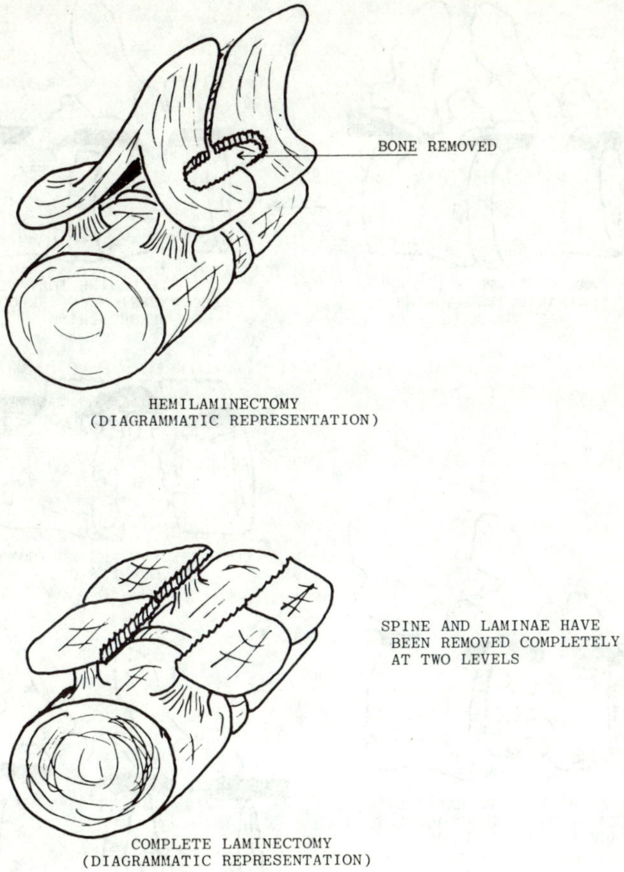

back of the spine. All displaced fragments are removed and the spinal cord is decompressed (Figure 7-3).

When the displaced bone fragments are a part of the vertebral body that has been fractured and thrust backward against the spinal cord, one of two surgical remedies may be chosen (Figure 7-3). One option is a complete laminectomy. This will decompress the spinal cord from behind, permitting the cord to ride over the displaced fragments. Two problems must be faced if the posterior approach is selected.

First, the cord may remain tightly tethered over the fragment with continued cord pressure in spite of the complete laminectomy.

Figure 7-3

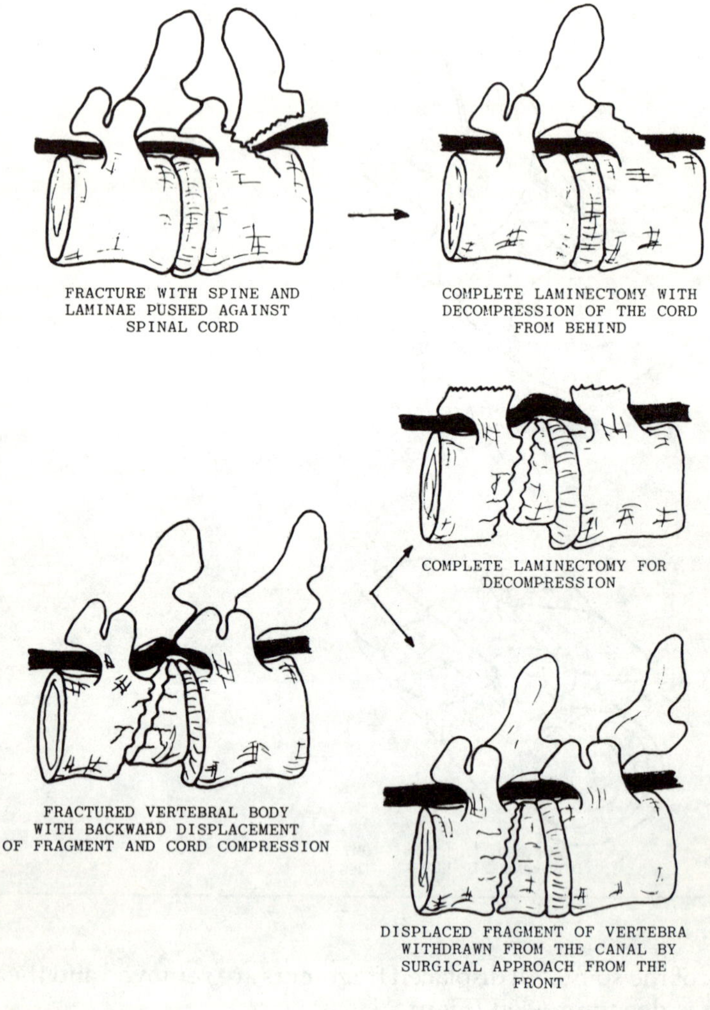

Pressure of this nature can lead to cord infarction because the anterior spinal artery may be occluded.

Second, a complete laminectomy when the vertebral body is fractured increases instability of the spine at the level of the fracture. If the body of the vertebra is severely fractured, the only intact parts of the vertebra will be the spine and laminae. Therefore, if these are removed for decompression, nothing is left to maintain stability. For this reason it may sometimes be necessary to do a fusion when a decompressive laminectomy is performed. Many large trauma centers perform fusions.

The fusion may be done with metal rods that bridge the fracture site and are anchored to stable vertebrae above and below. The rods used are the same ones commonly used by orthopedic surgeons to correct the deformity of scoliosis (curvature of the spine). A fusion of this type permits early mobilization of the patient because adequate spinal stability is achieved at the time of surgery. A fusion that is done with a bone graft takes 3 to 4 months before stability is achieved. The patient must be immobilized by a cast or kept on a frame until bony fusion is accomplished.

The other option in the management of posteriorly displaced, fractured vertebral bodies is to approach the fracture from the front of the spine. In this manner the fragments could be pulled out of the spinal canal, thereby decompressing the spinal cord. Access to the front of the spine is the major problem in this type of an approach. If the fractured vertebral body is in the thoracic spine, the approach to the front of the spine would have to be through the chest. In like fashion to approach a fractured lumbar vertebra from the front, one would have to go through the abdomen. It is, however, relatively easy to reach the front of the cervical vertebrae.

Mechanisms of injury. Until recently, the mechanism of spinal cord injury was believed to be entirely mechanical. To be sure, with severe fractures or dislocations, the cord is injured by direct pressure and, at times, by complete transection of the cord. In seemingly less severe bony injuries of the vertebral column without bony impingement, complete and irreversible cord paralysis can occur. In some instances, the cord injury occurs when there is a temporary dislocation at the moment of injury, with the bony elements returning to their normal, anatomic position immediately thereafter. Yet many severe cord injuries occur for which there is no obvious explanation.

Experimentally produced spinal cord injuries in laboratory animals indicate that there is a progressive process of cord injury for 24 to 48 hours following injury. Thus an injury of mild-to-moderate degree may serve to initiate this destructive process. Experimental evidence reveals that there is a markedly decreased blood flow in the spinal cord at the site of injury, and this is especially true in the gray matter of the cord. The diminished blood flow occurs because of constriction of the blood vessels in the area. Chemical analysis indicates that the concentration of norepinephrine increases locally and in direct proportion to the amount of blood vessel spasm. Future treatment may include the administration of drugs that block the formation of norepinephrine.

If the experimental evidence is applied clinically, it would indicate that similar vessel spasm occurs in injured spinal cords of humans. If spasm is severe, the blood flow permitted will not supply the needed oxygen and glucose to the tissues. The nervous elements of the spinal cord will be injured or will die.

Treatment considerations. Our present methods of treatment of spinal cord injuries are woefully inadequate. Thus there is controversy regarding treatment. Not every patient who has a spinal cord injury should have a complete laminectomy for decompression. The operation may even be detrimental, to say nothing of the needless pain and additional expense involved. It is the consensus of opinion that, if a patient has a complete cord lesion (no neurological function below the level of injury) with no motor or sensory function for 24 hours, recovery will never occur. Some neurosurgeons advocate a laminectomy with complete cord lesions if there is a complete block to the flow of dye with a myelogram. This criterion would include the most severe injuries, with exploded fractures and wide dislocations in which the cord is often totally transected. A laminectomy in these cases is obviously of no benefit to the patient. Therefore each case must be considered individually. If there is reasonable suspicion that the neurological deficit is because of continued pressure on the cord by bony fragments or dislocated vertebrae, then a laminectomy should be done. However, in the light of the experimental data mentioned above, it is probably impossible to judge whether bony compression is significant.

Surgical stabilization of the spine by fusion at the fracture site has the advantage of permitting early mobilization. The patient can be gotten up, thereby avoiding the complications of prolonged bed rest. These complications (discussed in Chapter 5) include decubitus ulcers, pneumonia, kidney stones, and osteoporosis. Good nursing care, however, should enable most patients to tolerate an extended period of bed rest while fractures heal and stability is achieved.

In summary, the following situations may warrant surgery, although each case must be considered individually:

1. If the spine (especially with cervical injuries) is so unstable that further cord injury is possible
2. If it is important that the patient be mobilized rather than wait for stability to be achieved by bed rest and traction
3. If the patient who has a partial cord injury shows signs of deterioration

4. If the cord injury is partial and bony fragments appear to be impinging upon the cord
5. If, with fracture dislocations of the cervical spine, satisfactory alignment cannot be accomplished by cervical traction

Degenerative Changes

The natural aging process results in certain changes in the bony vertebral column. People who have done heavy work or who have sustained trauma will have the process accelerated, and it is likely to be more severe. The results of this process may or may not by symptomatic. In some instances surgery is necessary to accomplish relief. Figure 7-4 illustrates some of the features of this process.

Figure 7-4 Degenerative Changes of the Spine, Collectively Referred to as Degenerative Disc Disease

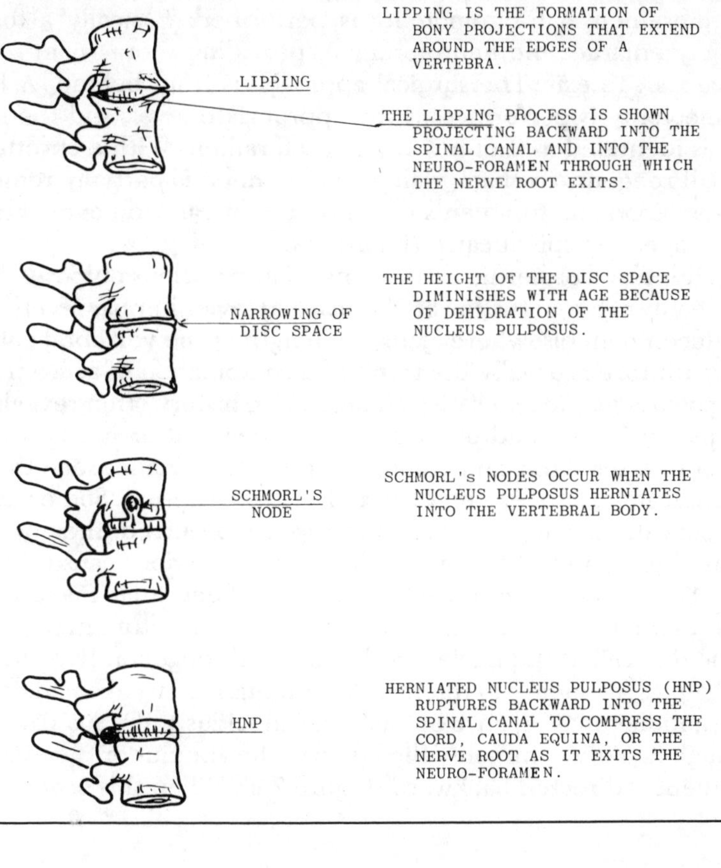

The degenerative change called lipping can become a surgical problem in two situations: (1) If lipping is prominent and projects into the spinal canal, it may impinge upon the spinal cord. When it extends across the width of the canal, it is called a spondylotic ridge or bar. The tight squeeze of the cord between the spondylotic ridge and the back wall of the spinal canal produces slow but progressive cord injury. The common site for this process to be manifested clinically is the cervical region of the spine. Patients with this condition may suddenly be rendered quadriplegic should they be in a car hit from the rear or receive trauma that forces their heads backward. The sudden backward thrust of the head causes the cord to be pinched at the level of the spondylotic ridge. (2) If lipping is prominent in the neuroforamen, the nerve root exiting at that point is tightly pinched. The bony lip in the neuroforamen is called a spur.

A complete laminectomy is performed when the spinal cord is pinched between a spondylotic ridge and the back wall of the spinal canal. This permits the cord to pass over the ridge without pressure from behind. When a spur impinges upon the nerve root in the neuroforamen, a foraminotomy is performed. Basically a foraminotomy enlarges the neuroforamen, providing more room for the nerve root to exit. The surgical approach is from behind. A hemilaminectomy is performed at the appropriate level, and the nerve root is identified as it enters the neuroforamen. With a curette and a small rongeur, the back wall of the foramen is partially removed. This enlarges the foramen so the nerve root can ride over the spur as it leaves the spinal canal (Figure 7-5).

Ruptured or herniated discs (herniated nucleus pulposus, HNP) commonly occur at the lower cervical and lower lumbar levels. They are uncommon elsewhere along the length of the vertebral column. Their rupture is usually the result of a combination of acute trauma and preexisting degenerative changes. The history often reveals that the patient's pain and other symptoms begin after lifting a heavy object or after significant trauma. On the other hand, something as insignificant as a sneeze may cause the disc to rupture. Some patients can provide no clue as to why the rupture occurred; they describe an insidious onset of the symptoms with no obvious cause.

The normal disc has strong, circular fibers that make up the annulus (Figure 2-8). The annulus surrounds a structure in the center of the disc called the nucleus pulposus. With degenerative changes, or changes secondary to trauma, the annulus may weaken and bulge. The annulus may even tear, with the nucleus pulposus extruding through it. Very commonly the bulge in the annulus or the extruded fragment is directed backward (Figure 7-4). When this occurs, pres-

Figure 7-5 Foraminotomy

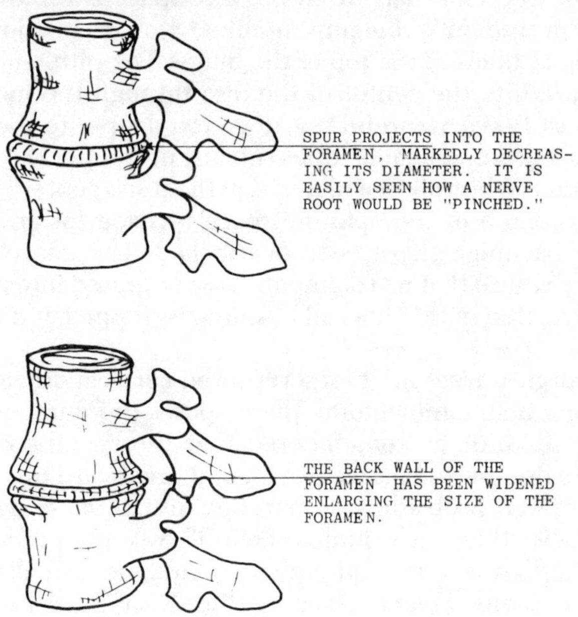

sure is put on the dura and the nerve root at that level. The patient complains of pain in the back or neck with pain radiating into the involved extremity. Certain fingers or toes may be numb, and some of the muscles in the limb may be weak. In addition, the neurological examination reveals a decreased or absent reflex.

The diagnosis of a ruptured disc is made on the basis of the history and the neurological examination; it is confirmed by a myelogram. Before surgery is done, each patient should, in most cases, receive several days of physical therapy, with bed rest, muscle relaxant medication, and pain medication. A significant number of patients will respond to this conservative treatment, so that surgery can be avoided or at least postponed.

The surgical treatment for a herniated lumbar disc begins with a hemilaminectomy that exposes the dura and the exiting nerve root (Figure 2-8). The nerve root is gently retracted toward the midline by a handheld nerve root retractor. This exposes the back side of the disc and any extruded fragment of disc that is present. The fragment is then grasped and removed by an instrument such as a pituitary forceps. After the extruded fragments have been removed, the forceps is inserted through the hole in the annulus into the center of the disc, and all free material within the disc space is removed. When there is a prominently bulging annulus, a short incision is made through the annulus at the top of the bulge. The pituitary forceps is then inserted into the center of the disc through the incision. The surgeon must be very careful not to go too deep into the disc with the forceps, because major arteries run just in front of the disc in the lumbar region. When all free material in the disc's center is removed, a thorough search of the epidural space is made for any extruded fragments that might have been overlooked. The neuroforamen is explored to be sure that no fragments have migrated into it. Next the wound is irrigated with saline; all bleeding is stopped and the wound is closed.

The surgical treatment for a ruptured cervical disc is begun by performing a hemilaminectomy that exposes the dura and existing nerve root. It must be remembered that the spinal cord lies just beneath the dura in the cervical area, and great care must be taken not to injure it. A protruding or extruded disc in the cervical region is much smaller than in the lumbar area. The exposed cervical nerve root is very slightly retracted and protected, as a small incision is made in the dome of the protruding disc. Next, pressure is applied around the base of the protrusion. When this is done, disc material easily extrudes through the incision in the annulus. No instrument is inserted into the disc space. The epidural space is carefully explored for fragments of disc that may have been missed. Next, the neuroforamen is checked to be sure it is large enough to permit the nerve root to pass through it. It is often necessary to do a foraminotomy in the cervical region, whereas it is less common to perform one in the lumbar area.

Many neurosurgeons use an anterior approach to manage foraminal encroachment by spurs and ruptured discs. They incise the disc in the front and remove a portion of it to provide exposure. When the disc protrusion or spur is removed, they place a piece of bone in the space created when the disc was removed. The two adjacent vertebral bodies fuse to the bone graft, producing a firm fusion. The patient must wear a brace for a few months until the fusion is completed.

Tumors

Tumors occur in the epidural space in four different ways:

1. *Metastasis or infiltration.* Carcinoma of the lung, breast, prostate, and kidney commonly spreads to the blood vessels in the

epidural space. There it grows and becomes symptomatic. Malignancies of some of the blood-forming elements also commonly invade the epidural space. These include leukemia, lymphosarcoma, and Hodgkin's disease.

2. *Primary tumors.* Meningiomas and neurofibromas may arise in the epidural space. They produce spinal cord compression as they enlarge.

3. *Bone metastasis.* Carcinoma of the lung, breast, prostate, and kidney also spreads initially by metastasis to the vertebrae. Here it enlarges by destroying bone. Eventually the tumor reaches a size to encroach on the epidural space and press on the spinal cord.

4. *Primary bone tumors.* Occasionally primary tumors arise locally within the vertebrae. Multiple myeloma and chordoma occur in this group. They become symptomatic as they grow and compress the spinal cord.

The patient with a tumor in the epidural space experiences back pain followed by progressive weakness and numbness of the lower extremities and difficulty controlling the bladder and bowel. When a patient is elderly and has very severe back pain without obvious cause, always consider epidural metastasis.

Epidural tumors occur most commonly in the thoracic spine, but they also occur in the lumbar and cervical spine. If there is bone destruction it will probably show on plain X rays. A bone scan very commonly will pinpoint the site of bone destruction by tumor. A myelogram locates the level of spinal cord compression. It is always helpful if the radiologist who does the myelogram marks the skin that overlies the location of the tumor. This enables the surgeon to make an incision at the proper level. When a myelogram shows a complete block of the flow of dye, surgery should be done soon thereafter. It is well known that a patient with a spinal cord tumor may rapidly become paraplegic following a myelogram. Arrangements should be made prior to the myelogram to follow with surgery if a complete block is revealed.

There are three reasons to operate on a patient who has spinal cord compression because of a malignant tumor in the epidural space. The major reason is to prevent the patient from becoming paraplegic. Even though life expectancy is relatively short, the prevention of paraplegia makes the remaining days much more pleasant. Second, surgery also may relieve much of the pain the patient experiences. The third reason for surgery is that a tissue diagnosis can be made. This means that the pathologist can tell what kind of tumor is present, information that is important in deciding which cancer drugs to use and whether X-ray therapy should be given.

A complete laminectomy is the operation performed. This decompresses the spinal cord. When the tumor is like a napkin ring, much of it can be stripped off the dura and removed (Figure 7-6). When the tumor involves bone, the surgeon may decide that the laminectomy is all that needs to be done, in which case only a small portion of tumor is removed for the pathological diagnosis. It is often helpful to insert radioactive gold seeds into the remaining tumor within the bone. This, coupled with X-ray therapy postoperatively, may provide local control of the tumor. Many of these tumors are extremely bloody at surgery, so blood must be available. The surgeon must maintain control of bleeding. The wound should never be closed until bleeding has been stopped. A postoperative hematoma will act like any other mass and can compress the spinal cord, producing a paraplegia. If there is any question about the possibility of a hematoma developing, a drain should be placed in the epidural space. This will permit any blood that accumulates to drain into the bandage.

Infections

Infections occur in the epidural space, but fortunately they are not common. In the past, tuberculosis of the spine was common, but with our present-day antituberculous drugs, its occurrence is uncommon

Figure 7-6 Malignant Tumors in the Epidural Space

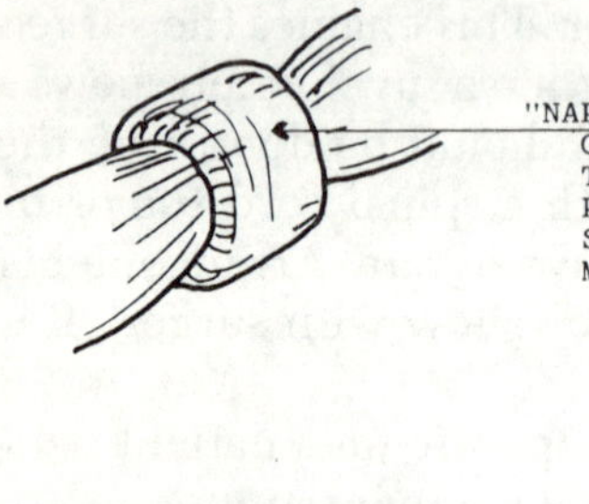

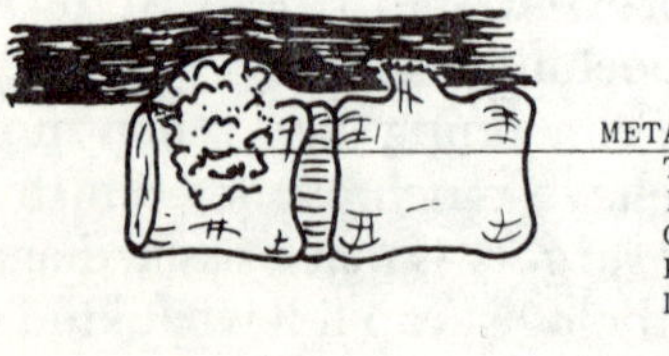

in the United States. Infections of the disc space can occur following a lumbar laminectomy.

Acute epidural abscesses may occur when the bacteria spreads in the bloodstream from a focus of infection elsewhere in the body. The *Staphylococcus* is the most common bacteria. It produces pus that may compress the cord, resulting in paraplegia. The treatment of epidural abscesses is to perform a laminectomy, thereby draining the abscess. Cultures and sensitivities are taken to identify the bacteria and to determine the antibiotic to use.

Infections of the intervertebral disc space usually respond to bed rest and high doses of antibiotics.

The Subdural and Subarachnoid Spaces

The subdural space in the spinal canal is a potential space because the arachnoid, distended by spinal fluid, lies against the inner surface of the dura. The two membranes are, however, easily separated. Commonly a myelographic dye will enter the subdural space rather than the subarachnoid space. Therefore any pathology inside the dura actually occurs in the subarachnoid space or within the spinal cord itself.

It is necessary at this point to discuss certain terms used to designate the location of a disease process. A process that occurs within the spinal cord is said to be intramedullary. If it is not in the cord but within the dura (in the subarachnoid space), the process is described as being intradural and extramedullary.

Tumors

A tumor is the major surgical problem that occurs intradural and extramedullary. The common tumors in this catagory are the meningioma and the neurofibroma, and the thoracic spine is where these tumors most often occur. Lipomas (fat cell tumors) and ependymomas are found also but are more common in the lumbar spine, where they are among the elements of the cauda equina. Because the dura in the spinal canal is relatively impervious to the passage of tumor cells, occurrence of metastatic tumors either extra- or intramedullary is uncommon.

A complete laminectomy is performed to provide access to the intradural extramedullary space. All bleeding is stopped by using electrocautery and gelfoam. The dura and arachnoid are next incised. This exposes the spinal cord and the subarachnoid space. Stitches are placed along the edges of the incision to act as traction sutures (Figure 7-7).

The symptoms of tumors that are intradural extramedullary in location are those indicative of spinal cord compression (Figure 7-8). The patient may have some back pain but not as severe as that occurring with malignant tumors in the epidural space. The patient notes weakness in the legs. The gait becomes spastic. The legs become numb, and bladder control is impaired.

In most cases surgical management of the neurofibroma is relatively easy. When it is exposed, the surgeon identifies the root from which the tumor arose. A metallic clip is placed across the nerve root proximal and distal to the tumor. The root is then divided at both points, and the tumor is lifted from its bed. It is usually otherwise unattached, but care must be taken to divide any adhesions that are present between the tumor and the pia mater of the cord. Next a watertight dura closure is done to prevent a CSF fistula. The wound is then closed in the manner of any laminectomy.

When the tumor is a meningioma the surgical approach is similar to that used for a neurofibroma. The tumor may lie in front of the cord, to one side of it, or rarely, behind it. The tumor usually is easily separated from the cord, but the surgeon should watch for adhesions between the tumor and the cord. The dura that is attached to the base of the tumor must be excised along with the tumor, because otherwise the tumor may recur. The excised dura must be replaced by a graft that is sewn in the deficit in a watertight manner. The dural incision made for exposure is next closed tightly, and a routine laminectomy closure follows.

Surgical treatment of an ependymoma or lipoma involving the cauda equina may be very difficult. The nerve roots of the cauda equina usually run through the bulk of the tumor. They often adhere densely to the tumor, which makes it impossible to dissect the tumor from them. In most cases the surgeon has to accept less than total removal, because to persist may injure the nerve roots. The procedure, therefore, is to use the microscope to remove as much tumor as possible and then follow up with X-ray therapy postoperatively.

The intradural extramedullary space is also surgically exposed to perform pain-relieving procedures such as a cordotomy or a rhizotomy (Chapter 10).

Intramedullary Pathology

Tumors occur in the spinal cord just as they do in the brain. The ependymoma and the astrocytoma are the common ones. Patients with intramedullary tumors show signs of cord compression as the

Figure 7-7 Complete Laminectomy at Three Levels, Exposing the Spinal Cord

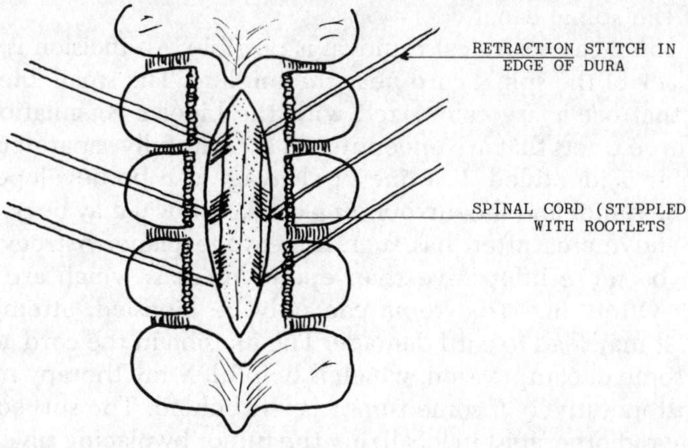

Figure 7-8 Common Intradural Extramedullary Spinal Cord Tumors

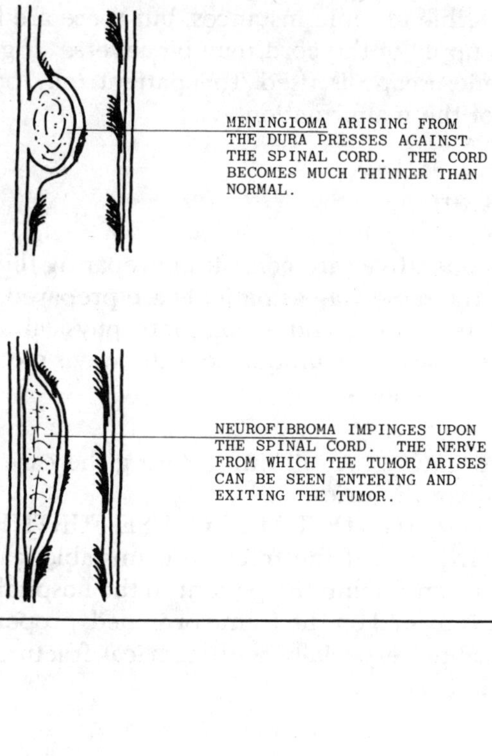

tumor expands, pressing the surrounding nerve tracts against the sides of the spinal canal.

In some cases surgical removal is possible. An incision is made in the back of the spinal cord near the midline. The small, bleeding vessels that occur are cauterized with the bipolar coagulation forceps. Nerve tracts that are encountered are carefully separated until the tumor is identified. If a line of cleavage can be developed between the tumor and the surrounding cord, removal may be possible. The ependymoma often has such a cleavage plane. Astrocytomas tend to be more infiltrative than ependymomas, which are more defined. Often an astrocytoma can only be biopsied; attempts to remove it may lead to cord damage. The incision in the cord accomplishes some decompression, which is helpful. X-ray therapy may be used postoperatively if some tumor is left behind. The surgeon can assist the radiotherapist in localizing the tumor by placing silver clips around the edge of the remaining tumor.

Arteriovenous malformations occur on the surface and inside of the spinal cord. They may bleed acutely or the patient may have symptoms suggestive of insidious cord disease. Arteriograms of the malformation's circulation are done with a catheter in the aorta. Dye is injected into vessels going to the spinal cord from the aorta. Surgical removal is possible in some instances, but there are hazards because the blood supply of the cord may be adverse. If great care is taken and the microscope is used, the patient may benefit from partial removal of the malformation.

Preoperative Care

Generally the preoperative care consists of preparing the patient for surgery in much the same way as patients are prepared for a craniotomy. A complete history, and a complete physical and general evaluation are necessary. The unique considerations dictated by the specific lesion are as follows:

I. Spinal cord injuries. At all times during the care of patients with spinal cord injuries:
   A. DO NOTHING THAT MAY CAUSE FURTHER SPINAL CORD INJURY. If the fracture is unstable, care must be taken in transferring the patient to the hospital. When the patient is turned on the frame or in bed, proper alignment of the spine (especially with cervical fractures) must be assured.

B. Prevent decubitus ulcers by good skin care.
C. Provide good bladder and bowel care (see Chapter 5).
D. Watch carefully for pulmonary problems. The quadriplegic patient breathes only with the diaphragm and cannot cough; therefore atelectasis and pneumonia are common.
E. Psychological support must be provided at all times. These patients must be encouraged.

II. Herniated nucleus pulposus.
A. It must always be remembered that ruptured discs are not the only cause of neck or back pain. Other causes include:
1. Muscular and ligamentous strains or sprains
2. Bony abnormalities of the spine such as spondylolisthesis
3. Neoplasms of the spine, particularly metastatic carcinoma
4. Disease of the abdominal and pelvic organs

B. The preoperative period for a patient with a suspected herniated nucleus pulposus is, therefore, a time for observation and diagnosis. If the pathological process is eventually identified as a neoplasm, or an intra-abdominal disease, or pelvic disease, the appropriate, specific treatment is provided. If the pain is due to a ruptured disc, muscular or ligamentous injury, or bony abnormalities, a period of conservative therapy is wise. Many patients will respond to the conservative efforts, thereby avoiding surgery. Such a conservative program includes:
1. Bed rest. The patient is permitted up only to go to the bathroom.
2. A firm mattress with a piece of plywood between the mattress and springs.
3. Pelvic or cervical traction. Pelvic traction with small weights used (20–30 pounds) does little other than keep the patient in bed. Cervical traction (8–12 pounds) may help to lessen spasm of the neck muscles.
4. Physical therapy. Heat, massage, and diathermy help to lessen the pain of muscle spasms.
5. Muscle relaxants. Several different medications are available that are supposed to have muscle-relaxing capabilities. It is doubtful, however, that they are very effective. Many seem to sedate the patient somewhat, thus perhaps providing some benefit.
6. Analgesics. When the patient is in acute pain, as is often the case at the onset, narcotics may be needed. Because

the problem is likely to be chronic and recurring, the medication should quickly be changed to nonnarcotic analgesics when the pain lessens.

C. When the patient fails to respond to an adequate period of conservative treatment, surgery is then considered, taking into account:
   1. Psychological factors. Is the patient overly reactive to pain? Is the patient hysterical or a malingerer? Is a lawsuit involved?
   2. Patient rapport. Is the surgery to be done because the surgeon is at the end of her or his rope? Is the patient insisting that something more be done? Never let the patient dictate his or her own treatment. This is a good time to get another consultation from a neurosurgeon or orthopedic surgeon.
   3. Informed consent (operative permit). Relief of pain and other symptoms should never be guaranteed. The patient will not have a normal back or neck following surgery, may continue to have difficulties, and may in the future need more surgery. Discuss the problems of future employment and insurance that might occur because of having had neck or back surgery. The patient should be told of the possibility of paraplegia. This should include not only a discussion of paralysis of limbs but also of problems occurring with sensory loss, bladder and bowel dysfunction, and the loss of sexual functions.

D. Preoperative medical preparation.
   1. If the patient has taken a lot of aspirin, the bleeding and clotting factors should be checked.
   2. If the patient is a smoker or has lung disease, it is wise to give intermittent positive pressure breathing (IPPB) along with mucolytic agents, bronchodilators, and expectorants. In this way the tracheobronchial passages are cleaned out. This helps to prevent postoperative pneumonia and atelectasis. The postoperative pain makes the patient reluctant to cough and deep breathe.
   3. Elastic stockings should always be used to prevent thrombophlebitis.

III. Spinal cord tumors. The major concern with spinal cord tumors (epidural, intradural, and intramedullary) is the possibility of rapidly developing paraplegia. The following points are made with this in mind:

A. The patient needs to be watched carefully by the medical team for signs of developing paraplegia; note motor, sensory, and bladder function.
B. If a myelogram is to be done, have contingency plans to do any definitive surgery thereafter. This is especially true if a complete block to the flow of dye occurs with the myelogram.
C. If the cord is under pressure from the tumor, dehydrating agents and cortisone may prevent or slow down spinal deterioration for awhile. It is of help to do this during the time between the myelogram and surgery.

Postoperative Care

Most of the points made in Chapter 6 about postoperative care of the craniotomy patient also apply to the postoperative care of a laminectomy patient. One additional factor is the problem of pain following a laminectomy. The pain is severe, and the patients are, therefore, reluctant to move and deep breathe. Active steps must be taken in the postoperative period to prevent pulmonary complications and thrombophlebitis.

Complications

The complications following a craniotomy may also occur after a laminectomy. Remember that a postoperative hematoma following a laminectomy can cause spinal cord compression and, therefore, quadriplegia or paraplegia. Check the movements of the extremities as a part of the neurological vital signs after a laminectomy.

CHAPTER 8

Peripheral Nerve Surgery

The peripheral nervous system, unlike the central nervous system, has regenerative capabilities. In spite of this the surgical results from peripheral nerve surgery are often less than ideal. Peripheral nerve surgery may be on peripheral nerves themselves or for the relief of the various compression syndromes.

In Chapter 1 the peripheral nervous system was discussed in terms of the sensory organs and the terminal effector organs of the motor system, leaving discussion of its anatomy until now. Remember that the dorsal and ventral nerve roots leave the spinal cord and fuse together. At the thoracic levels of the cord, this fused structure becomes the peripheral nerve. In the chest wall such a nerve runs along the lower edge of the rib at that particular level. Those nerves that run along the 8th through 12th ribs enter the abdominal wall at their respective rib ends. At the cervical, lumbar, and sacral cord levels, the fused neural structure joins similar structures above and below it. In this manner a plexus is formed. The brachial plexus is formed in the cervical area. In the lumbar region the lumbar plexus forms, and the sacral plexus is formed at the sacral level (Figures 8-1, 8-2, and 8-3).

A plexus provides a way by which nerve fibers arising from different cord levels can mix with each other. When the appropriate mixing and separating of nerve fibers is accomplished, specific peripheral nerves arise and leave the plexus. Each peripheral nerve then goes to its particular destination to provide motor supply to

Figure 8-1 Brachial Plexus, Showing the Origins of the Major Peripheral Nerves of the Upper Extremity

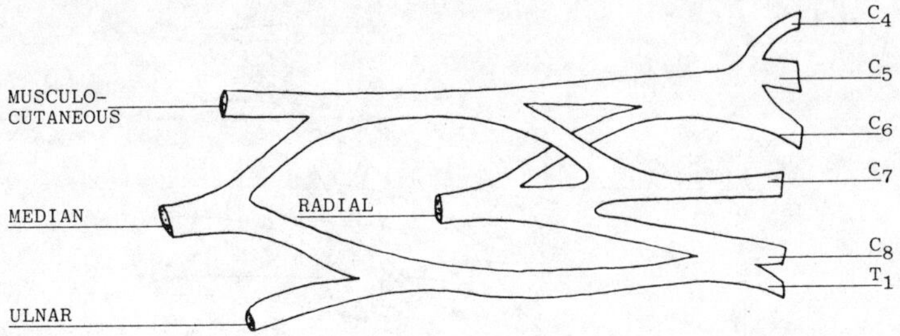

muscles and to join sensory organs in the skin, joints, muscles, and tendons.

A peripheral nerve is composed of a connective tissue framework that forms small tubules in which the nerve fibers run. The perineurium surrounds several nerve fibers. The endoneurium runs between adjacent nerve fibers. It is the endoneurium that makes the endoneural tubules. The perineurium and the axons it contains are called a fascicle. Some nerves contain several fascicles. Adjacent fascicles are bound together by the epineurium, which is a loose connective tissue outside of the perineurium (Figure 8-4).

Figure 8-2 Lumbar Plexus, Showing the Major Peripheral Nerves that Arise from the Plexus

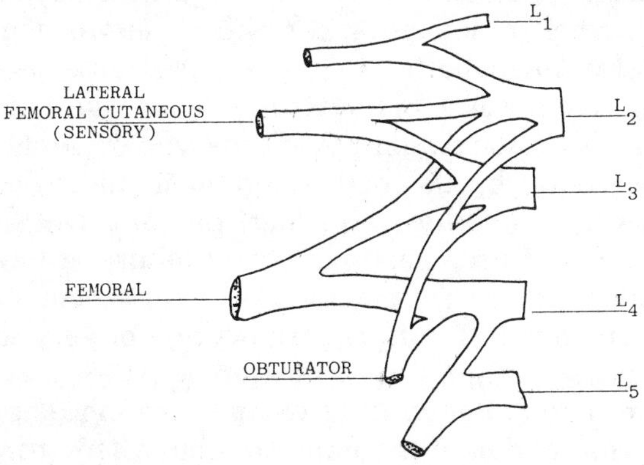

Figure 8-3 Sacral Plexus, Showing the Major Nerves that Arise from the Plexus

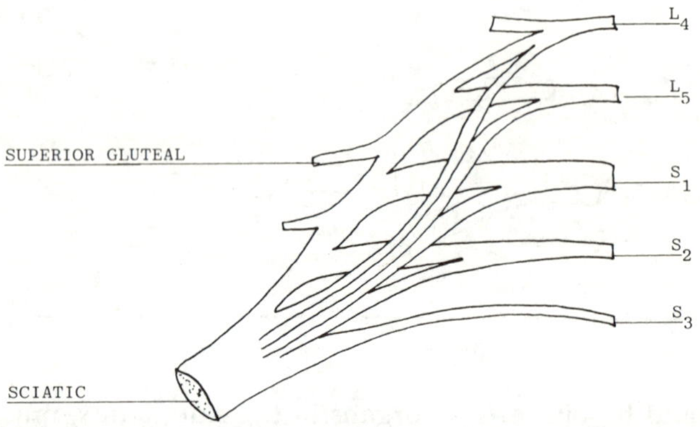

In Chapter 2 the many diseases that affect the peripheral nerves were discussed. Treatment in most instances is either the management of the basic medical problem or the elimination of toxic factors. The surgical problems that concern peripheral nerves occur as a result of trauma or entrapment of the nerve at some point along its length.

Trauma

Peripheral nerves may be completely or partially transected by sharp, penetrating objects or they may be contused by blunt trauma. Immediately after trauma to a peripheral nerve, it may be very difficult to determine whether the nerve was transected or whether it fails to function because of a contusion or because of pressure on it by adjacent soft-tissue swelling. Patients who present this dilemma are seen frequently by the neurosurgeon in the office. It can be expected that a mild contusion or local pressure will soon improve and function will return. This short-lived failure of function of the nerve is called neuropraxia. If recovery does not occur after a reasonable period, one begins to suspect transection or very severe contusion. A good history of the injury will often help the surgeon to decide which is more likely. Penetrating wounds are more apt to be associated with transection than blunt trauma where the skin is not penetrated. The electromyogram (EMG) and nerve conduction stud-

Figure 8-4 Cross-section of a Peripheral Nerve

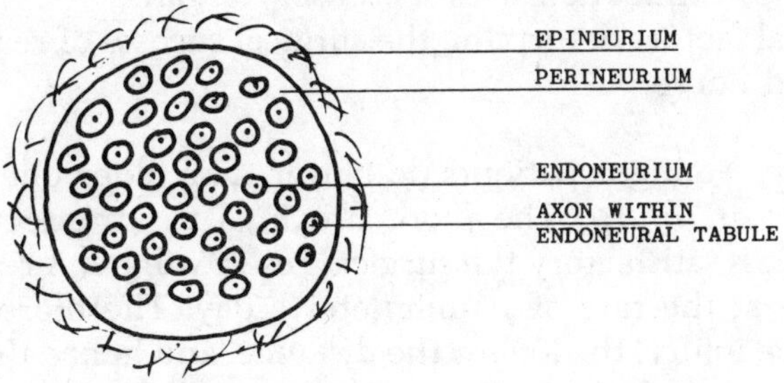

ies can also assist in evaluation of the extent and type of injury. In spite of contrary clinical factors and laboratory data, if recovery does not occur the nerve should be explored.

Many neurosurgeons believe the optimal time to repair a transected nerve is approximately 3 weeks after the injury. This is especially true if there was significant crushing of the nerve at the time of injury. The nerve has largely recovered from the insult of the injury at 3 weeks, and the axon is ready to grow. On the other hand some neurosurgeons will proceed with repair of the nerve at the time of injury if the nerve was severed by a sharp, penetrating object and tissue contusion was minimal.

A discussion of the changes that occur after a nerve is transected will reveal why 3 weeks after the injury may be the ideal time for surgical reanastomosis of the divided nerve ends. Within a few hours after a nerve is transected, changes occur in the nerve distal to the transection. The axons and their myelin sheath break down. Macrophages from the endoneurium enter the endoneural tubules and remove all debris by phagocytosis. Next Schwann's cells (the cells that produce myelin in the peripheral nerve) divide to produce cords of cells in the endoneural tubules. The Schwann's cells then grow out of the endoneural tubules toward the proximal end of the divided nerve. In this way the gap between the two divided ends of the nerve is bridged. Some degenerative change also occurs in the proximal end of the transected nerve, but it extends only a short distance from the end.

Next, regeneration begins with the axon in the proximal end elongating. When it reaches the site of transection, it sends out fibrils. Many of the fibrils are guided to the distal endoneural tubules by the

Schwann's cells that have grown across the gap. Subsequently the axon grows into the distal endoneural tubule and remyelination is begun. Eventually the axon reaches the motor end plate in muscle or establishes connection with its sensory organ.

Several factors determine the surgical success of reanastomosis of a divided nerve:

1. *Age.* Younger patients do better than older ones.

2. *Site of injury.* The more proximal the transection of the nerve, the less satisfactory the surgical result will be. A regenerating axon grows at the rate of 1 millimeter a day. Therefore, the more proximal the injury, the longer the distance, and hence the time, the axon must grow before function can be restored. Atrophy of a muscle may be considerable before the motor fiber can reach it.

3. *Mixed nerves.* Surgery on nerves that contain large numbers of both motor and sensory fibers is less successful than if the nerve contains primarily motor fibers or primarily sensory ones. This is because the regenerating axon that grows from the proximal end of the transection may enter the wrong endoneural tubule in the distal end of the transection. Thus a regenerating motor fiber may enter the endoneural tubule that was intended to contain a sensory fiber. Therefore the surgical repair of a transected radial nerve, which is largely motor, will be more successful than repair of a transected median nerve, which is mixed.

4. *Length of injury.* If a long segment of the nerve is injured, the surgical result will be less satisfactory than if the nerve was merely transected by a sharp object. Injuries to long segments occur with gunshot wounds. When long segments of a nerve are missing, it is often impossible to obtain length enough to join the remaining ends. If this happens the following steps may be tried:

a. The nerve, both proximal and distal, to the transection is freed from all surrounding tissue. This may permit the ends to be approximated more easily. It may, however, adversely affect the blood supply of the mobilized nerve.

b. Sometimes the elbow or knee can be bent to enable the anastomosis of the separated ends of the nerve. The flexed extremity must be kept in a splint until the nerve heals. A long period of immobilization may lead to the limitation of movement of the flexed joint. When healing occurs and the splint is removed, extension of the flexed elbow or knee will cause the nerve to stretch and may hamper the nerve's regeneration.

c. The other remedy for the large gap between nerve ends is a nerve graft (discussed below).

5. *Associated injury.* Significant injury to surrounding muscles, tendons, ligaments, and bone will adversely affect recovery. Severe local injury may lead to scar formation and possible involvement of the nerve. Local blood supply may be compromised. Infection will undoubtly lessen the chance of a satisfactory surgical result. Fractured bones may increase the amount of stretch injury suffered by the nerve.

Surgical Techniques

If the nerve at surgery is found to be bound tightly within scar tissue, the neurosurgeon will perform a neurolysis. An external neurolysis is done when the nerve is dissected free of the surrounding scar tissue. Scarring of this type occurs when there was local hemorrhage as well as injury to the tissues that lay adjacent to the nerve. If the nerve itself was also injured by blunt trauma, scarring may occur within the nerve. Recall that the framework of a peripheral nerve is composed of connective tissue. It heals, when injured, by forming scar tissue that may act as constrictive bands around fascicles of the nerve. When this occurs an internal neurolysis is required. An old technique of performing an internal neurolysis was to inject saline into the nerve at the site of suspected internal scarring. The saline supposedly dissected along the fascicles of the nerve, disrupting encircling bands of scar tissue. It is now believed that this technique is probably not very effective in relieving the constrictive pressures imposed by the scar. The increasing use of the dissecting microscope and the advent of microsurgical techniques have made it possible to incise the nerve and cut bands of scar under direct vision. The individual fascicles can be freed of scar in this manner.

When the nerve has been transected, a neurorrhaphy is performed. The dissecting microscope should be used if all possible; 6–10 power magnification is usually sufficient. If the transection is a clean one, no trimming is needed. If not, a few millimeters can be trimmed from each end. Both ends are viewed in the microscope in an effort to match the ends of nerve. It is usually possible to find a blood vessel on the nerve's surface that has also been cut and, with it, match the two ends of the nerve. By marking this and by looking at the individual fascicles of the nerve, proper alignment is accomplished. Each divided fascicle is next sutured to its matching member. Very small stitches are placed through the epineurium of the two ends of the divided fascicle. The two ends are pulled together, and the knot is tied. Similar stitches are placed in the perineurium around the circumference of the fascicle. Interrupted stitches are used because a running stitch could be constrictive. The fascicles in the center of the nerve are sutured first, and those laterally situated are done last. Eventually the perineurium of the entire nerve is sutured with multiple interrupted stitches.

When a long length of nerve is lost at the time of injury, nerve grafts can be used. Nerves grafted from other humans or cadavers are not well tolerated, so until the rejection problem is solved, the nerve used in the graft will have to come from the patient. This means there will be a neurological deficit at the donor site. The only nerves that can be used are, therefore, the smaller sensory nerves like the sural nerve in the calf; and these nerves are not large enough to graft the larger peripheral nerves such as the median nerve or the sciatic nerve.

Traumatic Entrapment Neuropathies and Compression Syndromes

Traumatic entrapment of peripheral nerves can occur at any point along a nerve's path. Entrapment of a nerve by scar tissue was discussed above. Now the discussion turns to entrapment that occurs other than by scar, to the more common traumatic neuropathies, and to compression syndromes.

Carpal Tunnel Syndrome

The carpal tunnel begins at the wrist and extends to the middle of the palm. The tunnel contains several tendons and the median nerve. Figure 8-5 should be noted to understand how compression can occur. Compression within the tunnel occurs either if the tunnel is made smaller or if there is swelling of the structures in the canal. It is easy to see that a fracture of one or more of the bones of the tunnel may cause the canal to be smaller. Rheumatoid arthritis may also decrease the size of the carpal tunnel. The carpal tunnel syndrome is often associated with pregnancy. In most cases the symptoms of median nerve compression disappear when the pregnancy is terminated. It is probably fluid retention with swelling that produces the syndrome in pregnancy. The carpal tunnel syndrome also

Figure 8-5 Cross-section of the Carpal Tunnel

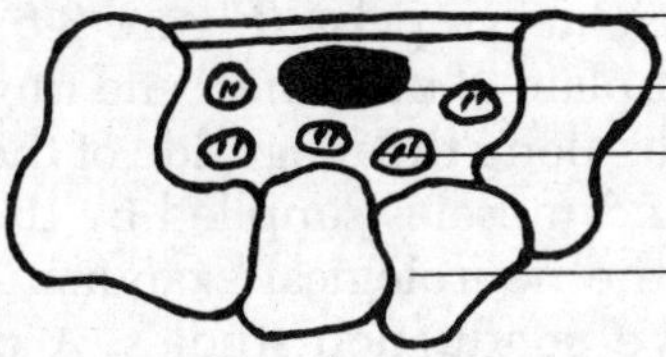

occurs when the palm of the hand and wrist receive undue pressure such as occurs with the use of a jackhammer or the like. The syndrome may also occur without any obvious cause.

The patient complains of numbness of the thumb, forefinger, and middle finger. There is also weakness of the muscles supplied by the median nerve. In addition to numbness the patients also complain of pain in the wrist or hand. The pain, often described as an ache, may extend up the arm a variable distance.

The diagnosis is made clinically and can be confirmed with an EMG and nerve conduction times. There is slowed conduction through the carpal tunnel. If the examiner taps the wrist with his or her finger, the patient will feel the radiation of numbness and tingling in the involved fingers. When this occurs, the patient is said to have a positive Tinel's sign.

Treatment

1. The wrist should be splinted so the patient does not bend it.
2. Corticosteroids may be injected into the canal; this sometimes provides good relief.
3. If all conservative efforts fail, surgery is performed. The carpal ligament is divided. The division should be done with direct vision, and it should be a complete division. Failure to get relief often means the ligament was not divided in the palm.

Entrapment of the Ulnar Nerve

The ulnar nerve is commonly entrapped at the elbow where it runs in the ulnar groove. A fracture of the epicondyle may compress the ulnar nerve that swings around it. The new bone growth may actually surround the ulnar nerve. The nerve is very superficial at this point, which makes it vulnerable both to blunt trauma (e.g., funny bone sensation) and to penetrating injury. People who sit at a desk or in an armchair will often rest their elbows on the desk or chair arm for long periods of time. This may lead to chronic ulnar nerve compression and eventually to an ulnar nerve palsy (Figure 8-6).

Clinically the patient will complain of numbness and tingling of the fourth and fifth fingers as well as along the ulnar side of the hand. There will be weakness of the hand muscles supplied by the ulnar nerve. The diagnosis is made by the neurological examination and confirmed by the EMG and nerve conduction studies. A positive Tinel's sign can be elicited at the elbow, but normally tapping of the ulnar nerve will cause radiating paresthesia.

Treatment

1. Eliminate the cause, for example, by padding the elbow, and refrain from resting it on the desk, etc.
2. If the nerve is involved by bone growth, it must be freed by surgery.
3. If the nerve is repeatedly bumped or involved in scar, it is usually removed from the ulnar groove to a position forward of the epicondyle. Some neurosurgeons will merely remove the medial epicondyle with a bone rongeur. This permits the ulnar nerve to be pulled a bit forward of its normal position when the elbow is bent.

The Radial Nerve

The radial nerve lies next to the humerus and spirals around it at about the midpoint of this bone. Therefore fractures of the humerus very often are associated with a radial nerve palsy. It is not uncom-

Figure 8-6 Ulnar Nerve in the Ulnar Groove Swings around the Medial Epicondyle at the Elbow

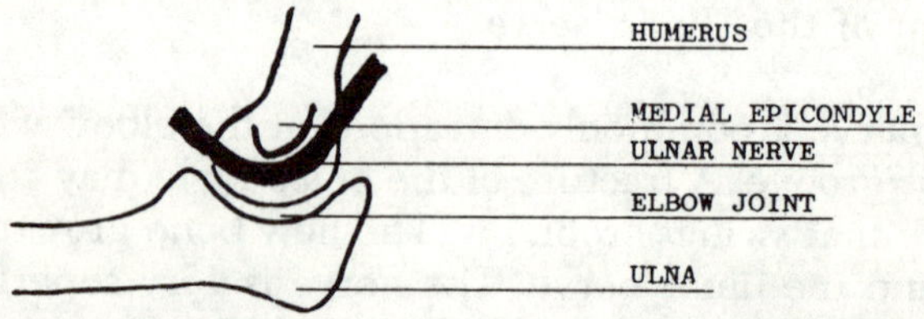

mon to have the radial nerve incorporated within the callus of the healing bone. Because the radial nerve is located close to the bone, it is vulnerable to compression. Compression may occur when the patient rests an arm upon the back of a chair; hence, radial nerve palsy is also called the Saturday night palsy. One can visualize a drunken person on Saturday night coming home and passing out with an arm hanging over the back of a chair. Clinically a patient will have a wristdrop, which means an inability to extend the wrist. The patient will also have a little numbness on the back of the hand.

Treatment

1. If the palsy has occurred because the nerve is incorporated in callus, surgery is done to free the nerve.
2. If the palsy is the result of compression by position (e.g., arm on back of chair), nothing is done. The chance of recovery in this instance is quite good. It is advisable to place the wrist in a splint, holding it in a functional position. The wrist should be slightly extended when in the splint. Range of motion must be maintained until the nerve's function returns.

The Brachial Plexus

Injuries of the brachial plexus are common in this age of the automobile and mechanization, and they occur in a variety of ways. The brachial plexus is very susceptible to traction injuries. The use of forceps to pull on a baby's head at birth may injure the brachial plexus. In an accident or fall the plexus may be stretched and may occasionally be avulsed from the spinal cord. Injuries to the plexus occur when patients get their arms pulled violently as a result of accidentally catching them in various types of machinery. Entrapment or compression of the brachial plexus may occur with fractures of the clavicle or first rib, two structures between which the plexus runs; the callus, or malalignment of a healed fracture, may significantly reduce the space between the clavicle and rib. Compression of the brachial plexus between the clavicle and rib is called the costoclavicular compression syndrome. The brachial plexus is also thought by some neurologists and neurosurgeons to be vulnerable to compression at the point where the plexus runs between the scalenus anterior and the scalenus medius in the neck. This is called the scalenus anticus syndrome. Metastatic tumors often spread to the supraclavicular area and compress the brachial plexus. Clinically a patient will have neurological complaints and deficits that depend on how severely and completely the plexus is involved by the disease process.

Treatment

1. In general the surgical results of brachial plexus surgery are less satisfactory than surgery on individual peripheral nerves.
2. If the plexus is transected by a penetrating instrument, it is worthwhile to reapproximate the divided ends, but the results will probably be disappointing.
3. The costoclavicular syndrome is treated by removing a portion of the first rib.
4. The scalenus anticus syndrome was previously treated by merely dividing the anterior scalene muscle, but results were often poor. Now many neurosurgeons resect the first rib, including the point where the anterior scalene muscle attaches.
5. When the plexus is bound down by scar, an external neurolysis may be done. If tumor involves the plexus, X-ray therapy is given to temporize function and relieve pain.
6. Usually nothing can be done if the plexus is avulsed from the cord.

Compression Syndromes of the Nerves of the Leg

Many of the nerves of the leg may be trapped by scar tissue or are anatomically entrapped. The two nerves most commonly so involved are the common peroneal nerve and the sciatic nerve.

Common Peroneal Nerve

Running very superficially around the head of the fibula just below the outer side of the knee, the common peroneal nerve is vulnerable to pressure; and when it is injured, the patient has a foot drop. This causes patients to have to lift the afflicted leg high in taking steps to avoid stubbing the toes. The nerve may be injured when sleeping, when crossing the legs while seated, and from pressure of a tightly applied cast.

Treatment:

1. Avoid pressure on the nerve if that is the cause of the palsy.
2. If divided or entrapped by scar, the appropriate surgical procedure is done.

3. The patient with foot drop should be fitted for a brace. This will aid walking and lessen the tendency of heel cord shortening. Full range of motion of the ankle must be maintained until the nerve's function returns.

Sciatic Nerve

The sciatic nerve can be injured deep within the buttocks as it crosses the sciatic notch. Common causes of injury include severe external trauma, an improperly administered hypodermic injection, and a dislocated hip.

Treatment:

1. If there is probable transection or entrapment of the nerve, surgical exploration is in order.
2. External and internal neurolysis may be needed.
3. If the nerve is divided, an anastomosis of the divided ends is worth trying.

Preoperative Care

Preoperative efforts are to prepare the patient for surgery; they are like those to prepare for a craniotomy, because the same general considerations apply. If the surgery is done with local or regional anesthesia (block), a complete history and a complete physical and general evaluation are still necessary. The following considerations are more unique to peripheral nerve injuries:

1. Range of motion of the involved limbs is necessary.
2. Avoid injury to the involved extremity. The loss of sensation that may be present makes injury more likely. The patient can not feel the pain of a tight cast or pain from excessively hot water.
3. Minimize atrophy of muscles that have lost their nerve supply. Massage and electrical stimulation are both helpful.
4. Treat all skin lesions. It is unwise to operate on any patient who has infected skin lesions.

Postoperative Care

The same postoperative principles apply to peripheral nerve patients and to craniotomy patients. The following points need to be mentioned in addition:

1. It is still necessary to maintain joint range of motion, avoid injury to the injured extremity, and minimize atrophy of muscles.
2. Mobilize the patient as soon as possible to avoid the usual postoperative complications (see Postoperative Care in Chapter 6).
3. If the patient is to use crutches, be sure they fit and the patient is instructed to use them properly. Excessive pressure in the axilla can hurt peripheral nerves.
4. If a splint is applied to an extremity, be sure it is applied properly. Inspect the wound daily if possible.
5. If a joint was flexed to permit the anastomosis of the divided nerve, a splint must be applied. Remember the range of motion of that joint will be adversely affected. Mobilize the joint as soon as possible and give active treatment. When a joint is flexed and in a splint, periodically make a new splint that decreases the angle of flexion each time.

CHAPTER 9

Neurosurgical Procedures for Miscellaneous Disorders

In addition to the major categories of neurosurgery discussed so far, there are several neurosurgical procedures that are somewhat difficult to classify. A general understanding of them is essential to a broad understanding of neurological surgery.

Hydrocephalus and Congenital Malformations

Hydrocephalus

Recall from earlier discussions of the causes and pathology of hydrocephalus that there are two general types: (1) Obstructive or noncommunicating hydrocephalus occurs as the result of some process that blocks the normal flow of CSF from its site of origin in the lateral ventricles to the subarachnoid space; and (2) Nonobstructive or communicating hydrocephalus occurs when the CSF is not absorbed by the arachnoid granulations after it has reached the subarachnoid space.

A review of the evolution of surgical procedures used to treat hydrocephalus is instructive. One of the first efforts of surgical treatment was the excision of the choroid plexus. It was reasoned that if the source of the spinal fluid was eliminated, hydrocephalus would not occur. The fact of the matter is that, in spite of removal of the choroid plexus, the disease usually continues.

Dr. Walter Dandy described an operation called the third ventriculostomy to be used to treat obstructive hydrocephalus. A hole was made in the wall of the dilated third ventricle. A fistula was thereby created through which CSF would then flow into the subarachnoid space of the basal cisterns and then over the cerebral hemispheres to be absorbed by the arachnoid villi.

An ingenious operation called the ventriculocisternostomy was devised by Dr. A. Torkildsen. In this procedure one end of a catheter is inserted into one of the lateral ventricles through a burr hole. The tube then runs under the scalp, the other end being placed in the cisterna magnum. CSF flows from the ventricle through the catheter into the cisterna magnum. The Torkildsen shunt is still used to treat obstructive hydrocephalus in children and adults. It does not work well in most infants who have obstructive hydrocephalus as a result of congenital malformations. The reason for this failure is probably because the subarachnoid space has not formed completely in these infants.

Because a large percentage of hydrocephalus occurs in infants with various congenital malformations, better surgical solutions were still needed. Several types of shunting devices were next used to divert the flow of spinal fluid. Shunts were tried that carried the CSF to virtually every organ or space of the body. The fluid was shunted to the kidney, gall bladder, pleural cavity, peritoneal cavity, and heart—among many others—the heart and the peritoneal cavity becoming the most common choices.

The brain-to-cardiac shunt is one in which one end of a catheter is inserted into the right lateral ventricle through a burr hole in the skull located behind the right ear. The catheter is then attached to a pump device. The other end of the shunt then runs from the pump device to the heart. This is accomplished by tunneling the catheter under the skin to the internal jugular vein in the neck. The catheter is then inserted into the vein and advanced until the end is in the right atrium of the heart. Several types of pumping devices have been developed. They are designed to be pumped manually or to passively permit the flow of the CSF when the pressure in the ventricles increases. Manual pumping is done by pressing on the skin that overlies the pump. When the pump is pressed, CSF is pushed into the heart; when it is released, CSF is drawn into the pump from the ventricle. The end of the catheter in the heart is designed so CSF can escape into the blood but so blood cannot enter the catheter.

The brain-to-cardiac shunt works nicely and is applicable in obstructive hydrocephalus in both infants and adults. When used in infants, problems arise as the infant grows. As the body of the infant lengthens, the catheter going to the heart becomes too short. The cardiac end of the shunt consequently is withdrawn into the superior vena cava. When this occurs, the shunt does not work well, and often a clot forms around the end of the shunt. Frequent revisions are, therefore, necessary during the first few years of life.

The brain-to-peritoneal shunt is preferred by some neurosurgeons over the brain-to-cardiac shunt. The same shunt device is used commonly, but the end that comes from the pump device is inserted into the peritoneal cavity rather than into the heart. A long length of catheter can be coiled up in the peritoneal cavity so that as the body grows the end of the catheter remains in the peritoneal cavity. This shunt works well but, as with the brain-to-cardiac shunt, various problems arise.

The lumbar subarachnoid–to–peritoneal shunt is a useful shunt for treatment of communicating hydrocephalus or pseudotumor cerebri, a disease that usually occurs in obese females. For some reason (possibly hormonal) diffuse swelling of the brain occurs. The patient has headache, nausea, vomiting, and often visual complaints, like a patient with a brain tumor—therefore the term *pseudotumor.* These patients may become blind if treatment is not provided. A lumbar subarachnoid–to–peritoneal shunt functions by carrying CSF from the lumbar subarachnoid space through a small catheter under the skin to the peritoneal space.

There are two problems that occur with all shunts: infection and mechanical malfunction of the shunt device. Meningitis, or infection along the length of the catheter, may occur. When this happens the entire shunt must be removed becaused the infection will never be irradicated if the shunt remains in place. The mechanical problems that occur are many and varied. For example, if the protein content of the CSF is high, the catheters may be plugged. There is also the chance that the catheters can be kinked, preventing CSF flow.

Although shunting techniques and their designs change frequently, certain principles in their use do not. The use of a shunt should satisfy the following criteria:

1. It should shunt the CSF from the ventricles or subarachnoid space, preventing progressive ventricular enlargement.
2. The CSF should be shunted to a space, like the peritoneal cavity or the blood, where it is not lost by the body. For example, in the past, CSF has, on occasion, been shunted to the ureter, where it is lost in the urine.

3. The shunt should be contained within the body where infection is minimized.
4. If possible the shunt technique used should be able to compensate for growth in body length.
5. The shunt should be installed with a minimum amount of surgery.
6. The design and materials should minimize the chances for mechanical failure and the need for revision.

Craniosynostosis

Craniosynostosis (craniostenosis) (see Chapter 2 for the pathology), the premature closure of the suture lines of the growing skull, produces two problems. The more common problem is a cosmetically unacceptable head shape. The more serious one is the possible prevention of brain growth because closure of the suture lines prevents expansion of the skull.

The objective of the surgical treatment is to open the closed suture line. There are several variations in the technique used (Figure 9–1). A bone rongeur is used to make a channel in the bone the full length of the closed suture line. It is not enough merely to open the suture line, because new bone growth is rapid at this stage of life, and fusion between the two edges of the channel will occur rapidly. This is prevented by folding a strip of silastic over the bone edge and by suturing it securely. When multiple sutures are closed, each one must be opened. The procedure will not succeed if the full length of the suture is not opened.

Blood loss and infection are the hazards of this operation. It must be realized that infants have a small blood volume, so that shock may occur if bleeding is not strictly controlled. Infection is disastrous because it will spread the full length of the silastic strip. A brain abscess or meningitis may occur. Once infection occurs, the silastic strip must be removed before the infection can be controlled; it is virtually impossible to cure an infection if a foreign body is present.

Meningomyelocele

The meningomyelocele is a malformation that most commonly occurs in the lumbar area but that can occur at any point along the length of the spine. It results because of failure of the development of the bone over the back of the spinal canal, failure of midline fusion of muscles and fibrous tissue, and failure of proper skin coverage. As

Figure 9-1 Surgical Treatment of Craniosynostosis

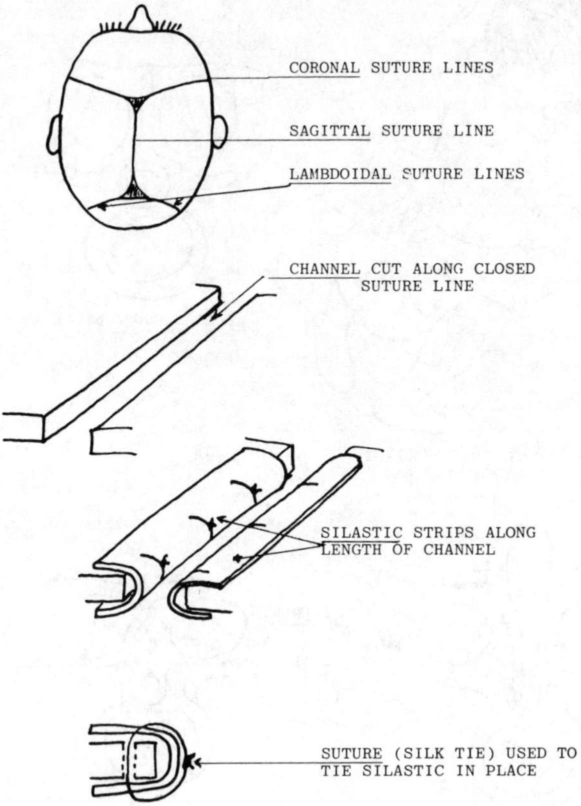

a result the dura and elements of the cord or cauda equina herniate outward, presenting a dome-shaped mass on the back. The skin seems to fuse with the dura around the edges, but it seldom covers the entire mass (Figure 9–2). At birth, a meningomyelocele presents a thin-walled structure that contains spinal fluid. It is often ruptured as the baby passes through the birth canal, and spinal fluid can be seen draining from it.

Early closure of a meningomyelocele is important for two reasons. If the sac has ruptured, there is a hazard of infection. There is also evidence that neurological deficits will be less severe with early closure. It is believed that pressure in the meningomyelocele stretches the nervous tissue in it and causes further injury.

Figure 9-2 Surgical Treatment of a Meningomyelocele

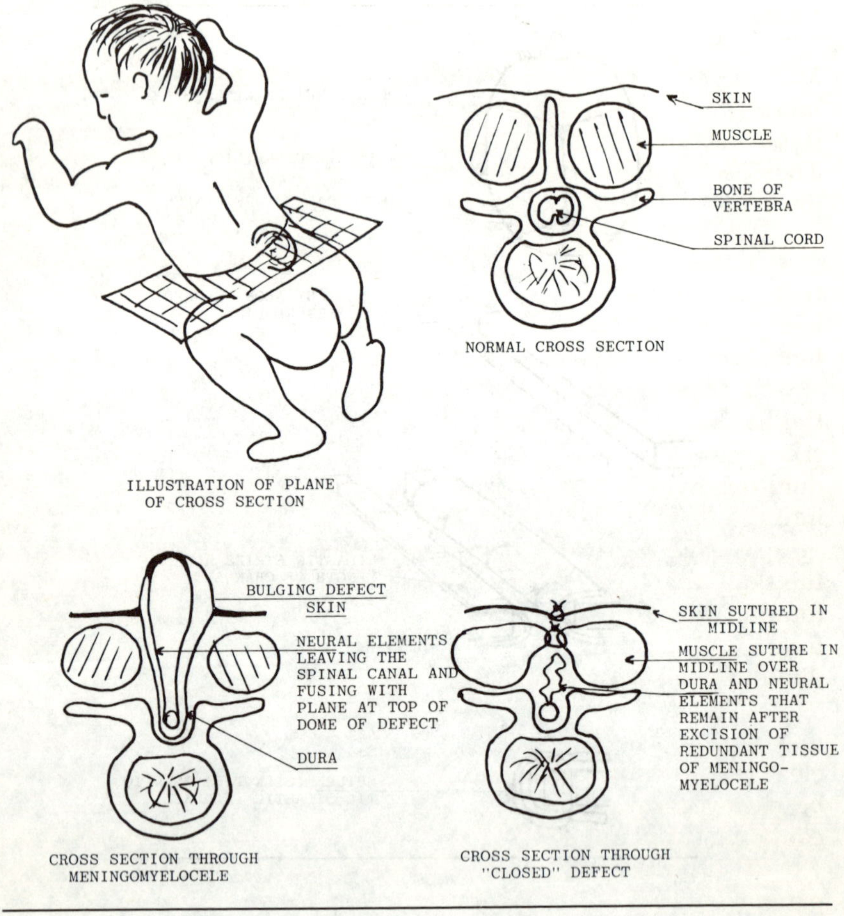

The closure of a meningomyelocele is accomplished by excising as much redundant dura and skin as possible. Often the neural components fuse in a tangle at the top of the defect's dome. In that case, the defect is buried under the muscle and skin closure.

The closure of a meningomyelocele usually will not improve the neurological status of the infant. Very often the baby is paraplegic and will remain so for life. There is also likely to be no voluntary control of bladder or bowel function. As if that were not enough, these patients often have associated neurological problems such as hydrocephalus as well as various orthopedic problems including clubfeet.

Skull Fractures and Skull Defects

Simple Fractures

Most skull fractures require no surgical treatment. They are seen merely as simple, linear shadows on a skull X ray and are usually stable, healing in a few months without ever causing any symptoms. The following are instances when fractures may require surgical intervention:

1. Sharp edges of the fractured bone may lacerate blood vessels that run in the dura or brain and thereby cause bleeding and hematoma formation. The management of epidural and subdural hematomas was discussed in Chapter 6.

2. The fractured bone may lacerate the dura, which permits the leakage of CSF through the ear (otorrhea) or the nose (rhinorrhea). Healing usually occurs spontaneously, but on occasion the dura may require suturing or a graft of fascia may need to be sewn into the defect.

3. Fracture lines very frequently run to foramina in the base of the skull. When this occurs, the cranial nerves that exit through the foramina may be injured. Rarely, it may be necessary to open the foramen if it can be shown that the size of the foramen has been diminished. The facial nerve is often injured in this manner.

4. If a laceration of the scalp is associated with a skull fracture, it is wise to take the patient to the operating room to debride, cleanse, and close the wound. It is imperative that all dirt and hair be removed because an infection will occur if the wound is closed containing contaminants.

5. If portions of fractured bone are driven into the brain, the patient is taken to the operating room to elevate or remove the fractured pieces of bone. If there is an associated laceration of the scalp, surgical treatment should be rendered immediately to lessen the chance of infection.

Compound Depressed Skull Fractures

All compound depressed skull fractures are by definition contaminated wounds. They must be thoroughly cleansed as soon as possible. Many of these wounds will contain hair, fragments of clothing, paint, grease, and most any other contaminant imaginable. In addition, the scalp laceration may be extensive, and much of the tissue may have been so severely injured that it cannot survive, making it necessary to cut away injured tissue that has been devitalized.

The management of the fractured bone requires judgment on the part of the surgeon. In most cases any bone fragments that have been completely detached and that lie free within the wound should be removed. They have lost their blood supply and are therefore devitalized. If not removed, they act as a haven for bacteria. If, however, the bone is fractured through the outer table only and it is driven inward, it may be all right to elevate the fragment to its normal position. If the wound is grossly contaminated, even this may be unwise. Once bone is infected (osteomyelitis) the infection is almost impossible to control with antibiotics, so adequate debridement must be accomplished inititially. If fragments of bone are driven through the dura and into the brain, they must be removed. If there is any question about some fragments of bone remaining within the substance of the brain, an X ray should be obtained in the operating room before the wound is closed.

Any one of the hematomas discussed in Chapter 6 (intracerebral, subdural, and epidural) may be encountered with a depressed skull fracture. Bleeding from lacerated dural sinuses commonly occurs with depressed skull fractures. Very often a fragment of bone is driven into a dural sinus, so that, when the surgeon removes or elevates the fragment, massive bleeding occurs. This eventuality must be kept in mind, and blood should be available should it be needed.

Finally, when the bleeding is under control, closure of the wound is begun. The wound is thoroughly irrigated with saline solution. If the brain is exposed, solutions containing antibiotics should not be used. A watertight closure of the dura should be done if at all possible. Failure to achieve this greatly increases the risk of the occurrence of a brain abscess or meningitis. Often in extensive skull fractures, the dura is so badly shredded that any closure is impossible. In this instance one should debride the dura and then sew a graft in the dural defect. The fascia lata, which is a strong membrane obtained from the outer aspect of the patient's thigh, makes an ideal graft for this purpose. The graft is sewn into position using a monofilament, synthetic running stitch. Braided stitches, such as silk or cotton, are less desirable because bacteria get between the filaments of the stitch material and are thereby inaccessible to antibiotics.

The scalp is closed when a watertight dural closure has been accomplished. It is usually better to do a single-layer closure of the scalp when gross contamination is present. Buried stitches and their knots may harbor bacteria. A monofilament, synthetic stitch or small-gauge wire works very well. A sterile dressing is then applied after coating the suture line with antibiotic ointment.

Repair of Skull Defects

Cranioplasty is the term applied to the surgical procedure by which a bony skull defect is repaired. A deficit of skull bone occurs when bone fragments of a depressed skull fracture are removed or when the bone flap is removed for some reason at the time of a craniotomy. A cranioplasty is done to protect the brain against penetrating injuries and to remove unsightly (especially on the forehead) scalp depressions that result from the absence of underlying bone.

The defect in the bone can be filled or covered with several different materials. A flat piece of sheet metal called tantalum may be cut to cover the defect. Holes are drilled around the edge of the plate, and the plate is then secured tightly to the skull with small screws. Pieces of rib can be removed and placed in the bony defect. The rib acts as a graft, forming, ideally, a strong bony union with the exposed edges of the skull.

More recently substances have become available that can be mixed at the operating room table and molded to the exact configuration and size of the skull defect. When completed, the result is a strong, contoured plate that is tied to the surrounding skull by suture material or wire.

Infection is the big hazard following a cranioplasty. If the wound was infected at the time the skull defect was created, a cranioplasty should not be performed for a year. This should provide time for complete healing and removal of any foci of bacteria that might remain. If a cranioplasty becomes infected, the artificial material must be removed before healing will occur.

Epilepsy

Most patients with a seizure disorder are not candidates for surgery; instead the seizures must be controlled as well as possible with anticonvulsant medication. The candidate for the surgical treatment of epilepsy is the patient who is incapacitated in spite of adequate medical treatment and whose seizures originate from a single, surgically accessible focus in the brain. Such a focus is usually in the cortex, and it can be accurately located by the EEG.

The surgery is done by performing a craniotomy that exposes that portion of the cortex where the epileptic focus is located. When the brain is exposed, small sterile EEG electrodes are placed on the cortical surface. The electroencephalographer can in this way be very precise about the location and size of the epileptic focus. When the focus has been pinpointed, that portion of the cortex is excised.

In the average neurosurgical practice, patients who are candidates for cortical resection are not frequently encountered. In most instances surgery of this nature should be done by a neurosurgeon who has frequent access to patients of this type. The volume permits him or her to perfect both the diagnostic and operative techniques.

Spasticity

Patients who have suffered spinal cord injuries frequently develop severe flexor spasms of the lower extremities. The legs will suddenly and uncontrollably flex in a violent manner. Such patients may be injured when they are thrown against bed rails or from their wheelchairs. Violent spasms also make skin care difficult because of bruising. If decubitus ulcers have developed, it is almost impossible to get them to heal if the patient has significant flexor spasms.

It has been shown that good nursing care will often prevent or minimize flexor spasms. If the full range of motion of all joints in the lower extremities is maintained, the spasms are less severe. If the bladder is not permitted to become distended and if bowel function is maintained, spasms are also less likely to occur. In spite of all efforts, however, some patients will be troubled with flexor spasms. Because nursing care and rehabilitation are difficult when spasms occur, often specific effort is required to treat them.

It has long been realized that, if the reflex arc is interrupted, flexor spasms will not occur. This is most easily accomplished by cutting either the dorsal or the ventral roots. The technique of cutting the dorsal root is the same procedure that is done when a dorsal rhizotomy is performed to achieve pain relief (see Chapter 10). The dorsal root is cut, not to divide the entering pain fibers, but instead to divide fibers that carry impulses from the muscle's spindles and joint position sense receptors. In other words, cutting the dorsal root divides the sensory portion of the gamma loop system. If the ventral root is cut instead of the dorsal root, we have divided the motor portion of the gamma loop as well as the motor fibers that arise from the anterior horn cells and go to muscle fibers.

If it is desirable to stop flexor spasms in the legs, the reflex arcs must be divided at all levels of the spinal cord that are concerned with function of the legs. Therefore the dorsal or ventral roots must be divided from T_{12} or L_1 to S_1 inclusively and bilaterally. This is done by performing complete laminectomies exposing cord segments T_{12}–S_1. The dura is then opened, and the dorsal roots or ventral roots are cut over the segments selected. Experience has shown that if the dorsal roots are cut, the relief obtained may not last; just why is not clear. Thus it is probably better to cut the ventral roots to achieve a lasting result.

Spasticity can also be relieved on occasion by injection of absolute alcohol or phenol intrathecally (into the spinal fluid). These substances are extremely noxious when they come into contact with neural tissue, so they can in effect produce a chemical rhizotomy. A chemical rhizotomy is done by performing a spinal tap with the patient lying on his or her side. The foot of the bed is elevated on blocks so the buttocks are higher than the head. CSF is permitted to drip until it stops, which means the fluid level is at the point of the needle. Alcohol is then injected slowly through the spinal needle. The chemical rhizotomy will be done on all neural structures that pass through the alcohol layer. The problem with the chemical rhizotomy is that nerves going to the bladder are also chemically divided. This may be unacceptable if the patient has been able to achieve reflex emptying of the bladder.

Other surgical procedures can also be used to reduce or eliminate spasticity. Because spasms of the muscles that adduct the legs are especially bothersome, the obturator nerve, which goes to these muscles, can be divided. Similarly the sciatic nerve could conceivably be divided to eliminate spasms in the lower extremities.

Mental Disorders

Observations of people with brain injuries and experimental evidence led to the concept of surgical treatment of mental disease in the latter part of the nineteenth century. Initially surgery was done on patients who were psychotic; especially those who had schizophrenia. A critical review of the results in those patients led generally to the opinion that the surgery was not particularly helpful. To be sure, many experienced relief of their schizophrenia symptoms, but many manifested personality changes and behavior patterns that were equally undesirable.

The initial operations were procedures in which most of the fiber tracts going to and coming from the frontal lobes were divided. In effect the cortex of much of the frontal lobes was isolated from the rest of the brain. The operations were called prefrontal lobotomies or prefrontal leucotomies.

The undesirable effects of the operations were those attendant on any frontal lobe destruction or disease. The patients were often apathetic, showing little concern for their physical appearance or for the feelings of others. They were disruptive in the family situation, often causing embarrassment to other family members and friends. Although the undesired effects tended to lessen with time, many patients required continual custodial care.

As experience broadened, it was realized that if certain general regions of the frontal lobe's white matter were disrupted and other regions were left alone, the desired results could be achieved while the undesired results could be minimized. It was also appreciated that the limited and more specific techniques worked better on patients who had nonpsychotic illnesses; compulsive and anxiety neurosis, anxiety states, depression, and drug addiction seemed to be reasonably improved with the more limited techniques.

At present there are no hard-and-fast rules about where cuts should be made. It appears, however, that, in patients with nonpsychotic illness, undercutting of the cortex of the orbital surface (the underside) of the frontal lobes is most effective. It is probable that the effects realized result because tracts from the hypothalamus and thalamus going to the orbital cortex are divided.

Surgical treatment of mental disorders has dwindled from its more common use in the 1940s. The major strides in treatment have been in the realm of medical treatment, although the modifications in techniques and the selectivity in their use has earned surgery a legitimate place in the treatment of mental disorders.

Involuntary Movements

The various involuntary movements that occur in neurological disease were discussed in Chapter 3. In spite of the fact that involuntary movements occur with diseases of the basal ganglia, historically the initial surgical attempts to stop these movements were concerned with the interruption of motor pathways. A portion of the motor cortex was excised or else the corticospinal tract was divided. To be sure the movements usually ceased, but paralysis was the price usually paid.

Inevitably attention turned to the basal ganglia. Various destructive procedures were tried with questionable success in relieving the unwanted movements. In 1952 Dr. Irving S. Cooper found that occlusion of the anterior choroidal artery relieved the tremor and rigidity in a patient with Parkinson's syndrome. Inasmuch as the anterior choroidal artery provides the blood supply to some of the basal ganglia, Cooper's observation indicated that a lesion in the basal ganglia could relieve tremor and rigidity while avoiding paralysis. The problem was that one could not be sure that occlusion of the anterior choroidal would always produce the desired effects. The uncertainity was due to some variation in the areas supplied by each anterior choroidal artery. To make use of Cooper's observation and other accumulating information, a method was needed by which a predictable lesion could be made at a predetermined site in the basal ganglia.

A workable technique using a special apparatus had been used for some time to make lesions in the brains of experimental animals. The apparatus and technique was adopted for use on humans. Surgery of this type is called stereotaxic surgery. The apparatus or stereoencephalotome is a rigid instrument that is fixed securely to the skull of the patient. It acts as a guide to hold electrodes, cannulas, or other instruments that can then be inserted into definite targets deep within the brain. The stereoencephalotome has fine adjustments that permit insertion with precision.

To determine the location of a specific target in the patient's brain, a ventriculogram is done to outline the third ventricle and adjacent structures. X rays are taken after the air is injected into the ventricles. Various anatomic structures are outlined by the air, and certain ones are selected as landmarks. Using the landmarks as a frame of reference, the surgeon can, by measuring, pinpoint the site where the lesion is to be made. With the site selected, the stereoencephalotome is adjusted, and then the instrument that is to make the lesion is inserted into the brain through a burr hole.

The instrument making the lesion may be one of several different types depending on the kind of lesion to be made. An insulated electrode may be inserted, which has an uninsulated tip. When an electrical current is applied, a lesion is made in a spherical shape around the tip of the electrode. A special instrument called a leucotome may also be used to make the lesion. This instrument has a wire snare that is pushed out of the instrument's end. The leucotome is then twisted and the snare cuts a lesion. A cryogenic probe is sometimes used to make a lesion by freezing the brain at the end of the probe. Several other means have also been used, such as ultrasound and implantation of radioactive metallic seeds.

The site where lesions are made will vary somewhat with the prejudice of the surgeon. Lesions have been made in the globus pallidus, in the ventral-lateral nuclei of the thalamus, and in certain adjacent nerve tracts. Most of the abnormal movements including tremor, athetosis, and chorea respond favorably to lesions in these areas.

Parkinsonism is the most common disorder with involuntary movement, and it is therefore the most common one to be treated surgically. The tremor, and to a lesser degree the rigidity, are often satisfactorily relieved by surgery. The slowness of movement seen in patients with Parkinson's syndrome remains to a degree. The drug L-dopa has been very successful in the treatment of parkinsonism, lessening the frequency of surgery.

Intracerebral hemorrhage that occurs when the lesion is made is the most common complication of stereotaxic surgery. Infection and hemiparesis may also occur.

CHAPTER 10

Treatment of Pain

There is no problem in the practice of medicine that is more challenging or more frustrating than the treatment of pain. It might appear that all the physician needs to do to stop it is to prescribe medication. There lies the problem, because such a naïve expectation by a patient or such a casual effort by a physician will usually result in failure.

In Chapter 1 the anatomy of the pain pathways was discussed in detail. Recall that a painful stimulus activates receptors that initiate a nerve impulse. The impulse travels to the central nervous system through specific spinal or cranial nerves. In the CNS the impulse travels in definite tracts to the thalamus. From the thalamus the nerve impulse goes to the sensory cortex of the cerebrum. It is probable that we are conscious of a painful stimulus when the impulse reaches the thalamus, but it is in the sensory cortex that qualitative and quantitative characterization of pain is achieved.

Evaluation

Pain is entirely subjective because we have no way to measure it. If we had a "pain meter," things would be greatly simplified. Until we have one, pain syndromes must be evaluated by the history. Why did the pain occur? Was there an injury? If so, what were the circumstances of the injury? If there was no trauma, can the patient relate anything that might have caused the pain? How did the pain start? Was it initially mild, becoming more severe? Is the pain constant or intermittent? Can anything be done to lessen the pain? What might make it worse? What does the pain feel like? Is it sharp or dull? Is it like a colic or just an ache?

When taking the history, find out if possible how it started and what caused it. Next try to get some idea of the course of the pain since its onset. Ask the patient to describe the pain. Notice the terms she or he uses, such as knifelike, horrible, or gnawing; it is a good idea to ask what is meant by certain words. For example, patient and interviewer may have entirely different understandings of the word *knifelike.* Find out how the patient gets relief. In general learn all there is to know about the pain and in so doing learn a great deal about the patient and how she or he copes with pain.

Pain can be considered as a protective phenomenon, and to a degree this is true. The pain resulting from a broken ankle prevents the person from walking on the ankle, which protects the ankle against further injury. On the other hand, the pain that continues after the cast has been applied serves no useful purpose. The pain of a patient who has cancer is for the most part harmful. It causes physical suffering, which prevents rest. It may completely demoralize and abolish the will to live.

Much has been written about the concept of a pain threshold. Such a threshold should not be considered to be a predetermined, constant level above which there is pain and below which there is no pain. There is the occasional person who experiences no pain in spite of severe painful stimulation. Certain primitive people who have been conditioned by enduring physical and emotional hardships can tolerate pain with relative ease. The excitement of the moment may permit an athlete to continue in the game in spite of painful injuries. All of these factors are positive factors and elevate the pain threshold. Unfortunately, in most instances, the negative factors anxiety, fear, depression, and emotional and physical fatigue are more prevalent. Much of the treatment of a patient with pain should be efforts to eliminate or minimize the negative factors.

In addition to psychological factors that have either positive or negative influences on the perception of pain, there are psychological factors or mechanisms that play a role in the origin of pain. These include malingering and psychoneurosis. Malingering is the deliberate feigning of an illness. The motive is often secondary gain. A person claims severe injury or pain as the result of an auto accident or an on-the-job injury, perpetuating complaints in hopes of obtaining a big cash settlement. This of course is grossly fraudulent, but unfortunately it is a common occurrence. Other malingerers are more subtle, presenting themselves at an emergency room or doctor's office complaining of severe pain and asking for narcotics. These unfortunate individuals are master manipulators who are often forced by their habit to assume an itinerant life, going from town to town. They commonly will submit to repeated operations by unsuspecting physicians.

There is no sharp line between the malingerer and the neurotic patient. Whereas malingerers know their illnesses are fraudulent they often start to believe their own stories; psychoneurotics are unaware of the motives behind their illnesses. Pain is very often the prominent feature in the illnesses of neurotic patients. In many cases there is true pain, but psychoneurotic illnesses are often deep-seated and complex problems that require intensive psychiatric therapy. The important thing is that the physician recognize that there are strong psychoneurotic tendencies in a neurotic patient and not dispense unlimited narcotics. A good rule to follow is that no medication stronger than aspirin be given until the cause of the pain is determined. In most cases of legitimate pain there will be some objective evidence of disease or injury. An X ray will show a fracture or a destruction of bone. The physical examination will reveal bruising, swelling, or some objective finding. If all else fails, the history will present reasonably firm evidence of authentic disease.

Members of the medical team must resist the temptation to be judgmental toward patients who complain of pain. Concern and compassion toward these people will be more successful in treatment than questioning the severity of pain or the need for strong pain medication. The discussion that follows is presented to provide insight into the psychodynamics of pain, not to provide clues to be used in searching out and exposing the malingerer or the neurotic. There are two broad aspects of pain that must be understood before thorough evaluation of a pain syndrome is possible and, therefore, before appropriate treatment can be rendered.

The first is the physical aspect of pain. This consists of the physical response of the body to the noxious sensation caused, for example, by a broken bone, an ankle sprain, or invasive cancer. The body's response is to limp, cease using an extremity, or act in some other way to preserve or protect the injured part.

The other aspect of pain is the psychological or emotional aspect. Pain is, by its nature, a threat. It is not, however, only a physical threat but also a psychological threat. The patient's ability to manage the psychological threat depends on several factors, among them: the ability of the patient to manage anxiety, uncertainty, and fear; and the support the patient receives from family, friends, clergy, and the medical team.

The average person with pain is able to contend with both the physical and emotional aspects of pain. The physical aspect responds to mild analgesics as well as to specific measures such as heat, massage, or immobilization. The psychological aspects are usually effectively managed by mild sedation and emotional support from the medical team, clergy, family, and friends.

Most of the problems that arise in managing pain syndromes result from the patient's inability to cope with the psychological threats of pain. This does not mean however that the patient is aware of his or her emotional dilemma; in fact the psychodynamics may function entirely outside of the sphere of consciousness. For example, a patient may be unable to cope with the threat of fear that occurs because of his or her disease. He or she may find it impossible to express these feelings; they seem inappropriate or unacceptable to a person with a self-image of an objective, mature adult. Nonetheless the feelings persist and must be met in one manner or another. In order to find a psychologically acceptable solution to this dilemma, a patient very often complains of pain or discomfort. Pain, which is acceptable, is substituted for fear, which is unacceptable. It is readily apparent in this instance that, although the complaint is of pain, narcotic analgesics will have no effect; it is probable that their use will even worsen the situation.

A patient who has an unsatisfactory relationship with a parent, spouse, or friend may consciously or unconsciously use pain to alter the relationship. The patient has certain emotional or physical needs that have not been met satisfactorily by this other person, so hypochondriasis and pain are used to manipulate and change an unsatisfactory relationship into one that adequately fulfills the needs of the patient. Again, although pain is the complaint, treatment with narcotic analgesics will in most instances fail.

Note that pain and suffering are not the same. Pain may be the major part of the suffering but not necessarily. As a general rule the more dramatic the patient is when telling about his or her pain, the more likely it is that the pain has a malingering or psychoneurotic basis. A patient may complain, for example, of a headache like "a thousand jackhammers working inside my head." Another feature that may be encountered with psychoneurotic patients is the tendency to be vague in their descriptions. They easily stray in their description of the pain to seemingly irrelevant topics. Often in the history such patients will have derogatory comments to make about physicians they have had. They may say they are worse since an operation or that the physical therapy aggravated their back pain. Very commonly when malingering or neurotic patients are about to leave the doctor's office, they will make the comment: "Doctor, I do not like to take medicine of any kind. In fact, I rarely even take an aspirin, but I wonder if you could give me something strong to take if the pain gets real bad?"

When the history and physical examination are completed, the physican will have a good idea about the cause and severity of the pain and some idea about any psychoneurotic tendencies that should be considered. Efforts are now made to treat the pain.

Treatment

The basic effort should be the simplest method available to achieve the desired result. In the context of the above discussion, the goal is to relieve the patient's pain. In most instances medical therapy should be tried before considering a surgical solution to the pain. Of course if the patient's pain is due to appendicitis, surgery is done as soon as possible.

Medical therapy is of two types. First, if possible, the cause of the pain is treated or eliminated. Thus a patient with a duodenal ulcer is treated with antacids, antispasmodics, and a bland diet. Pain resulting from an infection is treated with antibiotics. If pain is due to a foreign body in the eye, the foreign body is removed.

The second part of medical therapy is administration of pain medication. Certain things must be considered in prescribing pain medication. How severe is the pain? We want to give medication that will relieve the pain if possible. If the patient is not in the hospital, usually the only practical mode of administration is oral. In cases of lesser pain, aspirin or Tylenol will suffice, but with more severe pain, a narcotic will be needed. The prognosis and expected course of the patient's disease must be taken into consideration. If the patient has a chronic disease producing pain, a long-term administration of narcotics is likely to result in addiction. In these instances the milder forms of pain medication should be used. The patient should be told to expect some pain. With psychological support such patients can do reasonably well.

If the pain is moderate but expected to be short-lived, narcotics can be given orally. When pain is very severe, hospitalization is necessary so narcotics can be given parenterally (intramuscularly or intravenously). Pain caused by cancer presents particular problems. Such patients should be provided enough analgesic for relief. Habituation or addiction should be no great concern in such cases. To be sure, close supervision is needed to prevent overdose or abuse. Only responsible family members or appointees should have access to the drugs. If the medication is given parenterally at home, the patient and family should have adequate instruction in technique to prevent infection and overdose.

If the patient has more than one physician, it is wise for only one of them to prescribe the narcotics. To avoid embarrassment to the patient and family, the druggist should be told the reasons for the frequent narcotic prescriptions. This is simply done by a phone call from the doctor or by a note written on the prescription pad that the doctor uses.

Medical Treatment

Mild Analgesics

Salicylates. The salicylates—aspirin and sodium salicylate—are probably the most valuable of all medications. They are the drug of choice when a mild analgesic is needed. They are most effective against headache, joint, and muscle pain. Salicylates are less effective for relief of abdominal pains but may be worth trying for the pain of cancer. The salicylates work by direct action in the CNS and by direct effect on the peripheral pain receptor. In addition to their analgesic properties the salicylates have an antipyretic effect (they lessen fever) and an anti-inflammatory effect.

The adverse reactions are usually related to gastrointestinal complaints such as heartburn, nausea and, in a small percentage of people, gastric bleeding. In a small number of patients actual allergic reactions can occur with urticaria or anaphylactic reactions.

The salicylates are often combined with codeine. The analgesic effect is greater with this combination than if one of the drugs is used alone.

Para-aminophenol derivatives. The *para*-aminophenol derivatives acetaminophen and phenacetin are equivalent to the salicylates in their analgesic and antipyretic characteristics. They are useful in treating mild to moderate headache and muscle pains, but they have little anti-inflammatory activity and therefore are of little help in treating arthritis.

Adverse reactions are not common, and thus these drugs are indicated if the patient is unable to take the salicylates.

Acetaminophen is more commonly known by the trade names Tylenol and Tempra. It is available in combination with codeine, which gives a greater degree of pain relief than if used alone.

Codeine. Codeine is an opiate (a derivative of opium) that is useful in mild to moderate pain. It is significantly less effective than morphine and probably less effective than meperidine (Demerol). Although it can be given intramuscularly it is more valuable as an oral medication. Most often it is given in combination with aspirin or acetaminophen. Codeine is also used as a cough suppressant.

Codeine is less addictive when given orally and especially when combined with aspirin or acetaminophen. Nausea, constipation, and sedation occur with codeine use. In high doses it has the same disadvantages as morphine, including respiratory depression.

Oxycodone. Oxycodone (Percodan) is a codeine derivative, but its analgesic potency is greater than that of codeine. It is a good analgesic, but development of dependence is similar to morphine.

Propoxyphene. Propoxyphene (Darvon) is available alone or as a combination with aspirin (Darvon with ASA) or with APC (Darvon Compound). The combinations are intended to be as effective as codeine with aspirin, but it has not been shown that equal effectiveness is achieved.

Strong Analgesics

Strong analgesics are reserved for severe pain such as renal or biliary colic and myocardial infarction. Like the mild analgesics they alter pain perception, but they also alter the psychological response to pain by decreasing fear and anxiety. The strong analgesics may be classified in the following manner:

1. *Opium preparations.* Opium occurs naturally as a resin obtained from the opium poppy. The majority of the resin consists of oil, sugar, and protein. Morphine is the major analgesic present in the resin and accounts for approximately 8–12 percent. Codeine also occurs but makes up less than 1 percent of the opium resin.
2. *Semisynthetic modifications of morphine.* Heroin does not occur naturally but is a semisynthetic product of morphine. It has stronger analgesic properties than morphine but also stronger addicting properties. Hydromorphine (Dilaudid) is also a semisynthetic product of morphine that is used as a strong analgesic.
3. *Synthetic analgesics.* These act like morphine but are different in their basic molecular structure. This group includes meperidine (Demerol) and methadone (Dolophine).

Morphine. Morphine is the strong prototype with which all other strong analgesics are compared regardless of their basic molecular structure, and this discussion of morphine applies to all strong analgesics as well. Morphine can be administered in different ways but generally it is absorbed less well when taken orally than when given subcutaneously or intramuscularly. It can, of course, be given intravenously if needed, but this should be done with great care to prevent respiratory depression.

Morphine is carried in the blood in a fat-insoluble form; therefore it does not cross the blood brain-barrier easily. It is metabolized by the liver and then excreted in the urine. The metabolism of morphine is rapid, so the duration of drug action is only 3 to 4 hours.

The precise physiological effects of morphine are not fully understood, but it probably has some effect on the metabolism of serotonin, dopamine, and norepinephrine. More recent neurochemical research, however, has discovered the presence of naturally occurring (endogenous) morphine-like substances called *endorphins.* In addition, specific receptor sites for the endorphins have been identified in the spinal cord and brain. The endorphins which have potent analgesic qualities are probably produced by the pituitary gland. In view of this new information it is likely that the analgesia produced by morphine occurs when it is coupled at the receptor sites of the endorphins. Some of the clinical manifestations of morphine effects can be identified:

1. In the CNS, morphine produces analgesia, alters the mood and produces drowsiness. The strong narcotics also depress the respiratory center in the brain stem.
2. In the eye, morphine causes pinpoint pupils.
3. In the gastrointestinal tract, morphine acts to decrease peristalsis. In chronic use the opiates cause constipation, and it is this effect that makes them valuable in the treatment of diarrhea.

The analgesic qualities of morphine are related to its psychological effects. When given in sufficient doses, opiates may produce a euphoric state. The patient experiences a feeling of well-being and a great sense of peacefulness and contentment. Some patients become very energetic whereas others enter a dreamy state. The intravenous use of opiates (especially heroin) may produce such a pleasant euphoria that there is an overwhelming urge to continue their use.

The urge to reexperience the euphoric state quickly leads to dependence. If the opiates are abused with regularity, the patient becomes addicted to them. Tolerance rapidly develops, higher and higher doses being needed to produce euphoria. This is because the liver metabolizes the drug faster and the brain tolerates higher concentrations of it.

The person addicted to morphine has both a physical tolerance and a psychological tolerance. If the drug is not available the addict experiences withdrawal symptoms. The physical symptoms include chills, nausea, vomiting, and severe aches and pains. The psychological symptoms are those of extreme anxiety and an almost unbearable craving for the drug. The patient who develops tolerance for morphine will have a cross-tolerance for the other strong analgesics. This includes not only those with a molecular structure similar to morphine but also those with an entirely different molecular configuration.

In spite of the problems of tolerance and addiction, morphine remains invaluable for the treatment of severe pain, so it is essential to be aware of the adverse reactions that might occur with its use as well as of the precautions one should take in its administration:

1. Morphine depresses respiration, leading to an increase in the carbon dioxide content of the blood. This leads to dilatation of the cerebral vessels and thus causes an increase in the intracranial pressure.
2. Morphine causes drowsiness and clouds mental processes.
   a. It should therefore be avoided when a patient is being observed for an expanding intracranial mass. This includes patients with head injuries and those who have had a craniotomy.
   b. The patient should not be allowed to drive or do anything that requires clear thinking and sound judgment.
3. Morphine, in most cases, should not be given to patients in shock.
4. Morphine should be used with caution when a patient has liver or kidney disease.

Other strong analgesics. Certain strong analgesics have unique features when compared to morphine:

1. Hydromorphine (Dilaudid)
   a. Semisynthetic derivative of morphine.
   b. 2–4 milligrams of Dilaudid has the analgesic effect of 10 milligrams of morphine.
   c. Onset of drug action is faster than morphine but is of shorter duration.
   d. Probably has better absorption orally than morphine.
2. Meperidine (Demerol)
   a. Molecular structure different than morphine.
   b. Probably not as effective as morphine in relief of severe pain.
   c. Well-absorbed orally but rapidly metabolized.

3. Methadone (Dolophine)
   a. Prevents the withdrawal symptoms that occur with morphine abstinence.
   b. Used for narcotic-addict maintenance.
   c. Has good analgesic qualities for moderate to severe pain.
4. Pantopon
   a. Mixture of purified opium alkaloids.
   b. Analgesic effects are due to the amount of morphine present in the mixture.
5. Pentazocine (Talwin)
   a. Benzomorphan derivative.
   b. Not as effective as morphine in analgesic characteristics.
   c. Initially considerd to be free of addiction tendency, but experience has proved otherwise.

Surgical Relief

The use of a surgical procedure for the relief of pain should in most cases be considered only when all else has been tried and failed. The ideal candidate for a surgical procedure to relieve pain should have "real pain" and a documented disease with objective findings from X rays or from a physical examination. If the disease is a pain syndrome without objective signs, the syndrome should resemble recognized pain syndromes as classically described. The disease as it presents itself should be the reasonable and apparent cause of the pain. There should be correlation between the magnitude of the pain and the degree of involvement of the disease process.

Operating for pain syndromes that have a psychoneurotic origin is to be avoided. When surgery is done on a psychoneurotic patient, the pain may be relieved initially but almost invariably returns, and on its return, the pain is often more severe than it was before surgery. Generally it is a good practice to reserve surgical pain relief for pain that is due to malignant disease. This requires documentation and helps avoid operating for psychoneurotic pain syndromes. Realistically this cannot be strictly followed because there is legitimate pain that is benign in origin. Sometimes benign pain relieved by surgery will return after several years. The reason is not usually apparent, but it may be that the pain follows pathways not normally used for pain transmission.

Surgery for pain relief is actually destructive because the general concept requires interruption of normal pain pathways. A peripheral nerve, dorsal root, or spinal cord pathway is cut. This destruction is permanent because the pathways for the most part cannot be reestablished. The patient may need to accept numbness, even weakness in some instances. This is why it is a good idea if possible to use local anesthetics to block the nerve to be cut. The patient is thereby given the opportunity to see what she or he will have to live with (or without).

Some of the operations to relieve pain are major surgical procedures that have the risks inherent in any major operation. They are, themselves, painful, requiring several days or weeks of recuperation. In addition the cost of hospitalization and surgical fees make them no mean consideration. With these factors in mind the physician presenting the alternatives to a patient must be honest and straightforward. If the patient has a malignancy, is life expectancy long enough to warrant the operative pain and the convalescent period? Would the quality of remaining life be improved enough to justify the risk and the expense?

Pain-relieving Procedures

Neurectomy. The division of a peripheral nerve or a cranial nerve to relieve pain is called a neurectomy (Figure 10–1). A neurectomy can be performed with a knife, or in some cases, absolute alcohol can be injected to kill the nerve fibers. The neurectomy cannot be widely used throughout the body to relieve pain because most peripheral nerves carry motor fibers; others sensory fibers and sympathetic fibers as well as pain fibers. If all these nerves are cut, the patient will have paralysis of the muscles supplied by that nerve.

A neurectomy can be done when the pain is in the chest wall. Pain of this nature is usually the result of cancer invading the chest wall. The intercostal nerves, which run under each rib, are divided. In most cases several intercostal nerves must be divided because the disease process usually involves a wide area of the chest wall.

Rhizotomy. A rhizotomy involves the cutting of the dorsal roots just before they enter the spinal cord (Figure 10–1). Remember that the sensory fibers in the peripheral nerve enter the cord through the dorsal root, whereas the motor fibers are in the ventral or anterior nerve root. Although the rhizotomy has the advantage of not cutting motor fibers, it cannot be used extensively for pain relief because of what is called deafferentation. Remember that those fibers that bring information to the CNS are called afferent fibers. The information consists of not just pain but touch, temperature, and joint position sense as well. When all afferent information from a limb is interrupted, the limb is useless. The patient could move the limb if she or he looked at it, but it would not be able to function as a part of

Figure 10-1 Diagrammatic Illustration of the Spinal Cord, Nerve Root, and Peripheral Nerve in Cross-section, Showing Sites for the Performance of a Neurectomy, a Rhizotomy, and a Cordotomy

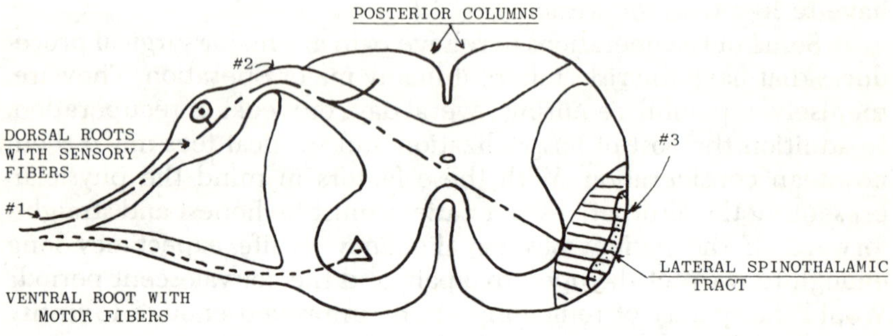

1. SITE OF DIVISION OF A NERVE FOR A NEURECTOMY
2. SITE OF DIVISION OF A DORSAL ROOT FOR A RHIZOTOMY
3. SITE OF CUTTING OF THE SPINOTHALAMIC TRACT FOR A CORDOTOMY

a coordinated unit. With eyes closed or in the dark, the patient would not have the slightest notion about the location of the limb relative to the rest of the body. A rhizotomy is useful in pain of the chest or abdominal walls. It is usually not used for limb pain except in the extreme case in which the limb is already useless.

Cordotomy. The most useful of all the pain-relieving operations is the cordotomy. It consists of cutting the spinothalamic tract in the spinal cord (Figure 10–1). Recall from Chapter 1 how the fibers that carry pain and temperature enter the cord through the dorsal root and then cross to the opposite side of the cord entering the lateral spinothalamic tract. The fibers that carry touch and joint position sense enter the posterior columns on the same side that they enter the cord. If we cut the spinothalamic tract we can interrupt pain fibers without causing complete deafferentation. We can therefore use the cordotomy to relieve pain that is on one side of the body including the trunk and the extremities. If the pain is in a leg or on one side of the pelvis or abdomen, we could cut the spinothalamic tract on the oppsite side of the cord and relieve the pain. In this instance the tract is usually cut in the high thoracic area at approximately the T_2 level. If the right spinothalamic tract is cut at T_2, the patient will have loss of pain and temperature sensation on the left side of the body from approximately T_7 and below. The sensory level is several segments below the level where the spinothalamic tract is transected. Pain in the upper chest, shoulder, and arm can be managed with a crodotomy, but the tract must be divided at C_2.

Pain that is on both sides, as is often the case with cancer of the female organs, is difficult to treat. Often the patient will say the pain is primarily on one side, but when a cordotomy is done and the severe pain is relieved, the other pain will become prominent. When the pain is bilateral, cordotomies can be done bilaterally, but it is unwise to do them at the same time. They should be done 2 to 3 weeks apart to lessen the chance of bladder problems. The patient usually needs a catheter for a few days when a unilateral cordotomy is done. When bilateral cordotomies are performed, and even though they are spaced apart, some patients will require a catheter thereafter. Bilateral cordotomies should not be done in the high cervical regions. This was learned through bad experiences. These patients were fine when awake, but when they went to sleep some of them stopped breathing. This phenomenon especially occurs during the first week or so after the operation.

The cordotomy is a major surgical procedure. It requires a laminectomy, opening of the dura, and an incision in the cord. There is the risk of paralysis or at least significant weakness because the corticospinal tract is very near the spinothalamic tract. Patients must be told of this possibility as well as of the possible need for a catheter.

A variation on this open cordotomy is called a percutaneous cordotomy, a similar operation performed by using a spinal needle and electrode. Various approaches and techniques have been described. In certain operator's hands, the technique is successful. The spinal needle is inserted into the subarachnoid space in the cervical region. It is inserted and oriented properly under X-ray control. When the position of the spinal needle is correct, an insulated, sharp-pointed electrode is inserted through the spinal needle with the sharp point entering the spinal cord. The electrode is then connected to a radio frequency generator. Under strict control the generator heats the end of the electrode in the cord. This creates a lesion in the spinothalamic tract that is just as effective as direct cutting of the tract. This technique has obvious advantages because there is little postoperative pain, and it can be done on high-risk patients. The disadvantage is the difficulty in perfecting the technique.

Spinothalamic tractotomy in the brainstem. The cutting of the spinothalamic tract higher in the brainstem has been tried in an effort to manage pain in the cervical regions. The tract has been cut in the medulla, the pons, and the midbrain. For the most part these operations are not done routinely. They have a high operative risk because the exposure is difficult. Many of the patients have experienced painful sensations that persist postoperatively when the tract is cut high in the brainstem.

Stereotaxic surgery. It seems only logical that a lesion in the thalamus should interrupt pain fibers. The termination of the spinothalamic tract, however, is so diffuse that it is unclear which nucleus of the thalamus should be destroyed to produce pain relief. Lesions in the posterior ventrolateral nucleus produce significant sensory loss on the opposite side of the body but no relief of pain; lesions elsewhere give pain relief but often for a short period only. The results are too inconsistent to make this technique of much practical value.

Cortical resection. Resection of the sensory cortex has been considered as a possible method to relieve pain, but experimental efforts have not really indicated that this would achieve success. The exact mechanism of pain perception is poorly understood, so cortical resection has no practical application as yet as a routine pain-relieving procedure.

Leucotomy or frontal lobotomy. Recall from Chapter 1 the function of the frontal lobes. It has been observed that those patients who have disease of the frontal lobes can tolerate more pain. In earlier days the technique of frontal lobotomy was used to treat various psychiatric disorders, and patients so treated were noted to tolerate pain quite well. It appears that, instead of diminishing the pain, the operation merely changes the way in which the patient reacts to it. In addition the anxiety and fear so commonly associated with pain are abolished. The use of a frontal lobotomy may be of help in severe intractable pain when there is associated anguish. The major problem with the operation is the profound change in the personality that usually occurs. Patients are not distressed in this regard, but the families who must care for them may be greatly alarmed. Patients' responses are flat and emotionless. They may be untidy and vulgar. In general they may play havoc with both family and home life. It is for this reason that the lobotomy should be reserved as a last resort. All concerned family members should be appraised of what might occur. Fortunately many of the disagreeable traits that are prominent during the first month or so following surgery disappear after a period of time.

More recently, modifications of the frontal lobotomy have been used for the surgical relief of chronic pain syndromes. The cingulumotomy has been relatively successful in relieving pain while minimizing undesirable personality changes. The cingulate gyrus is a part of each frontal lobe (Figure 10–2). Each cingulate gyrus is connected to other structures in the brain by the cingulum bundle. The objective of the cingulumotomy is to divide the cingulum bundle. This may be achieved either by direct surgical divisions, by way of a craniotomy, or by stereotaxic surgical techniques (see Chapter 9).

Other Techniques of Pain Relief

The recent interest in the ancient art of acupuncture has encouraged the development of new and promising techniques of pain relief. Traditionally acupuncture has been used in China for the relief of pain during minor surgical procedures. Western observers also report seeing it used as a substitute for general anesthesia during some major surgical procedures. Why acupuncture seems to work is not really known. It is probable that factors such as conditioning and suggestion play a role in its success. Certianly hypnosis seems to work in this manner. Efforts, however, have been made to explain the apparent success of acupuncture on a neuroanatomic and neurophysiological basis.

We have all at one time or another vigorously rubbed our shin bone after hitting it. We do it without thinking why, but obviously we rub the shin because it lessens the pain. The family cat, similarly, licks its paw because it helps the pain. These are examples of the concept of counterirritation. The stimulation at the painful site in some ways dampens the pain. The gate theory has been proposed to explain these observed phenomena.

Figure 10-2 Cross-section Showing the Cingulate Gyrus and the Cingulum Bundle

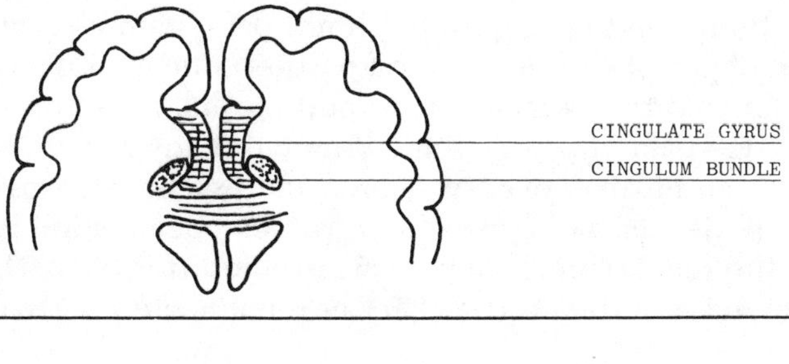

To understand the concept of the gate theory, envision a "gate" within the spinal cord through which all incoming sensory information must pass. Now imagine that the sensation that occurs when we rub our throbbing shin bone arrives in the form of an impulse at this gate. In some manner it is able to shut the gate so that impulses that arrive later, such as pain, cannot pass. In reality the gate is probably a second-order neuron that receives incoming sensory information and then transmits it on to higher centers (thalamus). Inhibition of this neuron by the incoming rubbing sensation in effect closes the gate to passage of the painful sensation.

The discovery of the endogenous opiate-like endorphins and their receptor sites in the CNS has led to the opiate theory of pain relief. In response to a painful stimulus, endorphins are released that attach themselves at specific receptor sites so that pain is not perceived. It is possible that analgesics, like aspirin, cause a chemical reaction that liberates endorphins. The many mechanical devices for pain relief that will be discussed later may also stimulate the endorphin activity.

Electrical Stimulation

Various mechanical devices and techniques have been developed that relieve pain by stimulation of either peripheral nerves or certain parts of the CNS. Some of these are now in widespread use; others are still in the developmental stages.

Transcutaneous electrical stimulation. A rather simple electrical device is widely used to relieve pain by transcutaneous electrical stimulation. The device is just a bit larger than a cigarette case and is easily carried on the belt or concealed in clothing. Electrodes are attached to it by wires and are taped to the patient's skin over the painful area or adjacent to it. The power source is a rechargeable battery in the packet, which delivers an electrical current to the skin. The device is adjustable so the pulse width, frequency, and amount of current can be altered. The transcutaneous stimulator has been most successful in relief of pain of peripheral nerve origin, so it works well for stump (end of amputated limb) pain, pain associated with neuromas of peripheral nerves, and postherpetic neuralgia. It works less well for pain that remains after multiple laminectomies. Initially it may "help" pain of psychogenic origin; but any relief is generally short-lived, and it may even worsen some psychogenic pains. Most clinical experiences in the use of the transcutaneous stimulator have been for the relief of chronic pain syndromes. It is likely that it will play an increasing role in the relief of some acute pain syndromes.

Its use is promising for relief of incisional pain following surgical operations.

The only serious limitation to the use of the transcutaneous stimulator is heart disease. Care is advised when a patient has an irregular heartbeat. Electrodes should never be placed near a pacemaker. There may be some skin reaction in isolated patients because of sensitivity to the adhesive used on the electrodes.

Direct peripheral nerve stimulation. Electrodes may be implanted surgically to provide direct stimulation to a peripheral nerve. The pain syndromes that respond most favorably are similar to those that respond to transcutaneous electrical stimulation.

Posterior column stimulation. Electrodes are placed against the posterior columns of the spinal cord after a laminectomy has been performed. The relief of pain is less predictable than with either transcutaneous stimulation or direct peripheral nerve stimulation.

Electrical stimulation of the thalamus. Small wire electrodes have been inserted into the thalamus, and by electrical stimulation pain has been relieved. It appears that pain is relieved by inhibiting the transmission of pain impulses.

Electrical stimulation of the posterior limb of the internal capsule. The posterior limb of the internal capsule contains the sensory fiber tracts going to the sensory cortex from the thalamus. Stimulation through electrodes implanted in the posterior limb of the internal capsule may help relieve pain of CNS origin. This technique may be helpful in treating pain of the thalamic syndrome, phantom limb pain, and pain of spinal cord origin such as may occur in traumatic paraplegia.

Electrical stimulation of the medial forebrain bundle of the hypothalamus. Studies in laboratory animals suggest that there are actual pleasure centers in the brain. The medial forebrain bundle of the hypothalamus is probably such a center. Whether electrical stimulation of a pleasure center would be valuable in pain control remains to be seen.

Injection

There are various injection procedures that may be of value in treating certain pain syndromes. By their nature, most provide short-term relief, but they are simply done and may be sufficient to relieve the pain of the terminal patient.

Local anesthetics. Local injection of anesthetics into painful areas or around nerves may provide temporary relief. In some cases the pain relief achieved may be significantly longer than the period of anesthesia produced by the local anesthetic. Why this occurs is not clearly understood, but in some manner a self-perpetuating pain cycle may be broken. It is always wise to do a local block before injecting alcohol or phenol to produce a long-lasting or permanent block. In this way it can be determined whether the block will be successful. The patient also gets a chance to see what he or she will have to contend with after a permanent block is performed.

Alcohol and phenol. A block of several month's duration can be achieved by injecting ethyl alcohol or phenol around a nerve. These agents are destructive and, therefore, injure both sensory and motor fibers in a nerve, so they must be used selectively. It would be a rare situation in which paralysis would be acceptable in order to achieve pain relief. The development of a painful neuropathy may occur following alcohol blocks, and the pain that occurs may be as severe as the pain for which the initial block was done.

Corticosteroids. Corticosteroids have an anti-inflammatory effect, and it is for this reason that they are used in certain pain syndromes. Injection of corticosteroids into painful joints or bursa is very successful in relieving pain. Corticosteroids are often injected into trigger points in painful muscles, apparently with some success. They are frequently combined with a local anesthetic. The empiric use of corticosteroid injections for any type of pain is, however, to be condemned.

Subarachnoid saline infusion. Saline (hypothermic-normotonic or hypertonic-normothermic) solutions injected into the spinal fluid through a lumbar puncture may relieve pain. The relief of pain is relatively short (1 to 3 months), but the procedure is simple and is ideal for terminal patients. Muscle weakness and sphincter disorders occur but are not common problems.

CSF barbotage. CFS barbotage has been found to be effective in relieving pain for short periods of time (days to a few months). A lumbar puncture is performed, and spinal fluid is withdrawn into a syringe. When the syringe is full, the fluid is forced back through the needle as rapidly as possible. This is repeated several times. The mechanism of pain relief is not well understood.

Pain Clinics and Rehabilitation Units

Our growing awareness of the need for a multidisciplinary approach to pain problems has led to the establishment of pain clinics and rehabilitation units. These are usually self-contained facilities with a specially trained staff performing the following functions:

1. Drug detoxification
2. Diagnostic evaluation, including psychological testing
3. Behavior modification
4. Pyschiatric therapy
5. Physical therapy
6. Family counseling
7. Neurosurgical pain-relieving procedures.

CHAPTER 11

Disorders of Communication

By Joyce Keen

The process of communication is one of the most complex functions performed by humans. Several areas of the brain must work together to receive, process, and produce speech and language. Disease or injury of any one or more of these areas will affect a patient's ability to communicate. It is important that the medical team have some understanding of the language problems that can occur inasmuch as communication with a patient is so basic in his or her care.

Hearing Loss

Hearing loss is not common following injury or disease of the brain itself. However it is common when either the structures of the ear or cranial nerve VIII is affected by a pathological process. If the medical team is observant during the initial contacts with a patient, they should be able to detect any hearing difficulties. The most accurate behavioral indications of hearing loss are seen when the patient:

1. Requests repetitions of what is said
2. Watches the speaker's face carefully
3. Listens to television or radio at loud levels
4. Talks in an abnormally loud voice
5. Follows requests well after they are repeated
6. Confuses similar-sounding words such as *tell* and *sell*

When loss is suspected, an audiological evaluation should be done to help determine the type, extent, cause, and possible treatment.

If a patient is known to have a hearing loss, the medical team should remember:

1. To make sure the patient is wearing her or his hearing aid (if she or he has one) and that it is turned on and has good batteries.
2. To face the patient and wait for the patient's attention before speaking.
3. Not to yell. Most patients do not profit from listening to loud voices, as sounds continue to be distorted at such levels.
4. To keep background noises to a minimum.

Aphasia

Aphasia, in simple terms, is the loss of ability to associate meaning with words. It is seen in patients with injury or disease involving particularly the dominant cerebral hemisphere (i.e., the left cerebral hemisphere in a right-handed patient). The aphasic patient is commonly recognized by the fact that he or she does not talk or that his or her words do not make sense.

The communication problems in this instance are far reaching and complex. Any or all of the following aspects of speech may be affected in the aphasic patient:

1. *Listening comprehension.* Although able to hear what is said, the aphasic person may be unable to understand it. A request may sound like a foreign language to the patient, or he or she may not remember parts of it.

2. *Reading comprehension.* As with problems of listening comprehension, the printed word *chair* may have no meaning to the person with aphasia even though he or she may read the word aloud correctly. The patient no longer makes the association, which should be automatic in normal adults. One patient may not be able to match the appropriate word to the object. Another may read the sentence "Place the fork to the left of the plate" and then err by putting the knife next to the glass.

3. *Verbal output.* The verbal responses of an aphasic patient may range from no speech or repetitive, meaningless words to fluent conversation with some misuse of, or loss of memory for, specific words. A few patients use frequent "jargon" words that have no

meaning or familiar sound. The patient may be totally unaware that his or her speech is abnormal.

4. *Writing.* The patient with aphasia often loses his or her memory for putting letters together to make meaningful words. He or she may begin to write a word that is well known but end up with something completely different (Figure 11–1). Thus, there is an inability to communicate in writing. Occasionally, a patient can write his or her name "automatically" but cannot write other words.

5. *Gestures.* Some severely aphasic patients are unable to understand or to formulate and use gestures. They may make no response to a simple gesture such as "Come here." They may be

Figure 11-1 The Writing of an 18-Year-Old Male after Craniotomy and Evacuation of Hematoma and Removal of the Left Temporal Lobe (Typed Words Were Dictated)

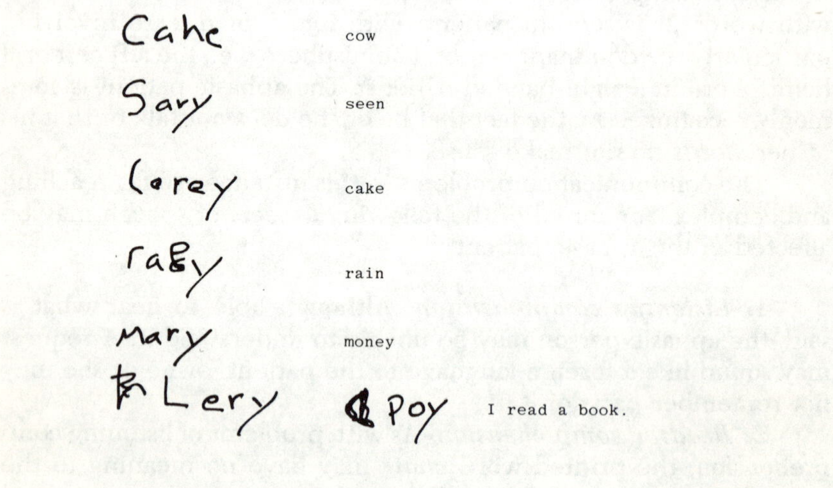

unable to think of a gesture to communicate with others. This type of person may be incontinent owing to the inability to communicate rather than because of lack of awareness. Other severely affected patients may not associate an object with its function. An example of this could be a patient who tried to use a comb to clean her or his teeth or "forgot" how to use a razor appropriately.

The communication loss from aphasia occurs in varying degrees and patterns but usually affects the areas discussed above. It should be realized that the person with aphasia may appear confused or unstable because of "strange" speech or speech errors. Because he or she often cannot understand or follow instructions, the patient may be thought uncooperative, hard of hearing, or demented.

Most often the patient's aphasia is missed entirely, either because behavior clues are not noted or because the patient is able to cover up for what he or she misses. Frequently a patient can get along in his or her environment if he or she " watches" what is happening, knows the daily schedule, and nods "yes" or "no" when addressed with questions. The patient with mild difficulty may not admit the problem in spite of being worried by it. It is understandable that a patient might be frightened by a sudden inability to follow a simple conversation or to read a letter from a friend.

The simplest way to recognize aphasia is to check the patient's comprehension informally by asking him or her to point to objects in the room or to follow unpredictable directions. When doing this, be sure not to give obvious cues. For example, a patient will often open his or her mouth if you come into the room with a thermometer, but he or she will not expect to be asked to touch his or her nose or to point to the window. Some estimate of the patient's verbal difficulty can be obtained if he or she is asked to name objects rather than simply to repeat them. Reading comprehension can be indicated by responses to written directions but not by what the patient can read aloud.

Once a patient is identified as having aphasia, there are some general ways to help the patient to communicate:

1. Converse with the patient naturally; but when the message is important, keep it simple, short, and slow.
2. Use gestures or props to help the patient get the idea of what is being said.
3. Emphasize the most meaningful words. Place them at the end of phrases.
4. Talk in a normal, adult tone of voice.

5. Give your message more than once and phrase it differently each time.
6. Make sure the patient is watching when you speak.
7. Let the patient know you understand the problem and difficulty.
8. Encourage any verbal or gestural attempts to communicate, but do not insist on such responses. (This makes it much more difficult for some patients.)
9. Give the patient plenty of time to respond.
10. Ask questions that can be answered by "yes" or "no."
11. Try giving the patient a choice of two things so he or she can indicate a preference.
12. Do not encourage unrealistic expectations by telling the patient his or her speech will return to normal or by comparing him or her to other patients you have seen recover.

Movement-planning Disorders

Some brain-injured patients are unable to speak for reasons other than true muscle weakness or poor word recall. They appear to have difficulty planning, initiating, and carrying out the correct movements needed for speech. This kind of problem may also be observed with movements of other parts of the body. This difficulty often occurs along with aphasia, but it may be seen as an isolated deficit.

A speech disorder of this type may be severely limiting. The patient may make sounds or even say words unconsciously, but voluntary production is difficult or impossible. Such a patient may phonate when laughing but be unable to produce the same sound when asked. Many of the suggestions previously listed to help the patient with aphasia also apply to the one with a disorder of movement planning.

Confusion and Dementia

Many patients with brain injury or disease exhibit confused language. Their communication problems cannot be ascribed to aphasia or perceptual problems. The major characteristics of such responses are:

1. Speech is fluent. There is no consistent halting or search for words, although some phrases may be repeated continuously.

2. There may be a general loss of memory for past events.
3. There is often a reduced ability to remember such things as events and names for even a brief period of time.
4. The patient may be disoriented as to who he or she is; his or her past life; where he or she is; or what month, day, year, or time of day it is.
5. The patient may confabulate of "make up" facts to explain a happening.
6. The patient's confusion can be noted in all phases of his or her behavior and is not limited to communication.

The confused or disoriented patient should be frequently oriented to reality. The members of the medical team who come in contact with the patient can do this each time they see the patient by reminding him or her of the time of day, where he or she is, and what is being done.

Reduced Responsiveness

The patient with extensive brain disease or injury may be unable to communicate because of a reduced level of overall responsiveness. He or she may respond only minimally to tactile, auditory, or visual stimuli. This kind of patient is sometimes confused with an aphasic patient owing to his or her inability to talk or follow directions. Such a lack of response does not mean, however, that the patient does not understand, only that he or she is unable to respond. In spite of lack of response, this patient needs frequent stimulation. Auditory stimulation, visual stimulation, or tactile and vestibular stimulation can be used.

1. Auditory stimulation
   a. Have a radio or television going for some period during the day.
   b. Carry on normal conversation with others in the room, but do not say things you would not want the patient to hear.
   c. Tell the patient what you are doing anytime he or she is repositioned or other care is administered.
2. Visual stimulation
   a. Try to get visual contact with the patient whenever possible.
   b. Open drapes; arrange flowers and other objects so that they can be seen by the patient.

3. Tactile and vestibular stimulation
   a. Raise and lower the head of the patient's bed frequently.
   b. Touch the patient; reposition and move arms and legs often.

Dysarthria

Brain disease or injury often results in weakness (or spasticity) of the facial and speech musculature. This affects the patient's ability to control the rate, force, and direction of voice and speech production. This causes a breakdown in the clarity of speech that may range from total lack of control to minimal slurring. Such speech impairments are called dysarthria. Recent research indicates several different types of dysarthrias. The characteristics of each are directly related to the site of the neurological damage. It often takes careful listening to understand the dysarthric patient. Requests to repeat what is said or frequent reminders to speak carefully and slowly help make speech clear enough to decipher.

Neurological damage that alters speech production also frequently affects the patient's ability to swallow liquids and solids. Such inability means important changes in nursing care. Initially a nasogastric tube is often used to give the nourishment necessary to the patient. However it is important to remove this as soon as possible and to get the patient to return to swallowing and, it is hoped, self-feeding. If a gag reflex is present, it may indicate that the patient will be able to learn to swallow again without great difficulty.

In stubborn cases, the nurses may need the aid of the occupational therapist, the speech pathologist, and the dietician to stimulate swallowing return. After determining what the patient can understand and which structures are involved, the speech pathologist can indicate techniques and help with facilitation to swallow. The occupational therapist may also provide facilitation and make suggestions that will make feeding easier. The dietician can provide food that will aid stimulation and make it easier for the patient to swallow.

Generally, suggested techniques for aiding swallowing are to:

1. Make sure the patient is sitting up and a little forward, if possible, and that the head is midline with the body.
2. Provide foods of varied texture, taste, and temperature. Begin with foods that do not have to be chewed. (Liquids are usually more difficult to swallow than other foods.)

3. Verbalize the action needed for swallowing so that the patient's concentration is completely on the task.
4. Help make the patient confident that he will have immediate help if he has any difficulty.

Impaired Perception and Judgment

Defective perception can affect the patient's communication function and overall behavior. Many people who have cerebral disease or injury have difficulty perceiving visual stimuli correctly in spite of normal visual acuity. The visual disturbance may be in interpretation of spatial and figure-ground relationships, in recalling what is seen, or in loss of portions of the visual field (hemianopsia).

The patient whose visual field is reduced on the left side may eat only foods on the right side of his or her plate. The patient may have difficulty making sense of what he or she reads because of omitting words printed on the left of the page. Writing may also be affected.

Other perceptual problems include the patient's awareness of his or her self and body. Correct interpretation of where one's body parts are and of one's own position in relation to other objects, as well as awareness of one's own abilities and limitations, are all involved in normal perception. Disturbances in any of these areas cause judgment problems and sometimes confusion.

Patients having perceptual and judgment deficits often profit from frequent verbal cues. Reminders to look to the side of the field loss, feedback regarding positioning, and stress on taking time to judge correctly, all help the patient function better and with less physical assistance.

Management of Communication Disorders

It is important to realize how necessary communication is to our daily lives. It is basic to our identity and our relationships with others. The patient with a communication deficit is suddenly isolated by inability to make needs and feelings known. The patient may be very frightened and frustrated and, at the same time, unable to ask questions or understand explanations. He or she is often in a strange environment and dealing with unfamiliar people . Those who come in contact with the patient can best help in the following general ways:

1. Be responsive to the patient's needs but help him or her maintain whatever independence possible.
2. Do not assume the patient understands everything.
3. Do not assume the patient understands nothing.
4. Treat the patient as an adult both by manner and tone of voice.
5. Encourage whatever responses the patient is capable of but do not insist on any specific response.
6. Help make referrals for appropriate help.

Whenever a communication problem is seen or suspected in a patient, it may be of assistance to obtain a consultation and the help of a speech pathologist. This is particularly important when the patient and family are concerned or when there is a question regarding medical diagnosis. There are several specific reasons for enlisting the aid of a speech pathologist during the acute stages of a neurological disease:

1. The speech pathologist can recognize and differentiate the patient's communication problem and may also explain the patient's exact level of function and whether or not the problem is treatable.
2. After evaluation of the patient's communication function, specific recommendations can be made as to how best to communicate with the patient.
3. The speech pathologist can explain the patient's problems to the family, along with what to expect and how to communicate.
4. The patient can be helped to better understand these problems and be assured of getting help.
5. The speech pathologist can provide follow-up service by beginning treatment, monitoring and documenting progress or regression, suggesting referrals to other professionals, and recommending treatment at a later time.

CHAPTER 12

Nonsurgical Disorders Encountered in Neurosurgical Patients

Certain problems, although not usually surgical, are frequently encountered by the neurological surgeon, and for this reason warrant discussion.

Headaches

There are many causes of headache. In order to make some sense out of such a broad subject, an orderly approach must be taken. The discussion that follows should enable the medical team to arrive at a reasonable diagnosis and assist in determining the therapeutic approach to take.

There are several pain-sensitive structures in the head and neck. They include:

1. Major arteries at the base of the brain—cerebral arteries
2. Meningeal arteries
3. Portions of the dura at the base of the brain
4. Dural and venous sinuses and the cerebral veins that enter them
5. Scalp and neck muscles and arteries
6. Certain cranial nerves including V, VII, IX, and X

Any process that in some manner involves or affects the above structures may produce headache or head pain. Head pains may be divided into catagories by the nature of their process: (1) vascular headaches, (2) headaches from actual pressure or traction on pain-sensitive structures, (3) headaches from irritation or inflammation of pain-sensitive structures, and (4) psychogenic pain or headache.

Vascular Headaches

There are several headaches or pain syndromes that are thought to be due to primary involvement of the blood vessels in the brain, dura, and scalp. Some of these syndromes are well defined, others just vague entities.

Migraine Headaches

Patients often use the term *migraine* to mean a severe headache. To be sure, the patient may have a severe migraine headache, but it is more likely that he or she has a severe headache based on psychogenic factors. The patient with classic migraine headaches often has an aura that precedes the pain. Visual phenomena are common and include such things as flashing lights, silvery lines, or some visual field defect that occurs transiently. Some patients experience a temporary numbness or weakness on one side of the body or the other.

The aura occurs because certain cerebral arteries go into spasm. If the spasm is significant, the blood flow is diminished, and the brain lacks the oxygen and glucose that it needs. The visual cortex is quite sensitive to diminished blood flow.

The aura usually lasts 20 to 30 minutes, and then the headache begins. The pain is probably due to vasodilatation of the cerebral and scalp vessels. The headache is often one-sided and pulsating. Nausea and vomiting are common. The patient experiences sensitivity to light (photophobia) and, therefore, seeks a dark, quiet room. The pain lasts a few days. Sometimes if the patient can sleep, he or she will awaken without the headache.

Migraine headaches are more common in females than males. They may begin in childhood or adolescence. They are said to occur in compulsive people, and there may be some inheritance tendency. The headache may be precipitated by stress from a job or by emotional turmoil. Some patients do well during the stressful time, only to get their headache after the problem is resolved. The headache may occur on weekends or vacations.

Treatment: If the headaches occur frequently, the patient takes ergotamine or methysergide daily to try and prevent them. If they are occasional the patient is provided ergotamine to take at the first sign of a headache (onset of aura). This approach is often successful in aborting the headache, but the patient must be cautioned not to take the medication too often.

Complications: Occasionally the neurological phenomena that occur with the aura may persist. Thus the patient may have a persisting hemiparesis, visual field defect, or some other neurological problem. In what is called ophthalmoplegic migraine the patient may develop an ocular palsy. The third nerve is most commonly involved, but palsies of the fourth or sixth cranial nerves do occur. Rarely, the vascular spasm of migraine involves the basilar artery. In this case the pateint has vertigo, unsteady gait, dysarthria, and visual changes.

Headaches Known as "Vascular Headaches"

A group of headaches commonly called vascular headaches are considered to be like migraines, but the patient does not experience an aura. These headaches are, therefore, nonspecific in their character, and differentiation from other types of headache may be impossible.

Headaches Secondary to Other Factors

Vascular headaches may occur with exposure to toxic substances like carbon monoxide, alcohol, and some insecticides. They may be caused by anoxia. Withdrawal from drugs such as amphetamines may also cause a vascular type of headache. So may arterial hypertension.

Cluster Headaches

The etiology of cluster headaches is obscure. There may be sensitivity to histamine that causes this pain of vascular origin. The pain tends to occur at about the same time each day and on successive days for a period of time—hence the term *cluster.* The patient experiences pain associated with nasal stuffiness as well as redness, tearing, and swelling of the eye on the side of the pain. Treatment is the same as that for classic migraines.

Headaches Caused by Pressure or Traction

Any type of mass lesion may, by pressure or traction, produce a headache. It is easy to visualize the stretching of the pain-sensitive cerebral arteries, veins, and dura by an enlarging mass in the head.

The mass lesions that commonly cause this type of headache are: (1) brain tumors, (2) spontaneous intracerebral or traumatic hematomas, (3) abscesses, and (4) diffuse brain swelling—pseudotumor cerebri.

The clinical presentation of the headache caused by pressure or traction depends on the lesion present. A sudden onset of headache would be seen with a spontaneous intracerebral hematoma, whereas an insidious onset would be likely with a brain tumor or a chronic subdural hematoma.

The headache of most mass lesions is often not severe; yet it is persistent and is frequently present in the morning when the patient awakens. The headache may be very severe if the mass develops rapidly, such as occurs with a spontaneous intracerebral hematoma or an acute epidural hematoma. Brain tumor headaches can be very severe if there is bleeding into the tumor or if the location of the tumor causes hydrocephalus. The latter occurs with tumors in the posterior fossa.

The location of headaches caused by mass lesions is not of much localizing value. Thus a right-sided, frontal headache does not mean the tumor is located there. Generally speaking, however, the headache caused by a cerebellar tumor is usually in the occipital region, and there is often associated neck stiffness. Coughing usually makes the headache worse.

The symptoms of mass lesions have been discussed elsewhere. In general, however, the patient has the symptoms of increased intracranial pressure (headache, nausea, vomiting, and visual change) as well as certain focal symptoms (hemiplegia, aphasia).

Treatment of the headache caused by a mass lesion depends on the nature of the lesion; for example, tumor removal or abscess drainage. In addition, the patient is given analgesic medication for the pain itself. Cerebral edema would be treated with steroids and diuretics.

Headaches Caused by Inflammation or Irritation

Subarachnoid hemorrhage and meningitis are the major causes of headaches stemming from inflammation or irritation.

Subarachnoid Hemorrhage

Blood in the CFS is irritating to many of the pain-sensitive structures in the head, so a subarachnoid hemorrhage causes a headache that is characteristically sudden and severe. The patient will complain bitterly of headache if his or her level of consciousness is not altered by an accumulating blood clot or vascular spasm. The patient also suffers a stiff neck (nuchal rigidity) and intolerance to light (photophobia) and to noise. There is often nausea and vomiting with the headache. These patients may require strong analgesics and possibly sedation. Some judgment is needed in prescribing narcotics because the neurovital signs may be altered by the drug.

Meningitis

The meningitis infection may be either viral or bacterial in origin. Headache onset may be rapid, but not sudden, as seen with subarachnoid hemorrhages. The pain may be very severe. The patient has nuchal rigidity as well as light intolerance, and there may commonly be nausea and vomiting. In addition the patient will usually have fever and will be toxic, appearing acutely ill. Appropriate antibiotics are given if the meningitis is of bacterial origin, and hydration and analgesics are prescribed as well.

Less Common Causes

Sinus infection. Headaches are often said to be due to sinus infections or disease, but actually this is an uncommon cause of headache. Sinus infections are usually confused with the very commonly occurring allergic rhinitis, which produces a runny nose, stuffiness, and so forth. Pain of sinus disease is commonly facial or frontal pain associated with fever, facial swelling, and redness, which is typical of bacterial infections.

Temporal arteritis. Inflammatory processes may occur in the walls of arteries in the scalp and brain. The most commonly recognized entity of this type is temporal arteritis. It is usually seen as a rather sudden pain in the temple of an elderly patient. The temporal artery in the scalp may be prominent, and the skin overlying it is tender to the touch.

The feared complication of temporal arteritis is blindness. The ophthalmic artery may be similarly involved, and the retina does not therefore receive adequate blood supply. Steroids must be given to prevent this complication. Similar arteritis may occur in the cerebral arteries, and the patient who has this process may suffer an infarction of the brain.

Psychogenic Headaches

Most psychogenic headaches (those due to tension) are relatively mild and respond to over-the-counter analgesics. The doctor usually does not see this type of headache in the office. The patient seeks medical help only when the headaches persist and fail to respond to therapy.

Depression is the major cause of psychogenic headaches. Among the causes of depression are: (1) marital and sexual problems, (2) dissatisfaction with a job, (3) family problems, and (4) inability to cope with life in general, with interpersonal relationships and situational problems.

Psychogenic headaches are usually generalized, but the patient may often describe them as being in the frontal area and behind the eyes. Frequently the patient feels as though a tight band is circling the head. There is also the sensation of tightness and stiffness of the neck. The patient may say that the headaches have been present for days, months, or even years. The patient may complain of tender knots in the neck muscles. He or she has usually seen various doctors and tried most medication, physical therapy, and even psychotherapy with no relief. The headache occurs any time during the day and is often present when the patient awakens in the early morning. They commonly occur on the weekends and during vacations. When told his or her headache is due to tension or depression, the patient will invariably say he or she has nothing to be tense or depressed about. It is hard for the patient to accept tension as the cause of headaches that are present on awakening and commonly occur on weekends and vacations—times the pateint should be relaxed. In spite of this, if the patient is questioned further, complaints indicating tension and depression will be uncovered:

1. The sine qua non of depression is the tendency to awaken early; patients awaken at 3 or 4 o'clock in the morning and cannot go to sleep thereafter. Less common is difficulty going to sleep; patients toss and turn for several hours before dropping off. Much less common is sleeping in excessive amounts.
2. The patient is melancholy and blue, will cry easily, and often for no apparent reason.
3. Memory and concentration are poor.
4. Dizziness is common.
5. Weakness and fatigue are frequent complaints. The patient just lacks the drive to meet the challenges of life.

Sometimes a depressed person will be able to "get along" until he or she experiences some kind of traumatic situation. The best example of this is the whiplash injury that occurs when the patient's automobile is hit from the rear. To be sure, serious injuries may occur from such an accident, but in most instances the injury is nothing more than a mild to moderate strain of the neck muscles that should respond to muscle relaxants, mild analgesics, and a little physical therapy. Often, however, this kind of an accident precipitates the psychogenic headache. The patient then embarks on a course of months and even years of severe headaches, lawsuits, and self-perpetuating depressions.

The treatment of psychogenic headache is very difficult. If the patient can gain some insight into his or her depression and thereby understand the cause of the headache, treatment is easier. Antidepressant medications are helpful in some cases. Narcotic analgesics should be avoided because the problem will probably be chronic, and drug dependency may occur. In an effort to reduce cervical muscle spasm, various forms of physical therapy can be used. Unfortunately some patients do not do well until their lawsuit is settled; then symptoms diminish. In many instances, however, the headaches continue because the basic depression continues.

Seizure Disorders or Epilepsy

The neurological surgeon frequently has patients who have convulsions. These may occur in both the preoperative and postoperative period. A complete understanding of seizure phenomena is needed if seizure control is to be achieved.

The incidence of epilepsy in the general population is not accurately known, but an educated guess whould be .5 to 1 percent. Many more people than that will have a single seizure or a few seizures with fever in the first year or two of life.

The reason why a seizure occurs is not well understood. There seem to be groups of neurons in the brain that are abnormally irritable for one reason or another. They will fire off electrically, initiating a seizure. The EEG may be able to localize this focus of increased irritability, but often it cannot be identified.

Seizures can be divided into two broad groups. There is one group in which a definite cause can be identified; this group is called acquired or symptomatic epilepsy. Almost any pathological process that involves the CNS either primarily or secondarily can have seizures as a part of its clinical presentation. The following are some of the more common causes:

1. *Trauma.* A significant number of patients who suffer open head injuries with depressed skull fractures, dural lacerations, brain contusions and lacerations will have seizures.

2. *Infection.* Seizures are common with meningitis, encephalitis, and brain abscesses.
3. *Tumors.* A seizure is often the initial symptom of a brain tumor.
4. *Cerebrovascular disease.* The compromise of cerebral blood flow caused by arteriosclerosis may cause seizures. Small, cerebral infarcts may become a focus for seizure activity.
5. *Arterovenous malformations.*
6. *Toxins and metabolic abnormalities.* Exposure to toxic chemicals and poisons may cause seizures. Electrolyte imbalance and low blood sugar are examples of metabolic abnormalities that can cause seizures.
7. *Degenerative diseases.*

The other broad group of seizures is the one for which no reasonable cause of the seizures can be found; this group is called idiopathic epilepsy. Although we are unable to identify specific causes for these seizures, the following factors are considered likely causes:

1. *Birth trauma.* Passage of the baby's head through the birth canal causes distortion of the head and the brain, which can cause injury to the cortex of the brain, leaving a scar that may develop epileptogenic capabilities. Seizures caused by birth trauma may begin at any age.
2. *Inheritance.* There is often a strong family history of seizures. Some of the patient's relatives may have "abnormal" EEGs without having had seizures.
3. *Metabolic derangement.* Metabolic disorders in certain neurons may be identified eventually.

Clinical Types of Seizures

Grand Mal

The most common type of seizure is the grand mal seizure. Many patients with grand mal seizures have a warning that a seizure is about to occur. This aura may be a strange sensation or some kind of emotional feeling, and it may give enough warning for the patient to protect himself or herself from injury during the seizure. The next phase, jerking of the extremities, follows rapidly. The head and eyes may deviate to one side as the trunk stiffens and the limbs jerk. This deviation may be a clue as to the location of the initiating seizure focus. For example, if the head and eyes are turned to the patient's right, the focus is likely to be in the cortex of the left frontal lobe near the frontal eye fields. The patient appears to salivate. The saliva may be bloody because the tongue and the inside of the cheeks are frequently bitten. The patient may also urinate and have a bowel movement during the seizure.

The seizure lasts a variable period of time; then the rate of jerking slows and finally ceases as the neurons fatigue. After the seizure the patient commonly sleeps. There may also be some confusion, and the patient may appear to be in a foggy state. The muscles of the body are frequently very sore after a seizure. If the seizure was a particularly severe one, the bodies of the vertebrae may even be collapsed. If a patient complains of significant back pain after a seizure, get an X ray of the spine.

Occasionally after a seizure the patient may be paralyzed on one side or in one extremity. This is called Todd's paralysis. It lasts for a few hours, and then recovery begins and strength returns rapidly. The paralysis occurs because of the fatigue of the rapidly firing neurons during the seizure. The neurons actually expend all of their energy and require a period of recovery before they function again.

Grand mal seizures may occur at any time. Commonly they occur during sleep. They may cease for months or years, only to recur without apparent cause.

Petit Mal

Petit mal seizures occur in childhood and adolescence. The classic feature is the occurrence of brief periods (a few seconds) during which the child stares blankly, being out of contact with the environment. Following this period the child resumes his or her activities as though nothing had occurred. The petit mal seizures may occur infrequently, or they may appear in rapid succession. Sometimes the child with petit mal also has grand mal seizures. Sudden jerks called myoclonic jerks occur in association with both petit mal and grand mal seizures.

Focal Seizures

The classic focal seizure is the focal motor seizure or Jacksonian seizure. It occurs when the lesion or focus is in the motor strip. A rhythmic jerking begins in the distal part of an extremity and then spreads up the extremity. This spread is sometimes called a Jacksonian march. For example, the jerking may begin in the fingers, then spread to the hand, and then progressively involve the entire arm. The seizure may remain isolated to a single extremity or it may spread, crossing eventually to the other side of the body. When this occurs, the patient will lose consciousness, and a grand mal seizure occurs. Occasionally a focal motor seizure begins on one side of the face.

A focal sensory seizure occurs when the lesion is in the sensory strip. Rather than jerking, the patient experiences a spreading sensation described as numbness or pins and needles.

Psychomotor or Temporal Lobe Seizures

Psychomotor seizures can occur in both childhood and adulthood. Sometimes the patient has an aura, which may be some type of sensation or emotional feeling such as anxiety or even fear. Occasionally the aura in temporal lobe seizures is an odor the patient smells. Seizures that begin with an odor are called uncinate seizures because the lesion is in the uncus of the temporal lobe.

After the aura the patient starts some kind of stereotyped activity such as sucking, chewing, or smacking of the lips. He or she may walk about the room in a dreamy state. Visual or auditory hallucinations may occur. The patient may feel detached, and dimensions of the room and its contents seem distorted. On occasion a patient may be destructive or combative.

Miscellaneous Seizure Phenomena

Drop Attacks

Drop attacks are probably seizure phenomena and are sometimes called akinetic seizures. The patient suddenly loses all body tone and falls. These attacks are associated with a short loss of consciousness. The entire attack lasts very briefly.

Hysterical Seizures

The neurosurgeon frequently encounters patients who supposedly have seizures, but the seizures are bizarre and unlike any of the types described above. The possibility of hysterical seizures should in such cases be considered. Of course hysterical seizures are not true seizures at all, instead they are episodes of inconsistent, wild flinging movements of the extremities, with movement of the body from one side of the bed to the other. The patient does not lose consciousness and does not bite the tongue or urinate spontaneously. The hysterical seizure usually follows emotional stress and always occurs in the presence of others. The patient is rarely, if ever, injured by such a "seizure."

Status Epilepticus

Constant or nearly constant seizure activity can occur and is known as status epilepticus. The siezure is usually grand mal in type, although the phenomenon may occur with all seizure types. The patient remains unconscious because he or she is never able to recover from one seizure before another occurs. Status epilepticus is considered a medical emergency requiring immediate attention and treatment. The major potential problem is possible brain damage because of cerebral anoxia. Because the constant jerking that occurs with a grand mal seizure prevents effective breathing, cerebral anoxia is very likely if the seizure continues. The seizure activity can generally be stopped by intravenous, anticonvulsant medication. Intravenous Valium and Dilantin usually will stop the seizure. Sometimes sodium Amytal or paraldehyde can be tried. In the difficult cases, general anesthesia may be required. In addition to medication in status epilepticus, an adequate airway must be established as soon as possible.

Sometimes a patient will remain unconscious after all visual signs of seizure activity have stopped, but an EEG will show evidence of continued seizure activity. Thus the patient is having subclinical seizures that keep him or her from regaining consciousness. This seizure activity will require treatment before the patient will awaken.

Treatment of Epilepsy

Basic Cause

If a cause can be identified, it should be eliminated. This, of course, applies only to acquired or symptomatic epilepsy.

Medication

There are many medications used to treat epilepsy. Among the more common ones are:

1. Phenobarbital. Useful in all seizures and especially effective when used with Dilantin.
2. Dilantin (diphenylhydantoin). Used for grand mal, focal motor, and psychomotor epilepsy.
3. Mysoline (primidone). Used for grand mal, focal motor, and psychomotor epilepsy.
4. Zarontin (ethosuximide). The drug of choice for petit mal epilepsy.

5. Tridione (trimethadione). Used for petit mal and drop attacks.
6. Mesantoin (methylphenylethylhydantoin). Used for grand mal, focal motor, and psychomotor epilepsy.
7. Celontin. Used for petit mal seizures.

The drug or combination of drugs commonly used for specific types of seizures are:

1. Grand mal and focal motor epilepsy: Dilantin and phenobarbital.
2. Psychomotor epilepsy: Dilantin and either phenobarbital or Mysoline.
3. Petit mal: Zarontin or Tridione.

If a patient is poorly controlled when using the drugs of choice for his or her seizure type, be sure the medication is being taken properly or if it is being taken at all. In the laboratory it is possible to determine the blood concentration of anticonvulsant medications. The therapeutic ranges of blood concentration that must be achieved for good seizure control are well established. These determinations should be made on the patient with poor seizure control.

Environment and Life-style Factors

Moderation should characterize the patient's life-style. Extreme fatigue must be avoided but, on the other hand, he or she should be encouraged to take part in most activities. Sound judgment is required regarding driving automobiles and other potentially hazardous activities. Good nutrition is necessary to prevent hypoglycemia and other depleted states. For the most part, alcohol should not be used.

Important Points to Remember

1. A single seizure should not serve to label a patient an epileptic, particularly if the seizure occurs with high fever in early life.
2. The diagnosis of epilepsy should not be made until there is no doubt about the accuracy of the diagnosis and never with only the hearsay evidence of an untrained observer.
3. Because some patients find the word *epileptic* very unpleasant, the patient suspected of having epilepsy might better be labeled

a convulsive disorder suspect, a term often found more palatable.

4. Never lose sight of the fact that the term *epilepsy* still engenders suspicion and mistrust on the part of many; the epileptic patient is still forced to endure prejudice born of ignorance.
5. The epileptic is likely to have difficulty obtaining insurance, employment, and various licenses necessary for a normal, secure life.

Syncope or Fainting

Syncope is loss of consciousness that in most cases is only transient. The patient rapidly returns to normal thereafter. Often the patient will only be light-headed or dizzy headed rather than totally unconscious. There are many causes of syncope, but all share the same basic mechanism of decreased cerebral blood flow.

Orthostatic or Postural Hypotension

The blood pressure drops when a person stands after being seated or lying down, a phenomenon known as orthostatic hypotension. With gravity, the blood drains into the legs and lower body so that there is not enough blood available to be pumped to the brain. The normal response of the nervous sytem when a person stands is to cause the vessels in the legs and lower body to constrict, lessening the amount of blood that drains into them and providing more to satisfy cerebral needs. In some people this response may be a bit slow, causing lightheadedness to occur almost any time they stand too rapidly. These people soon learn to stand slowly, and in this manner they function well. This ability of the nervous sytem to cause vasoconstriction when we stand is lost or severely affected with peripheral neuropathies and spinal cord injuries. When a patient remains at bed rest for extended periods, orthostatic hypotension can also occur the first few times he or she gets out of bed.

Vasovagal Syncope

Vasovagal syncope, one of the most common causes of syncope, is often precipitated by anxiety, pain, trauma, or fear. The patient starts to sweat, develops a pallor, and may be nauseated. The heart rate slows and blood pools into the lower trunk and legs. When this occurs the blood pressure drops and cerebral blood flow is diminished. The patient may become dizzy and faint after this.

Heart Disease

Any pathological process that involves the heart may cause syncope. When the cardiac output of blood decreases, the cerebral blood flow diminishes and syncope occurs. Cardiac arrhythmias, heart blocks, and some heart valve diseases may cause syncope.

Carotid Sinus Reflex

The carotid sinus is a structure that is in the neck at the origin of each internal carotid artery. The carotid sinus sends nervous impulses to the CNS by way of the glossopharyngeal nerve. Stimulation of the carotid sinus causes slowing of the heart rate and decreased blood pressure. Some patients, particularly the elderly, have very sensitive carotid sinuses, so that minimal stimulation, such as might occur when putting on a tie or necklace, can cause syncope.

Hyperventilation

Hyperventilation usually occurs with emotional states that cause the patient to breathe rapidly. The carbon dioxide is blown off, which causes the cerebral blood vessels to constrict. If extreme, cerebral hypoxia may occur. The patient usually only becomes dizzy but can faint.

Tussive or Cough Syncope

Prolonged episodes of severe coughing increase the intrathoracic pressure, which prevents adequate return of blood to the heart. Thus cardiac output falls and cerebral blood flow is diminished.

Cerebrovascular Disease

Elderly patients who have diffuse, arteriosclerotic cerebrovascular disease may faint. This is especially true with basilar artery insufficiency. The patient usually has some type of focal, neurological complaint in addition to the syncope.

Hysterical Fainting

Hysterical fainting is not the result of decreased cerebral blood flow. It is usually a dramatic swoon in which the person wilts to the floor and is never injured. These episodes only occur in the presence of others and are used to manipulate events or other people. There is no change in the heart rate or blood pressure.

Vertigo or Dizziness

Vertigo is the sensation of movement of the patient or the environment. In the strictest sense it is not the same as light-headedness or giddiness. Vertigo may be associated with nausea and vomiting. It has several causes, including disorders that affect the labyrinth or vestibular apparatus, the vestibular nerve, or the CNS. Those who have experienced car sickness realize that vision also plays a role in vertigo.

Ménière's Disease

Sudden, severe episodes of vertigo occur in Ménière's disease. If the patient is standing, he or she is literally thrown to the ground. Each episode lasts a few minutes to a few hours. There is associated hearing loss and often severe nausea and vomiting.

Vestibular Neuronitis

Acute vertigo that often occurs following a nonspecific viral disease is known as vestibular neuronitis or acute labyrinthitis. The patient has the tendency to fall or deviate toward one side when walking. When lying in bed, vertigo often will be very severe if the head is moved. Thus patients will be very still without moving, to lessen the vertigo. Vestibular neuronitis will last a few days in most cases, occasionally a few weeks.

Benign Positional Vertigo

Common following a head injury, benign positional vertigo or benign positional nystagmus also occurs after an infection or after exposure to certain toxins. The vertigo seems to occur when the patient assumes a particular position, such as looking upward or to a particular side quickly.

Cerebellopontine Angle Tumors

An acoustic neuroma or meningioma located in the cerebellopontine angle may cause vertigo. The process is progressive, with hearing loss, focal neurological symptoms, and eventually symptoms from increased intracranial pressure.

Cerebrovascular Insufficiency

The patient may feel light-headed with cerebrovascular insufficiency, but there are usually focal, neurological symptoms associated.

Other Causes

Vasovagal syncope, cardiac arrythmias, and postural hypotension (see discussion of syncope above) may bring about vertigo. Dizziness is often a prominent complaint of patients with depression. The whiplash syndrome often has prominent dizziness as a part of its clinical presentation.

Bibliography/Suggested Readings

Chapter 1: Neuroanatomy and Neurophysiology

Brodal, A. *Neurological anatomy in relation to clinical medicine* (3rd. ed.). New York: Oxford University Press, 1969.

Carpenter, M. B. *Core text of neuroanatomy.* Baltimore: Williams and Wilkins, 1972.

Chusid, J. G. *Correlative neuroanatomy and functional neurology* (16th ed.). Los Altos, California: Lange Medical Publications, 1976.

Eyzaguirre, C., and Fidone, S. J. *Physiology of the nervous system* (2nd ed.). Chicago: Year Book Medical Publishers, 1975.

Guyton, A. S. *Textbook of medical physiology* (5th ed.). Philadelphia: W. B. Saunders, 1976.

Krieg, W. J. S. *Functional neuroanatomy.* New York: Blakiston, 1953.

Mettler, F. A. *Neuroanatomy.* St. Louis: C. V. Mosby, 1948.

Chapter 2: Neuropathology

Baker, A. B., and Baker, L. H. (Eds.). *Clinical neurology.* New York: Harper and Row, 1975.

Blackwood, W., and Corsellis, J. A. N. (Eds.). *Greenfield's neuropathology* (3rd ed.). Chicago: Year Book Medical Publishers, 1976.

Chusid, J. G. *Correlative neuroanatomy and functional neurology* (16th ed.). Los Altos, California: Lange Medical Publications, 1976.

Davis, L., and Davis, R. *Principles of neurological surgery.* Philadelphia: W. B. Saunders, 1963.

Eisenbeiss, J. A. Classification of head injuries. *Arizona Medicine 25:* 129-132, 1968.

Geschickter, C. F., and Cannon, A. *Color atlas of pathology.* Philadelphia: J. B. Lippincott, 1963.

Jackson, F. E. The pathophysiology of head injuries. *Clinical Symposia 18:* 67-93, 1966.

Merritt, H. H. (Ed.). *A textbook of neurology* (6th ed.). Philadelphia: Lea and Febiger, 1979.

Russell, D. S., and Rubinstein, L. J. *Pathology of tumors of the nervous system* (2nd ed.). Baltimore: Williams and Wilkins, 1963.

Slager, U. T. *Basic neuropathology.* Baltimore: Williams and Wilkins, 1972.

Walton, J. *Essentials of neurology* (4th ed.). Philadelphia: J. B. Lippincott, 1975.

Zulch, K. J. *Brain tumors: Their biology and pathology* (2nd ed.). Translated by A. B. Rothballer and J. Olszeuski. New York: Springer, 1965.

Chapter 3: Clinical Evaluation of the Central Nervous System

Alexander, M. M., and Brown, M. S. Physical examination: part 17, neurologic examination. *Nursing 76*(6):38-42, 1976.

Alexander, M. M., and Brown, M. S. Physical examination: part 18, neurologic examination. *Nursing 76*(6):50-55, 1976.

Bickerstaff, E. *Neurological examination in clinical practice.* London: Blackwell Scientific Publications, 1973.

Chusid, J. G. *Correlative neuroanatomy and functional neurology* (16th ed.). Los Altos, California: Lange Medical Publications, 1976.

DeJong, R. N. *Neurologic examination: incorporating the fundamentals of neuroanatomy and neurophysiology* (3rd ed.). New York: Hoeber, 1967.

Chapter 4: Diagnostic Tests

Bates, B. *A guide to physical examination.* Philadelphia: J. B. Lippincott, 1974.

Bell, M. et al. Nursing involvement with monitoring of intracranial pressure. *Journal of Neurosurgical Nursing 6:*28-31, 1975.

Blount, M., Kinney, A. B., and Donohoe, K. Obtaining and analyzing cerebrospinal fluid. *Nursing Clinics of North America 9:*593-609, 1974.

Blount, M. and Kinney, A. B. What to remember about EEG. *Nursing 74* (4):36-40, 1974.

Caffey, J. Pediatric X ray diagnosis (5th ed.). Chicago: Year Book Medical Publishers, 1967.

DiChiro, G., Ashburn, W. L., and Grove, A. S., Jr. Which radioisotope for brain scanning? *Neurology 18:*225-236, 1968.

DiChiro, G., Reames, P. M., and Matthews, W. B., Jr. RISA ventriculography and RISA cisternography. *Neurology 14:*185-191, 1964.

duBoulay, G. H. *Principles of X ray diagnosis of the skull.* London: Butterworth, 1965.

Fishman, R. A. *Cerebrospinal fluid in clinical neurology.* Edited by A. B. Baker. New York: Hoeber Med. Div., Harper and Row, 1962.

Madeja, C. Computerized tomography, an introduction. *Journal of Neurosurgical Nursing 9:*87-89, 1977.

New, P. et al. Computerized axial tomography with the EMI scanner. *Radiology 10:*109-123, 1974.

Tarlov, E. M. *Intracranial pressure measurement: current techniques and role in clinical management.* In current techniques in operative neurosurgery, edited by H. H. Schneider and W. H. Sweet, pp. 67-86. New York: Grune and Stratton, 1977.

Taveras, J. M. and Wood, E. H. *Diagnostic neuroradiology.* Baltimore: Williams and Wilkins, 1964.

Chapter 5: Nursing Care of the Neurosurgical Patient

American Association of Neurosurgical Nurses. *Core curriculum for neüro-surgical nurses.* Baltimore: Amer. Assn. of Neurosurgical Nurses, 1977.

Bates, D., Caronna, J. J., Cartlidge, N. E. F., Knill-Jones, R. P., Levy, D. E., Shaw, D. A., and Plum, F. A prospective study of nontraumatic coma: methods and results in 310 patients. *Annals of Neurology 2*(3):211-220, 1977

Gebbie, K., and Lavin, M. A. Classifying nursing diagnoses. *American Journal of Nursing 74:*250-253, 1974.

Jones, D., Dunbar, C., and Jirovec, M. (Eds.). *Medical-surgical nursing.* New York: McGraw-Hill, 1978.

Olson, E. The hazards of immobility. *Amer. Jour. of Nursing 67:*779-797, 1967.

Plum, F., and Posner, J. *The diagnosis of stupor and coma* (2nd ed.). Philadelphia: Davis, 1972.

Taylor, A. Autonomic dysreflexia in spinal cord injury. *Nursing Clinics of North America 9*(1):717-725, 1974.

Chapter 6: Craniotomy

Allcock, J. M. and Drake, C. G. Ruptured intracranial aneurysms-the role of arterial spasm. *Journal of Neurosurgery 22:*21-29, 1965.

Alphen, H. A. M. and Dreissen, J. J. R. Brain abscesses and subdural empyema-factors influencing mortality and results of various surgical techniques. *Journal of Neurology, Neurosurgery, and Psychiatry 39:* 481-490, 1976.

Bonvette, J. M. Preoperative and postoperative care of patients with cerebral aneurysms. *Nursing Clinics of North America 9:*655-666, 1974.

Caverness, W. F. and Walker, A. E. (Eds.). *Head injury.* Philadelphia: J. B. Lippincott, 1966.

Gurdjian, E. S. and Thomas, L. M. *Operative neurosurgery* (3rd ed.). Baltimore: Williams and Wilkins, 1970.

Howe, J. R. *Patient care in neurosurgery.* Boston: Little Brown, 1977.

Jackson, F. E. Treatment of head injuries. *Clinical Symposia 19:*4-34, 1967.

Jacobs, G., Rubin, R. C., and Wille, R. The treatment of intracranial aneurysms. *Journal of Neurosurgical Nursing, 8:*149-154, 1976.

Locksley, H. Natural history of subarachnoid hemorrhage, intracranial aneurysms, and arteriovenous malformations. *Journal of Neurosurgery 25:* 321-369, 1966.

Mount, L. A. and Anturas, T. Results of treatment of intracranial aneurysms by wrapping and coating. *Journal of Neurosurgery 42:*189-193, 1975.

Mullan, S. *Essentials of neurosurgery.* New York, Springer, 1961.

Perret, G. and Nishioka, H. Arteriovenous malformations: an analysis of 545 cases. *Journal of Neurosurgery 25:*467-490, 1966.

Posner, J. B. and Shapiro, W. B. Brain tumors–current status of treatment and its complications. *Archives of Neurology 32:*781-784, 1975.

Rand, R. W. *Microneurosurgery.* St. Louis: C. V. Mosby, 1969.

Schmidek, H. H. and Sweet, W. H. (Eds.). *Current techniques in operative neurosurgery.* New York: Grune and Stratton, 1977.

Vieth, R. G. and Odom, G. L. Intracranial metastasis and their neurological treatment. *Journal of Neurosurgery 23:*375-383, 1965.

Youmans, J. R. (Ed.). *Neurological surgery.* 3 vols. Phila.: Saunders, 1973.

Chapter 7: Laminectomy

Greenwood, J. Intramedullary tumors of spinal cord. *Journal of Neurosurgery 20:*665-668, 1963.

Guttman, L. *Spinal cord injuries* (2nd ed.). Oxford: Blackwell, 1976.

Mulder, D. and Dale, A. "Spinal cord tumors and discs." In *Clinical Neurology,* Vol. 1, edited by A. B. Baker, and L. H. Baker. New York: Harper and Row, 1975.

Northfield, D. W. C. *The surgery of the central nervous system.* Oxford: Blackwell Scientific Publications, 1973.

Schmidek, H. H. and Sweet, W. H. (Eds.). *Current techniques in operative neurosurgery.* New York: Grune and Stratton, 1977.

Smith, R. An evaluation of surgical treatment for spinal cord compression due to metastatic carcinoma. *Journal of Neurology, Neurosurgery and Psychiatry 28:*152-158, 1965.

Youmans, J. R. (Ed.). *Neurological surgery.* 3 vols. Philadelphia: W. B. Saunders, 1973.

Chapter 8: Peripheral Nerve Surgery

Mayfield, F. H. and True, C. W. Chronic injuries of peripheral nerves by entrapment. In *Neurological surgery,* Vol. 2, edited by J. R. Youmans, pp. 1141-1161. Philadelphia: W. B. Saunders, 1973.

Nulsen, F. E. and Kline, D. G. "Acute injuries of peripheral nerves." In *Neurological Surgery,* Vol. 2, edited by J. R. Youmans, pp. 1089-1140. Philadelphia: W. B. Saunders, 1973.

Seddon, H. J. Three types of nerve injury. *Brain 66:*238-288, 1943.

White, J. C. Timing of nerve suture after gunshot wound. *Surgery 48:*946-951, 1960.

Yeoman, D. M. and Seddon, H. J. Brachial plexus injuries: treatment of the flail arm. *Journal Bone and Joint Surgery 43B:*493-500, 1961.

Chapter 9: Neurosurgical Procedures for Miscellaneous Disorders

Anderson, F. M. and Geiger, L. Craniosynostosis: a survey of 204 cases. *Journal of Neurosurgery 22:*229-240, 1965.

Andy, O. The neurosurgical treatment of abnormal behavior. *American Journal of Medical Science 252:*232-238, 1966.

Blackwood, W. and Corsellis, J. A. N. (Eds.). *Greenfield's neuropathology* (3rd ed.). Chicago: Year Book Medical Publishers, 1976.

Braney, M. L. The child with hydrocephalus. *American Journal of Nursing 73:*828-831, 1973.
Cooper, I. S. and Bravo, G. J. Chemopallidectomy and chemothalamectomy. *Journal of Neurosurgery 15:*244-250, 1958.
Elkins, C. W. and Cameron, J. E. Cranioplasty with acrylic plates. *Journal of Neurosurgery 3:*199-205, 1946.
Gurdjian, E. S. and Webster, J. E. *Head injuries.* Boston: Little Brown, 1958.
Issac, N. M. The surgical treatment of epilepsy. *Journal of Neurosurgical Nursing 8:*155-167, 1976.
Kriss, F. C., Taren, J. A. and Kahn, E. A. Primary repair of compound skull fractures by replacement of bone fragments. *Journal of Neurosurgery 30:*698-702, 1969.
Marcus, A. J. and Davie, J. C. Neurosurgical treatment of Parkinson's disease. *Journal of Neurosurgical Nursing 2:*41-50, 1970.
Mrozinski, C. M. Complications encountered in the course of shunt therapy for hydrocephalus in children. *Journal of Neurosurgical Nursing 2:* 41-61, 1970.
Northfield, D. W. C. *The surgery of the central nervous system.* Oxford: Blackwell Scientific Publications, 1973.
Purpura, D. P., Penry, J. K., and Walter, R. D. (Eds.). *Advances in neurology, Vol. 8: Neurosurgical Management of the Epilepsies.* New York: Raven Press, 1975.
Smith, E. D. *Spina bifida and the total care of spinal myelomeningocele.* Springfield, Ill.: Charles C. Thomas, 1965.
Youmans, J. R. (Ed.). *Neurological surgery.* 3 vols. Philadelphia: W. B. Saunders, 1973.

Chapter 10: Treatment of Pain

Casey, K. L. The neurophysiologic basis of pain. *Postgraduate Medical Journal 53:*58-63, 1973.
Foltz, E. L. and White, L. E., Jr. Pain relief by frontal cingulumotomy. *Journal of Neurosurgery 19:*89-100, 1962.
Lee, J. F. (Ed.). *Pain management: symposium on the neurological treatment of pain.* Baltimore: Williams and Wilkins, 1977.
Loeser, J. D., Black, R. G., and Christman, A. Relief of pain by transcutaneous stimulation. *Journal of Neurosurgery 42:*308-314, 1965.
Long, D. M. and Hagfors, N. Electrical stimulation in the nervous system: the current status of electrical stimulation of the nervous system for relief of pain, *Pain 1:*109-123, 1975.
Melzack, R. and Wall, P. D. Pain mechanisms: a new theory. *Science 150:* 971-977, 1965.
Northfield, D. W. C. *The surgery of the central nervous system.* Oxford: Blackwell Scientific Publications, 1973.
Schmidek, H. H. and Sweet, W. H. (Eds.). *Current techniques in operative neurosurgery.* New York: Grune and Stratton, 1977.

White, J. C. and Sweet, W. H. *Pain and the neurosurgeon: a forty year experience.* Springfield, Illinois: Charles C. Thomas, 1969.

Wycis, H. T. and Speigel, E. A. Long-range results in the treatment of intractable pain by steriotaxic midbrain surgery. *Journal of Neurosurgery 19:* 101-107, 1962.

Youmans, J. R. (Ed.). *Neurological surgery.* 3 vols. Philadelphia: W. B. Saunders, 1973.

Chapter 11: Disorders of Communication

Belt, L. H. Working with dysphasic patients. *American Journal of Nursing 74:*1320-1322, 1974.

Buck, M. *Dysphasia: professional guidance for family and patients.* Englewood Cliffs, N.J.: Prentice Hall, 1968.

Hardin, W. B. and Merson, R. "The higher-order dysfunctions: apraxia, agnosia, and aphasia." In *Neurological pathophysiology,* edited by S. G. Eliasson, A. L. Prensley, and W. B. Hardin, Jr., pp. 170-186. New York: Oxford University Press, 1974.

Kolb, D. Understanding aphasia and the aphasic. *Journal of Neurosurgical Nursing 9:*15-18, 1977.

Skelly, M. Aphasic patients talk back. *American Journal of Nursing 75:* 1140-1142, 1975.

Chapter 12: Nonsurgical Disorders Encountered in Neurosurgical Patients

Chusid, J. G. Correlative neuroanatomy and functional neurology (16th ed.). Los Altos, California: Lange Medical Publications, 1976.

Cooper, C. Anticonvulsant drugs and the epileptic dilemma. *Nursing 76* (6):45-50, 1976.

Engel, G. L. *Fainting* (2nd ed.). Springfield, Ill.: Charles C. Thomas, 1962.

Freedman, A. P. "Paroxysmal disorders: migraine and other types of headache." In *A textbook of neurology* (6th ed.), edited by H. H. Merritt, pp. 825-843. Philadelphia: Lea and Febiger, 1979.

Mullan, S. *Essentials of neurosurgery.* New York: Springer, 1961.

Nelson, J. R. "Vertigo." In *Cecil-Loeb textbook of medicine* (13th ed.), edited by P. B. Beeson and W. McDermott, pp. 163-167. Philadelphia: W. B. Saunders, 1971.

Plum, F. "Headache." In *Cecil-Loeb textbook of medicine* (13th ed.), edited by P. B. Beeson and W. McDermott, pp. 154-160. Philadelphia: W. B. Saunders, 1971.

Wiley, L. The stigma of epilepsy. *Nursing 74*(4):36-45, 1974.

Williams, A. Classification and diagnosis of epilepsy. *Nursing Clinics of North America 9:*747-759, 1974.

Wolff, H. G. *Headache and other head pain* (2nd ed.). New York: Oxford University Press, 1963.

Index